THE COMPLETE
DR. ATKINS

THE COMPLETE
DR. ATKINS

Includes three titles in one volume:

DR. ATKINS' NEW DIET REVOLUTION

DR. ATKINS' NEW DIET COOKBOOK WITH FRAN GARE, M.S.

DR. ATKINS' NEW CARBOHYDRATE GRAM COUNTER

ROBERT C. ATKINS, M.D.

BARNES
&NOBLE
BOOKS
NEW YORK

Published by MJF Books
Fine Communications
322 Eighth Avenue
New York, NY 10001

The Complete Dr. Atkins
LC Control Number 2003113221
ISBN 1-56731-640-9

Originally published as three separate volumes: *Dr. Atkins' New Diet Revolution*, *Dr. Atkins' New Diet Cookbook*, and *Dr. Atkins' New Carbohydrate Gram Counter*

This edition published by arrangement with M. Evans and Company, Inc.

Manufactured in the United States of America on acid-free paper

MJF Books and the MJF colophon are trademarks of Fine Creative Media, Inc.

QM   10 9 8 7 6 5 4 3 2

DR. ATKINS' NEW DIET REVOLUTION

REVISED & UPDATED

To my loving and lovely wife Veronica,
who has unfailingly provided me with
emotional, intellectual, spiritual,
and low-carbohydrate nourishment.

Contents

Part Three—Why the Diet Makes You Healthy

Part Four—How to Do the Diet for Life

Part Five—Menus and Recipes

Preface to the First Edition

Dozens of diets will take your weight off temporarily. But if you're in the market for weight loss plus health, I think you should go a step further. Ask yourself stricter and more interesting questions: *How many diets will restore that vigor and sense of wellness I had almost forgotten I could have? How many diets will positively reinforce my health, day by day and year by year?*

I think that's the type of diet you *need*—an unabashed feel-good diet, a full-energy diet, a lifetime-wellness diet.

As an old veteran of the diet wars, I write from a unique perspective. People come to me concerned for their health, aware that I know something about losing weight. But, I believe, they're even more vividly conscious of the fact that I have a reputation for helping men and women with serious health disorders. The Atkins Center for Complementary Medicine is a major outpatient facility on 55th Street in Manhattan, with a patient population nearly 10,000 strong. These are patients with diabetes and heart disease and multiple sclerosis, with arthritis and chronic fatigue and hypertension. Less than 5% of those patients were interested *primarily* in weight loss when they first knocked at my door.

Yet fame and came to me as a master of effective dieting. It was only after the Atkins diet made me famous that I moved into my life's work in nutrition medicine, using it to treat serious health problems. Why, then, am I writing another book on dieting?

Dieting is a crucial part of the health care I provide. Unless you eat right, you can't be healthy, and if you do eat right, then, generally speaking, you *won't* be overweight.

This is a basic truism that everything in my experience as a physician has reinforced.

Obesity and ill health, crankiness and exhaustion, sleepy days and sleepless nights—let me tell you, those are a familiar melody in the ears of any physician who has treated the fat, malnourished, ill-exercised modern American for long. Obesity is not an accidental accumulation of extra ounces, it is a basic *metabolic* disorder intimately related to ill health.

When I wrote my original bestseller, *Diet Revolution*, twenty years ago, I was chiefly concerned about showing people how to lose weight quickly, easily, and without much pain or bother. The principles I devised for doing that still hold. They are an effective way of discarding the excess pounds and inches and keeping them off. Indeed, I strongly doubt that a more surefire and hunger-free method of dieting has ever been proposed.

But the principles I've been working on ever since my early days as a diet doctor are concerned with *more* than weight loss. They involve a commitment to *complete wellness*—the metabolic basis of richly satisfying well-being.

ROBERT C. ATKINS, M.D.
April 1992

Preface to the Paperback Edition

In the four years since the hardcover edition of this book was published, there have been several developments that just might help make the rest of your life a lot more pleasant.

It wouldn't surprise me if your goal of being really slim is beginning to look like an impossible dream; and perhaps you are ready to give up trying. If so, you are not alone; the same thing has been happening to the majority of the population, and all in the last few years.

There have always been a considerable number of overweight Americans; one in four were significantly so. For generations, that 25% represented a constant, predictable measure of our obesity problem. But ten years ago, an epidemic started and spread across America like a brushfire. Every year, some two million new cases developed. When last quantified, the decade's damage was officially measured to be an increase of 32% in the number of Americans who were obese (20% or more above their ideal weight).

If you are one of this growing number of weight gainers, it may be that you have been following the wrong diet—the diet that created this epidemic. As the only physician who has steadfastly opposed the universal application of the high carbohydrate, 30% fat diet, I can state with authority that the obesity epidemic is in fact *caused* by those very instructions and by that very diet.

Think of it: the "solution" is really the problem.

Using simplistic reasoning, it would seem that reducing fat in our diet would reduce fat in our bodies. The adage "Lose weight, stay on a low-fat diet" has been repeated so often that most of us assume it is scientifically proved. But as you will learn in this book, science "proves" something quite the opposite. There is proof that obesity is due to a very specific metabolic defect. And once you have the key, a key that seems to elude even out health care policy makers, you will be able to excise obesity with the precision of a skilled surgeon who dissects away a tumor while leaving the healthy tissue intact.

Armed with this knowledge, the project of losing weight will be transformed from a hunger- and fatigue-provoking ordeal that only a handful of us can endure for life, to a surprisingly easy matter of eating abundantly, luxuriously, and healthfully, yet always selectively and wisely.

Our physical urges are hard to combat. Fighting the scale armed only with willpower and determination works, at best, for only five low-fat dieters out of a hundred. But we might instead use our intellect, in the manner this book will show you, and bypass our need to rely on willpower.

Learn to unlock the secret of easy weight loss and youÕll be able to lose while eating second and third helpings of traditional main courses.

Once you learn of the caloric richness and satiety that the eating program within these pages provides, its impact should hit you like a sledgehammer. "This is not dieting," you will feel, "this is a banquet." And as weight loss and improved well-being take place, you will feel exhilaration, relief, and confidence that getting and staying slim will be a breeze and that the end of your weight problem is clearly in view.

ROBERT C. ATKINS, M.D.
November 1996

Preface to the New Edition

I've never heard of an author redoing his book when it is still a number one bestseller, but this book has been a success for seven years, and some updating is in order. So much has happened since this book was written that I feel I must keep you abreast of how important these changes will prove to be, not only for your weight control project, but also for expanding your health and lifespan.

No, my diet recommendations are not different, although I'll be telling you about some very delicious special foods and some plateau-breaking vita-nutrients created exclusively for Atkins dieters. What has changed dramatically is the world in which the *New Diet Revolution* plays such a significant role.

When I first wrote this book, I had to convince an entire nation of people who, for a generation, have been systematically brainwashed into believing fallacious ideas about overweight. The unchallenged dogma was that carbohydrates are necessary for everyone, that white flour is good for you, that fats and protein undermine your health, that weight loss requires strenuous exercise or going hungry, and that appetite suppressants may be necessary.

But because the *New Diet Revolution* works so well, producing essentially automatic weight loss with little regard to quantities, millions of people learned, almost exclusively by word of mouth, that a diet directly opposed to what they have been taught would easily bring their weight problem under control. And they also learned that those who defied the prevailing dogma would improve their energy levels and lab values and would often overcome many medication-requiring illnesses. That is why this book has sold more copies each succeeding year of the six-year span it has been in print. In that time, more than 2 out of every 100 adults in America has obtained a copy of this book, and more have read it. All of these readers have been forced to consider the possibility that one person may be right and the rest of the world wrong. This serious accusation is not made from arrogance, but rather of deep concern that the errors of the "rest of the world" are so widespread as to threaten your health in many ways unless I can help you understand how and why you are being used to further certain economic interests.

You have been repeatedly told that meat, eggs, butter and cream are bad for you and that pasta, cereals, bread, low-fat milk, flavored yogurt, high carbohydrate energy drinks and the like are good for you. Scientific research points in the other direction, but economics explain the discrepancy. The maligned foods, curiously enough, are all those that bring minimal profits to the food industry, and the approved foods, all of which are built upon the least expensive raw materials, are the ones the industry finds most profitable. Although scores of scientific papers have been published showing that what we are taught cannot be true, the utterances from medical associations, the government, and the media never change. Once that sinks in, you may be more receptive to sharing my suspicions that you have been victimized.

In the updated version of *New Diet Revolution,* I have written three new chapters. One deals with recent scientific developments that may clarify the controversy over which diet is really best for you. Another deals with questions I am asked most frequently by my readers, and the third deals with the rather preposterous misconceptions that I have seen in print about the program.

In addition, since my colleagues and I at the Atkins Center have expanded our services to our readers, I have updated many chapters to integrate information about how you may interact with us to facilitate your weight loss, health restoration and dietary enjoyment.

Also, throughout the book, I have updated information when appropriate.° And finally, I am aware that this very book has profoundly changed people's attitudes toward dieting and this edition recognizes the different mindset that people now have—namely, the expectation of success. This optimism, based on the success of people like you have seen, should, I am confident, serve to be a wonderfully self-fulfilling prophesy.

ROBERT C. ATKINS, M.D.
January 1999

°The many case histories are unchanged from the way they were originally written, and their names have been changed to protect their privacy.

PART ONE

Why the Diet Works

1 | *Dr. Atkins' Diet Revelation*

Is this you?

Determined to lose weight, you vowed to do it the "right" way, until success was yours. You stopped eating red meat, had omelets made in a Teflon pan from egg whites only, took the skin off the chicken, ate lots of pasta and baked potatoes with no butter. Frozen yogurt and fruit sherbet for desserts, oatmeal and skim milk for breakfast, or else, granola and a banana. For lunch, white meat turkey on a roll, and a generous salad with no oil.

And you stuck with it. You knew it was the right diet because everyone was pleased to see you on it, and congratulated you on your good and healthy taste in eating. And yet somehow it never quite felt like the right diet, and it never worked the way you thought it would. You found that you weren't quite satisfied eating this way: sometimes you were hungry, you didn't feel the kind of physical pick-me-up you thought you'd get from the "right" diet, and—worst of all—permanent, significant weight loss proved elusive. *You never actually got what you went on a diet for in the first place.*

Well, if that description fits, the probability is that you're just a normal person who's been *had.* Had by the society we live in, which encouraged you to believe in a right way that was just plain wrong for you. Had by a mudslide of media propaganda that promotes the fads of the moment irrespective of the metabolism of the people who have to go on them. But, if the person I've been describing is you, these frustrations are about to end. I have helped more than 25,000 people who've come to me needing to lose weight and unsure of how to do it, and I will help you too.

Diets come and go, but what people hope to get from them remains fairly constant. Let your fancy run free. Wouldn't you rather be on a diet that:

- Sets no limit on the amount of food you can eat?
- Completely excludes hunger from the dieting experience?
- Includes foods so rich that you've never seen them on any other diet?
- Reduces your appetite by a perfectly natural function of the body?
- Gives you a metabolic edge so significant that the whole concept of watching calories will become absurd to you?
- Produces steady weight loss, even if you have experienced dramatic failures or weight regain on other diets?
- Is so perfectly adapted to use as a lifetime diet that, unlike most diets, the lost weight won't come back?
- Consistently produces improvements in most of the health problems that accompany overweight?

Too good to be true? Not at all. Simply true. Moreover, repeatedly demonstrable and scientifically unimpeachable. That's a revelation.

These are the results for better than 90% of the tens of thousands of people under my personal supervision who have adopted the diet explained in this book, and I assume a very large percentage of the millions that have done it on their own. If you're overweight, this prospect is of such a life-altering order of magnitude that I have no doubt that you feel tempted to regard it as pie in the sky. You'll soon realize that's a poor analogy. First, I'll be taking away your pie, and second, these dietary results—far from being somewhere up in the clouds—are based on a set of well-grounded scientific facts that hardly anybody in the weight-loss business is paying attention to right now.

Health Was the Major Goal

I've spent twenty-five years treating the overweight and yet, significantly, *most of my patients during the last fifteen years did not come to me primarily for weight loss*. The pounds they shed were a beneficial side effect of usually quite successful treatments for conditions considerably more serious than obesity.

As a doctor, it was their dawning wellness that impressed me. As a potential dieter it will be their newfound slimness that will impress you.

So forgive this chapter's title, but it fits. And, if the first half of the revelation is in the alluring promise of weight loss, the second half is in the science that backs it up. That science has overwhelming significance for people who have found through hard experience that staying at a desirable weight is not too simple.

Let me place these facts on the table from the beginning:

1. Almost all obesity exists for metabolic reasons. Most studies have shown that the obese gain weight on *fewer* calories than people without a weight problem.

2. The basis of the metabolic disturbance in obesity has been pretty well worked out by the scientists over the last ten to fifteen years. It doesn't have to do with the metabolism of the fat you eat but with hyperinsulinism and insulin resistance. The insulin hormone and its effect on your blood sugar levels (which are constantly rising and falling in response to the food you eat) is far more directly related to your general health picture and to your likelihood of being victimized by killers such as heart disease and stroke than was ever suspected in the past. It is also *the single most significant determinant of your weight*. That is why, by the fifth decade of their lives, 85% of Type II diabetics are obese.

3. This metabolic defect involving insulin can be circumvented by restricting carbohydrates. When you restrict it, *you avoid the food subdivision that causes you to be fat*.

4. This metabolic correction is so striking that many of you will be able to *lose weight* eating a *higher* number of calories than you have been eating on diets top-heavy in carbohydrates. The so-called "calorie theory" has been a millstone around the necks of dieters and a miserable and malign influence on their efforts to lose.

5. Diets high in carbohydrates are precisely what most overweight people don't need and can't become slim on.

6. A carbohydrate-*restricted* diet is so effective at dissolving adipose tissue that it can create fat loss *greater* than occurs in fasting.

7. Our epidemics of diabetes, heart disease, and high blood

pressure are very largely the products of the hyperinsulinism connection.

8. The Atkins diet can correct and has corrected these serious medical complications of obesity. Indeed, 35% of my patients come to me for help with cardiovascular problems. The Atkins diet is probably the most aggressively health-promoting diet you will ever have the opportunity to be on.

Now let's get back to the word "revelation." Its meaning and connotation is to make known truths that were always there. Well, if the facts I have outlined are accepted as truths by an important segment of the scientific community, and yet are not so much as suspected by the majority of the populace, then this book will indeed be an act of revelation.

During the past twenty years, it has been suggested to the public, by techniques nearly as intense as brainwashing, that the only proper and healthy diet for a human being is a *low-fat* diet. If this were true, then the course of action for each and every one of us would be obvious and direct. But it's not true: *For many of us, the bypassing of carbohydrates is our ultimate solution.*

Now let's just look at a few of the misapprehensions about diet that are still widely held.

I Thought People Gained Weight Because They Ate Too Much

Not so. Most overweight people do not overeat. When they do, there is almost invariably a metabolic component driving them on, most often a truly addictive craving for carbohydrates.

People eating the right foods eat what they want to eat and stay around their ideal weight. However, the normal experience as one gets older is to find that one *cannot* eat the remarkably unnatural diet of the modern world and stay slim and healthy.

Your body, which was meant to function for a long, vigorous lifetime on healthy foods, becomes more and more sensitive to the actions of unhealthy ones. Your metabolism begins to creak and groan. Not only the pounds get added on but also the pains. Crushing fatigue, headaches, lassitude, irritability, depression—these are not really part of the process of reaching middle age, even though in our society they seem to be, largely because of the way we eat.

Your tough and hardy prehistoric ancestors were not eating devitalized, long shelf-life, processed foods, junk white bread, and pizza around their campfires—and they most certainly were not consuming sugar (as in our soft drinks and juices) when their bodies told them they needed water. If they had been, we never would have made it to civilization.

Carbohydrates or Fat

It's convenient to start with overweight, not only because it's the first thing my readers want to fix but because overweight is the most visible symptom of diet. My experience in treating more than 25,000 overweight patients has shown me that 90% of the time the overweight was caused by a disturbed carbohydrate metabolism.

Working off my operational assumption that a disturbed carbohydrate metabolism underlies obesity, my record of success has been rip-roaring, record-rending, and remarkably reproducible.

I'd like to mention a little ancient history. Twenty years ago, on the heels of widespread and fairly accurate reporting of my unusual success in treating overweight, I sold six million copies of *Dr. Atkins' Diet Revolution.**

I'm writing this new book to explain to a *new generation* all the latest developments in what has been the most successful weight-loss diet of the 20th century. I'm writing it as well to explain to my critics—I never go anywhere without them—how much new scientific evidence has appeared (especially in the last ten years) supporting the basic insights of low-carbohydrate dieting, a form of dieting that has been pushed aside in recent years by the influential but, alas, ineffective school of low-fat/low-calorie dieting that I would wager every single one of you is familiar with. This has been the dominant trend in dieting for the past decade, but its dominance hasn't, by and large, done a thing to take the pounds off.

Let's Examine the Calorie Myth

A calorie is an interesting little word that simply stands for a unit of energy—precisely the amount of heat needed to raise 1 gram of

---

*By now the sales have exceeded ten million copies worldwide.

water 1 degree Celsius at 1 atmosphere pressure.

Now, it has always been supposed that gaining weight results from taking in more calories than you expend through exercise, thermogenesis (the body's own heat production), and all the body's other metabolic functions. And, in fact, this is quite true.

What isn't true is what many doctors have concluded from this and passed on to their hapless patients. I'm referring to the notion that the only way to lose weight is to strictly control your intake of calories. Doctors brought up in this school of thought will tell their patients that all diets are basically equal in regard to their weight-loss potential. The only thing that matters is how many calories you take in!

This just isn't so. Different kinds of diets can have different effects on the amount of calories a person's body consumed daily, and, by taking different metabolic pathways, can cause the body to *require* different amounts of energy to do its work. On a low-carbohydrate diet, there are metabolic advantages that will allow you to *eat as many or more calories as you were eating before starting the diet and still begin losing pounds and inches*.

And if you eat fewer calories—most people do on this diet—you'll lose weight very fast. It's not that calories don't count, it's just than you can, in fact, sneak them out of your body, unused or dissipated as heat.

How does all this work on real people with real problems? Consider Stanley Moskowitz, a vigorous 64-year-old sculptor, who had survived three heart attacks in the 1980s, two "minor" and one severe. Stanley was overweight, his cholesterol levels were too high, and he had a great deal of arthritis—a very long-term problem for him. Naturally we took him off his ice cream and his French fries, his "junkfood Americana," as he called it, and just as naturally we urged him to eat a lot of meat, fish, fowl, and eggs when he wanted them, nuts, salads, vegetables, and a little cheese. A typical low-carbohydrate diet which he thoroughly enjoyed. But what was he going to do about his body and his beleaguered heart?

Stanley soon learned to smile about his results there, too. His cholesterol went down from 228 to 157—by the standard method of calculating such things, a massive reduction of 64% in his risk for another heart attack. And his weight? That went down from 228 to 190, a pretty good weight for a powerfully built six-footer, who creates all-metal sculptures in his studio. Incidentally, as a side effect of his net diet and the accompanying vita-nutrients, the pain

Stanley was so accustomed to in the joints of his shoulders and arms improved until they felt better than they had in more than twenty years.

I asked Stanley what he thought about all this, and he said, "Well, Dr. Atkins, these are probably the most startling physical changes I've experienced in my lifetime, and, strangely enough, all I had to do was enjoy myself."

Right. Let me tell you about another patient in more detail.

Mary Anne Evans

Before she saw me, Mary Anne had given up. I asked her to tell her own story.

"I said to myself, 'I'm simply going to be a fat person for the rest of my life.' I weighed 209 pounds when I came to see you, and I had been putting on weight steadily for twenty years—especially after each of my kids."

At 5'5" tall and 42 years old, Mary Anne's two-hundred-plus weight load was a health hazard and a half, and I told her so. She said she had tried countless diets—low-calorie diets including Weight Watchers; a hospital-based program that measured calories; and a liquid protein diet on which she had lost more than thirty pounds in three months and gained it back, with interest, in four.

She had thought it made sense to watch calories in order to lose weight, but somehow it never worked. Besides, it was terribly painful. The pounds that slid off with agonizing effort slipped on again effortlessly, which didn't seem quite fair.

So what was the use? Besides, she hadn't come to me with weight loss in mind. Her problems were quite medical. Mary Anne's blood pressure was high (160/100), she had a number of allergies, and her chief complaint was the extreme fatigue she had endured for the past several years. Add her overweight to all that, and I knew she was heading into a very difficult, mid-life physical crisis. Better act now.

To begin with, I took her off all carbohydrates. At nearly zero grams of carbohydrate, the most fat-retaining body will develop ketosis/lipolysis, which simply means it will be burning its own fat for fuel. Ketosis is the secret weapon of supereffective dieting. A person in that state is getting energy from ketones—little carbon fragments that are the fuels created by the burning of fat stores.

Many doctors have an unfavorable picture of ketosis, but, in fact, used as you'll use it on the Atkins program, it's going to be just as safe for you as it has been for my first 25,000 overweight patients. It's an extremely desirable state to be in, and it fully deserves the name I've coined for it: Benign Dietary Ketosis (BDK). But remember, you can't be in ketosis unless you're eating hardly any carbohydrates. For most people this means less than forty grams a day. To get you oriented, remember that an average person consumes approximately 300 gms of carbohydrates a day. And, of course, some people eat much more than that.

So let's look at Mary Anne. I wanted her to be in ketosis. She was willing to try. What did she do?

Mary Anne abandoned the crackers she ate with lunch and the potato she had with dinner; she gave up the popcorn, cake, and pizza she was used to snacking on during the day; she didn't put sugar in her coffee; she eschewed the occasional soft drink; she relinquished her breakfast orange juice; and, temporarily, she even gave up the vegetables she ate at dinner.

She was eating ham and eggs for breakfast, tuna fish for lunch, and chicken, pork chops, or steak for dinner. After the first few days, it was evident that she had had no trouble getting into BDK, and we added a salad at lunch and a salad at dinner.

> "By the second week, I realized I felt really good. I had a lot more energy than I'd had on the old diet, and I wasn't hungry."

Not being hungry is a typical result of being in BDK and one of the great initial attractions of the diet.

There was soon another reinforcement to keep on the diet: Mary Anne was losing weight—ten pounds in sixteen days. After five weeks, she'd lost 21 pounds, and her blood pressure was 120/78.

It took nine months to get Mary Anne Evans to 139 pounds, which was pretty close to where she wanted to be. Leaving 70 pounds behind, she's discarded one-third of the person she'd been.

> "It was so easy to do this. I lost weight without any hassle, I was eating things I really liked to eat anyway, and I was never

hungry. You said if I was hungry then I should eat as much as I wanted and anything I wanted as long as it had no carbohydrates, and that's what I did. And the change in my life was incredible. Before, my favorite position had been sitting. Now I go out camping with my youngest son, who's in the Boy Scouts, and last summer I went horseback riding in the Rockies. The people at the lab where I work can't believe the new me. I go out to lunch with some of the other women who are on diets, and they can't seem to lose weight, and *they're hungry*. And I'm sitting there eating a hamburger and a large salad."

Another two years have passed. Mary Anne's weight hovers around 142. She has a glass of wine before dinner a couple of nights a week, and she eats two potatoes weekly. Her only other carbohydrates are vegetables and salads and plenty of them. She's on a luxury diet that she perfectly well enjoys. She's full of energy, and her blood pressure is normal. She's a typical Atkins dieter.

Is This Shocking to You?

If it is, you're entirely normal. It contradicts the mythology that says the only way to be fit, slim, and healthy is to pursue low-fat dieting first, last, and always. That mythology is based on some well-observed scientific facts poorly interpreted. This mythology is mostly harmful, because a low-fat diet, which allows you to eat sugar, white flour, and other processed junk food, isn't healthy at all. And a low-fat diet, which can be healthy if it excludes junk, when extremely low is simply too austere for most people and infinitely more austere than the Atkins diet.

I also shouldn't have to tell you that moderate low-fat dieting—like the low-calorie dieting that preceded it—is a total failure when it comes to weight control. The facts bear it out, providing mute testimony to the low-fat fanaticism's frightening escalation of the obesity problem. In the decade between the mid-80s and mid-90s the percentage of daily calories of fat fell from 40% to 33%. But in that same time span, significant obesity rose from the 25% level it had maintained for 30 years, to 33%. For a nation the size of the U.S., that's 20 million new cases.

Needless to say, an unacceptably small number of dieters have been able to use fat restriction to lose weight. But for those who do, it has proven to be a complete wipeout for permanent weight loss. So big a wipeout that it's a major national embarrassment. On calorie-restrictive and/or low-fat diets, *only three to five percent* of dieters succeed in keeping their excess pounds off.

All you experienced dieters know that the test of a good diet is *keeping* the weight off. Any diet vigorously pursued can take those ounces and inches off initially. But once a low-calorie/low-fat dieter can no longer tolerate the biological gap between hunger and fulfillment found on such diets, what a rebound follows!

Meanwhile, the vast majority of those committed to following the Atkins diet have had little or no difficulty in maintaining their ideal weight after weight loss.

Whenever I talk about diet on my daily radio show in New York City, people call me up to tell me they've been on the diet for five years, or ten, or twenty, and they feel great. Fat? No, it never came back. I smile and congratulate them. And inside, I'm chuckling merrily. What they're telling me is that it's not just my own patients who've succeeded on the Atkins diet.

But then, dieting success on a properly managed low-carbohydrate diet is almost inescapable.

What's Dieting All About?

The word "diet" comes from the Latin *diaeta* and the Greek *diaita*, meaning "way of life" or "regimen." Not something one does for two or three months and then stops but the way one eats always. That's how I'd like you to think of it, because that's the only way you'll succeed at weight loss.

Most Americans eat a typical modern diet. Over half of them end up overweight. Why?

The foods we eat are divided into three basic categories—carbohydrates, fats, and proteins. Proteins are found in their largest concentrations in animal foods such as meat, fish, fowl, eggs, and cheese. They are also found in vegetables, foods such as nuts and seeds, and in high-protein legumes such as beans. Fat comes in many varieties but exists in almost all animal foods and in many vegetables. Carbohydrates exist in all vegetables, fruits, starches, and grains and, in its purest form, in refined sugar.

If you've been fat for very long, it's almost certain you have a disturbed carbohydrate metabolism. That's what the vast majority of studies have consistently shown. This means that the sugars, the refined carbohydrates, the junk foods that are such a whopping proportion of the American diet are slow poison to you. Those foods are bad for your health, bad for your energy level, bad for your mental state, bad for your figure. Bad for your career prospects, bad for your sex life, bad for your digestion, bad for your blood chemistry, bad for your heart. What I'm saying is that they're bad.

Most of the overweight people in the world are carbohydrate sensitive—often they're true carbohydrate addicts. They need a metabolic solution, not a low-fat one. They've struggled and struggled with low-calorie/low-fat diets and consistently failed. Why do they succeed on this diet?

This Diet Must Have Special Advantages

Yes. That is, you bet it does. Here are six reasons why the diet works.

First: It creates more fat mobilization than any other diet you have ever encountered. It has been *proven* (repeatedly) that it takes off more *fat* than other diets on which you would be eating an equal number of calories.

Second: A low-carbohydrate diet is not austere. Sheer hunger is behind most diet failure. A lifetime diet needs to be palatable, pleasant, and filling. The major austerity on this diet is the abandonment of sugar and such refined carbohydrates as white flour. But most people find that once they shake off the sugar addiction, they feel no strong desire to go back to it. For them, a diet on which they can eat an almost limitless variety of meat and fish and salads and vegetables prepared in the most appetizing manner (i.e., with butter and cream and spices and herbs to taste) is anything but austere. The Atkins diet is a dream diet—luxurious, sane, healthy, and varied.

Third: This is the easiest diet on which to *maintain* weight loss. The trouble with losing weight on an ordinary low-calorie diet or on a liquid-protein diet is that the maintenance program is so very different from the weight-loss program. Thus the pounds return with astonishing speed as, unprepared for maintenance, you go back to your former way of eating. There are sound physiological reasons for this. When you restrict the calories you eat, the body tends to become metabolically committed to putting the weight back on.

Success at *maintaining* weight loss is the great plus of the Atkins diet. That's interesting, since what most people know about low-carbohydrate dieting is that you can lose a lot of weight on it rapidly. And you can. But that's *not* the point. The only useful weight lost is the weight that doesn't come back again.

For that reason, there are actually four Atkins diets. Diet 1 is the initial *Induction* diet, which crashes you through most weight-loss barriers and will generally introduce even the most metabolically resistant person's fat-retaining body to weight reduction. Diet 2 is *Ongoing Weight Loss*—it will carry you smoothly toward your goal. Diet 3 is *Pre-Maintenance*—it begins to teach you the lessons of a style of eating that, with a modest degree of diligence on your part, will keep you slim forever. Diet 4 is the *Maintenance* diet. Even as you read this, thousands of my old patients and hundreds of thousands of my readers from years back are practicing this diet so that they'll never be fat again.

Let me state one crucial fact that you should always keep in mind: *for people committed to the Atkins diet, failure in maintaining weight loss is almost impossible.*

Fourth: Not only is this diet not austere, it makes you feel good. It's a high-energy diet. It's a quick and lasting solution to many of the commonest annoyances that patients tell doctors about in the privacy of the counseling room. Fatigue, irritability, depression, trouble concentrating, headaches, insomnia, dizziness, many forms of joint and muscle aches, heartburn, colitis, water retention, premenstrual syndrome, even tobacco addiction. For the lion's share of patients, a low-carbohydrate diet is a specific against these ills. And that's definitely a factor in keeping the weight off, because few people are willing to go back to feeling lousy once they've re-experienced the joys of feeling good.

Fifth: The diet is healthy. I found this out very quickly when I first began to put patients on it over thirty years ago. They began to recover from illnesses that I had no realization I was going to be treating *that way*. I discovered that most of my patients were suffering from a condition to which I gave the name Diet-Related Disorder (DRD), a condition which I'll describe in Chapters 11 to 14, where I discuss hypoglycemia, yeast infections, food allergies/intolerances, and a number of other conditions.

Correcting DRD was the key to most of my patients getting a

new lease on health. In addition, hypertension, diabetes, and most cardiovascular conditions respond with extraordinary rapidity to this diet. Since I was a practicing cardiologist when I began to prescribe the diet and 30 to 40% of my large patient population is still made up of people with cardiovascular problems, you can imagine how much of my success is based on the diet's heart benefits.

Sixth: The diet works because, as an increasing body of scientific evidence shows, it hooks onto the basic factor in both the control of obesity and the control of most of the modern degenerative illnesses. That factor is the excessive levels of insulin, an essential hormone in the human body. Insulin governs the basic mechanism by which the body lays on fat. When found in excessively high levels—we medical folk call that state hyperinsulinism—it vigorously promotes diabetes, atherosclerosis, and hypertension.

Thus the Atkins diet—partly by serendipity, for I had no intention of attacking the modern degenerative diseases when I first developed the diet—finds itself at the center of health planning for long, vigorous life.

This Ought to Change the Way You Look at Your Body

Metabolic defect. Hyperinsulinism. DRD. You'll understand these terms soon enough. Already they give you a hint of why you have a weight problem. For now, simply remember this: Diets high in sugar and refined carbohydrates radically increase the body's production of insulin, and insulin, as one distinguished scientist remarked, is "the best single index of adiposity." That final word is medical jargon for *fat*.

I bet you know people who eat more than you do and exercise less and yet can't seem to put on a pound. They're not lying about the amount they eat, any more than you are. They eat a *lot*. Maddening, but true.

What a revolutionary fact! In some ways, a cause for celebration. If you're overweight, you're not greedy, not weak-willed, not lazy, not self-indulgent, not *awful* but, in all probability, metabolically unfortunate. Doesn't that make a lot more sense? Overeating? So rarely is that true. Most people eat when they're hungry and stop when they're full. Well, then, how could they be *over*eating? They're doing what their bodies tell them to do, and bodies have a sort of wisdom.

The critical factor is *what* you eat.

What's Wrong with Carbohydrates?

If you mean what's wrong with a spear of broccoli or a bunch of spinach, the answer is nearly nothing, they're magnificent foods. When I speak of carbohydrates, I'm referring to the unhealthy ones—sugar and white flour, milk and white rice, processed and refined foods of all kinds, junk foods and the like. But, at least during the weight-loss portion of the Atkins diet, even potentially healthy carbohydrates such as starches and most fruits must be monitored.

Once you're lost your extra pounds, you can return to starches and fruits to the degree that they won't upset your metabolic balance and cause you to start gaining weight again. But the refined foods I've just mentioned simply aren't good for you—*ever*. Am I advocating a high-fat diet? Not in the long run. As my critics twenty years ago were forced to acknowledge when they looked into the matter, and as Professor John Yudkin proved, this isn't a high-fat diet. The average person on a low-carbohydrate diet eats less fat than he was eating on his previous "balanced" diet—the average diet in America today.[1]

There are many reasons for that, which I'll be telling you about. But for the moment, let's consider the question of whether we are in trouble because we are gorging ourselves on steaks and hot dogs.

I hardly need to tell you about the way we eat. You've all seen the aisles in the supermarket crammed with cookies and crackers, ice cream, frozen cakes and pies, soft drinks, and junk white breads so repugnant to the metabolism that many forms of rodents—wiser than us—won't even eat them except as a last resort.

This is not real food; it's invented, fake food. It's filled with sugar and highly refined carbohydrates *and* with fat (not to mention a dreadful panoply of chemical additives). For thousands of years, human beings were in luck—none of this food existed. Now we're stuck with it. Because it's incredibly profitable, it's also widely distributed. But there isn't a person on this planet who should be eating it.

I'm ready to tell you that if you want to be slim and vigorous, you can't eat like that, but you can eat like a king or queen—and certainly a prince or princess. (When you look at the recipes in Part V and see some of the delights prepared for you by our master low-carbohydrate chef, Graham Newbould—who, in happier days, was chef to the Prince and Princess of Wales—you'll see how appropriate it is that I should make such a statement.)

On the Atkins diet, you can eat the natural, healthy animal and vegetable foods that people ate and grew robust on in centuries past. You don't have to be austere or peculiar. You don't have to eat like a rabbit; you can eat like a human being. You can enjoy salads and fish, roast rack of lamb and lobster, butter and broccoli, and even that dietitian's sturdy nightmare—bacon and eggs for breakfast.

Now to answer the question at the head of this section: *What's wrong with carbohydrates?* The answer is, nothing, if you're not trying to lose weight and, if they're the right carbohydrates. The Atkins diet is called a low-carbohydrate diet because during the first two stages of the diet, the only carbohydrates you eat are moderate helpings of vegetables and salads. Later, once you've reached your ideal weight, you can eat larger helpings of the healthy carbohydrate foods, as long as you stay below the Critical Carbohydrate Level for Maintenance (CCLM) that keeps you from regaining your lost weight.

The Atkins diet isn't a peculiar, exotic diet. It's *the* human diet raised to its healthiest pitch and stripped of the 20th century food inventions that are so economically delightful and so physiologically disastrous.

The suggestion that this isn't a perfectly healthy way to eat because I don't tell you to flee in terror from a steak is amusing but also sad. There are big lies lurking in the medical forests, and one of the things this book will show is how you can detect them.

What You Need to Do

I'd like to ask you to try the diet out for 14 days. That will be more than enough time for you to not only lose a surprising amount of weight, but to find out how wonderful you'll feel on a low-carbohydrate meal plan and how refreshing it is to lose pounds and inches even while *you eat as much as you like*.

There are lots of diets on which you can lose weight temporarily and feel lousy while you're doing it. This isn't one of them.

Of course, when I propose you try the diet out for 14 days, I'm sure you realize I don't expect you to stop there. I'm trying to lure you into your lifetime diet.

The second reason for keeping close track of what happens to you in the first 14 days is that it will help you learn the degree of your metabolic resistance to weight loss. (See the weight table in Chapter 17.)

Metabolic Resistance—A Little or a Lot

Not everyone loses weight with the same ease, even on a low-carbohydrate diet. People with a less than average degree of metabolic resistance will lose anywhere from 8 to 15 pounds in two weeks on the diet; people with an average level, somewhat less.

However, the person who is truly metabolically resistant won't lose much at all without getting more exercise or taking nutritional supplements that help weight loss, or even slightly restricting the quantity of food he or she eats—or some combination of the three. And, if you're that rare person with an enormous metabolic resistance to weight loss, I'll show you just what you need to do. For you the program will be a little more strenuous than for everyone else.

Interestingly enough, many people who have struggled with overweight all their lives and have never been able to succeed for long on other diets have only a very moderate degree of metabolic resistance to weight loss, and lose quite quickly and easily on the Atkins diet. No one is more surprised than a person in that condition who finds the pounds swiftly vanishing. As an old pro in this arena, I have to tell you it's a particular pleasure witnessing their joy.

To all my readers I want to say: *I hope to amaze you, as I amazed millions of dieters who have learned before you.* I want you to surprise yourself. Never think it can't be done. It *has* been done.

This is a proven diet—enlarged, refined, and, I think, made better. But still, in its essence, it is the same diet that has helped millions of people to lose weight. *No other diet in the world has its track record.*

Formerly called a "fad" diet, it has survived the test of time. The low-fat diet it has superseded is the one that will be remembered in history books as an unsuccessful experiment.

2 | *What This Book Will Reveal to You*

If you have a weight problem, I certainly have the qualifications to help you. I suppose no diet book has ever been written by a doctor with so many weight-loss successes to his credit, including the vast majority of over 25,000 overweight individuals I have treated in my office at the Atkins Center, a clinical facility that overflows a six-story building in Manhattan. There are also millions of successes among those who have read my books or newsletters or listened to my daily radio broadcasts.

This level of success could not have been achieved by using a system similar to everyone else's or even a variation on the theme. It could only have been achieved by offering a revolutionary departure from the conventional diet wisdom. We went against the grain, stuck to our scientific principles, and provided a diet quite unlike all the others you may have been exposed to.

My purpose is not to be critical of other diets, for with enough determination, all can be made to work for a number of persevering individuals. Unfortunately, in the past two decades there has been a tendency to disseminate *only one diet*, as if it were the be-all and end-all for everyone—the only diet that works.

Never before in my career have I heard so many patients say, "I know what I'm supposed to eat, but I just can't make it work for me." The trouble is, they *don't* know what they're supposed to eat, but they've heard the wrong answer so often, they think it's an unchallenged truth.

You've heard the expression "fad diet." "Fad" refers to that which achieves a widespread, if evanescent, popularity. It conveys no value judgment on the ultimate worth of the thing described. The current diet fad is the low-fat, high-carbohydrate diet espoused by virtually every nationwide chain of diet centers, by the monthly magazine articles, the media advice-givers, professional organizations, and even by federal government bulletins. Low-fat dieting works for some people. I know that's true; I've seen it happen. But the notion that it works for everyone is sadly misinformed. And, if you delve into the medical literature, you'll discover that the apparent unanimity about its benefits is *only* apparent. Moreover, if you're overweight, you may be living testimony to the fact that it doesn't work for you. My experience leads me to say that for scores of millions of people—the majority of the overweight in America—it does not readily work. It runs directly counter to scientific evidence about the human metabolism and the actions of carbohydrate foods.

You may recall that thirty years ago, Britain's preeminent nutritionist, Dr. John Yudkin, announced that the majority of British physicians recommended a low-carbohydrate diet, and that the majority of American dieters, having read books by me, as well as by Drs. Taller, Stillman, and Tarnower, had created such an awareness of the principle of carbohydrate restriction that such dieting was elevated to "fad" status. Before that, calorie counting had been the fad. But has there been any change in the physiology of obese humans in these years? I doubt it. The pendulum merely swings.

Another swing of the pendulum has been sorely needed. Fueled by this very book, I believe it has begun, but there is much to overcome. The current fad is based on the kind of simplistic logic that captures the fancy of the unsophisticated: "If you don't want to be fat, don't eat fat; if you don't want cholesterol, don't eat cholesterol." It's the "You-are-what-you-eat" argument, totally devoid of any reference to known metabolic mechanisms. And the results are dismal.

The danger of the low-fat fad is clearly apparent from the study of USDA statistics. The pendulum began to swing toward fat restriction in 1975. That's when per-capita consumption of red meat began its decline, and fish, chicken, and skim milk showed rather surprising gains. For the last twenty years, the movement in these directions has been steady. But the figures carry with them an ominous warning. In those twenty years the per-capita consumption of sugars (including corn syrup) has escalated from a world-leading 118 pounds a year to over 150 pounds![1] Let's translate that into terms you understand best: We're consuming nearly 750 calories of sugar a day. And that's the average man, woman, or child, not the sugar addict. This means that, by a conservative reckoning, over one-third of all the calories an adult puts into his or her body each day comes from nutritionally empty and metabolically harmful caloric sweeteners.

If I can't convince you that this much sugar is a major potential health risk, then I would probably have a tough time convincing you to wear clothes in the winter.

To make matters worse, our intake of that other overly refined nutrient—white flour—by being exalted to "must-have" status by government agencies that invented a new, untested Food Pyramid, has also been escalating at an alarming rate.

I'm not about to fall into the error of the low-fat dieting devotees who claim that their diet works for everyone. I would feel rather foolish if I did. No diet works for everyone. Human biological individuality is very marked. Nonetheless, for the past 30 years I've worked at perfecting a diet that experience has shown me is successful with the great majority of patients. And this is a diet that makes them feel better, that supports their long-term health, and that controls their weight without hunger or discomfort—sizable advantages.

Nature's Diet

I can't emphasize too strongly that nature really did provide for us very well. Even before the onset of agriculture, the human animal was able, for millions of years, to remain strong and healthy in conditions of often savage deprivation by eating the fish and animals that scampered and swam around him, and the fruits and vegetables and berries that grew nearby. Without medicine, without expertise, without insulated housing or reliable heating, we nevertheless survived.

We were immensely aided by the fact that the dietary side of our primitive lifestyle was enormously healthy.

The dietary side of our sophisticated, modern lifestyle is enormously *un*healthy.

I'm optimistic that you'll learn to fully appreciate the fact that fresh food—unrefined, unprocessed, unmanufactured, unim-proved, un-"enriched"—is splendidly right for you.

The Atkins diet that I have high hopes you'll be eating for the rest of our life contains, in its most liberal, lifetime maintenance form, most vegetables, nuts and seeds, some grains and starches to the extent that your metabolism allows, and occasional fruits. It also contains a sumptuous variety of delicious protein foods and some high-fat foods like butter and cream that you'll find stricken from nearly every other current diet.

This isn't because this is a high-fat diet. It isn't that, although heaven knows I've often had the accusation thrown in my face. At the moment, virtually everything is laid to the discredit of dietary fat, and yet its advantages for a dieter seem never to be mentioned. Fat satiates the appetite. Fat is the only one of the three food categories that can stabilize blood sugar. Fat stops carbohydrate craving. And fat, in the absence of carbohydrates, accelerates the burning of stored fat. The wise dieter can use fat to his advantage.

Still, the Atkins diet is not a high-fat diet, partly because some of the largest sources of fat in the modern diet are the junk foods and convenience foods I would never allow you to eat. On the Atkins diet you will be eating a large percentage of meat, fish, fowl, eggs, and butter than you consumed before you went on it, but you may well be eating less fat overall.

Even though I will be showing you the benefits of fat and protein, I must emphasize that the real source of health improvement on this diet will come from excluding the typically gargantuan modern consumption of junk carbohydrates. In Chapter 3, I'll explain hyperinsulinism and, as soon as you begin to understand this fundamental modern concept—one of the genuine, scientific/medical breakthroughs of the last two decades—you'll understand why a *low-fat diet* is not a necessity for a person who's on *this* diet. The health improvements, inseparable from a diet that excludes all the possible combinations of sugar and white flour, are more than sufficient to make the Atkins diet one of the healthiest eating programs you could ever embark on.

I must make this point here at the outset because it's fundamental to everything I want you to know. You may buy this book and I may have a publishing success because you want to be a health-club knockout, and that's fine with me, but it wouldn't be a sufficient reason for writing this book.

This diet is intended to be the basis for your good health along with the vita-nutrients that are part-and-parcel of it. I have *no doubts* it can be just that. My current patients aren't fools—very few people are when it comes to figuring out how they feel—and what works for them is what I'm offering *you*. The important thing is that it made them healthier. The fact that it took off their excess weight was, for most of them, merely a side benefit. But, if the emotional benefits were a side issue, the medical benefits were front and center. Overweight has complex but undeniable connections with ill health. I couldn't let my patients stay fat, *because* they had come to me to get healthy, and ideal health requires ideal weight.

In your case, you've made contact with me to get slim, and to do that I'm going to have to make you healthier too. On the Atkins program, I don't think you could separate those results if you wanted to.

But, Dr. Atkins, I Want to Have Fun Eating, Have Fun Living, and Lose Weight for Life

And so you shall. Do you believe that a man can go from gaining 0.5 pounds a week to losing 3.9 pounds a week without significantly altering the number of calories he consumes? Let me introduce you to Harry Kronberg then. There are lots of Harry Kronbergs in my practice, but I didn't have to scratch my head trying to figure out which one to use because Harry happened to come in for a visit the day I was writing this chapter. I want you to pay close attention to his story and try not to give way to disbelief, because these results are real. And I think I'm going to bring Harry back to take repeated bows at a number of places in this book.

Harry Kronberg, the 39-year-old manager of a lumbar yard, came to me with a heart arrhythmia and a desperate weight problem. He had been chubby even as a child, but now things were out of hand. A few years before, he had gone to a diet center and lowered his weight from 245 to 185 on a low-fat diet. And he kept it all off, except for 95 pounds.

That's right, when Harry came to see me, he tipped the scales at 280, and on a 5' 6½" frame that was ponderous. In the previous 35 months, eating a relatively starchy, low-fat diet of approximately 1700 calories a day, he had gained 70 pounds, exactly 2 pounds a month, clearly indicating that he had a metabolic problem. Then he went on my diet, the diet you're going to read about in this book. This diet has radically restricted his carbohydrates while allowing him to eat freely of meat, fish, fowl, and eggs. Harry was told to eat as much as he wanted. The calorie count was strikingly similar to what he had been eating on his previous diet, but he never missed a meal, and never suffered a moment's hunger. The result was that in the first three months (to the day) that he's been on the diet, he's lost 50.5 pounds (3.9 pounds a week), and he's still losing at a steady three pounds weekly. His heart symptoms have gone away, his cholesterol has gone down from 207 to 134, his triglycerides from 134 to 31.

I think I can fairly say that Harry was impressed. In fact, he said to me, "I'm not going to stop taking these vitamins you're giving me, doctor. There's something in them that makes me lose weight." Well, there was something in them that made his experience run smoothly, but I have to confess there was nothing in them that made him lose weight.

But Will I Be Able to Enjoy Eating on This Diet?

It will really surprise me if you can't. Let's take a look at Patricia Finley's menu. She's been on the Atkins *Induction* diet for three and a half months and she's lost 31 pounds. She has another 35 to go, but I think she'll get there. Incidentally, most of the patients I'll tell you about in the course of this book will have reached their ideal weight already, but I don't see any reason to restrict myself to them. I've had so many thousands of dieting successes that it isn't really that brazen of me to assume that a large majority of the still-in-the-process-of-losing dieters who I tell you about will also succeed.

Patricia, who used to eat quite a lot of starches and who would sometimes go on massive dessert binges when she was under pressure, has converted to a tasty low-carbohydrate diet.

For breakfast, she eats bacon and eggs, or a cheese omelet, or some vegetables with blue cheese. Lunch can be tuna fish or chicken with a sumptuous salad. But sometimes she'll have chopped sirloin, sautéed with onions, chili powder and peppers. Patricia enjoys having olives or asparagus spears for snacks, but she puts the greatest amount of energy and attention into dinner. She finds that it isn't possible to feel deprived when you're enjoying a meal consisting of guacamole (for the uninitiated that's mashed avocado mixed with tomatoes, onion, and seasoning) and strips of chicken and steak. Add to that her passion for grated zucchini in olive oil with butter and nutmeg, her liking for broccoli with lemon butter sauce, and her homemade recipe for chicken soup, and what do you get? Starvation? *Not*. Patricia also enjoys lamb shanks with chopped onions, cooked with olive oil, herbs, and "Crazy Mixed Up Salt."

And she assures me this is only a small sample of the food she finds it possible and delightful to eat—*on her diet*

Yes, that's a strict weight-loss diet I've been describing. A diet that you can adapt to your own individual tastes as long as you eat only permitted foods.

I think there's food for thought in such a food story. Now, let me mention some of the other things this book will show you:

DIET EXPERIENCE AND WEIGHT CHANGES

- How to create an edge for yourself, a metabolic advantage that allows you to lose weight at a higher calorie intake than you've ever lost on before.
- How you'll succeed even though you may have always been hungry, tired, depressed, and unsuccessful on other diets. You won't be any of those things on this one.
- Why you won't need willpower on the Atkins diet.
- How binge eating can be stopped in a day.
- How you can reach your ideal weight by burning your excess fat as fuel—the marvelous condition of Benign Dietary Ketosis.
- How to insure that what you lose is fat and not lean body tissue.
- How you can keep those excess pounds off forever by a lifetime diet change in which you keep the same diet you lost on as your basic diet and add to it some of your most desired foods.
- How you can determine your degree of metabolic resistance to weight loss, and how to modify your diet accordingly.
- How to use the novel Atkins Fat Fast if you have severe metabolic resistance.
- How you can use a vita-nutrient solution, the answers derived from nutritional medicine, to help overcome metabolic resistance, and to allow you to eliminate the medications that keep you fat.

HEALTH CHANGES

- How to overcome Diet-Related Disorder—this is the *evil* trio of hypoglycemia, yeast infections, and food intolerances.
- How you can avoid the health catastrophe of hyperinsulinism.
- How you can custom design your exercise program.
- How to improve your energy level.
- How, in conjunction with the diet, you can organize a program

of nutritional supplementation that will do wonders for your health.

- How to lower your cholesterol level on the diet and improve your other blood-lipid values.
- How to use the diet to overcome medical conditions, including diabetes, heart disease, and high blood pressure, that are so often associated with obesity.

FOOD CHANGES

- How to use the rich, sumptuous foods forbidden on other diets to make your new diet a luxurious eating pattern fit for a prince or princess.
- How to create super-palatable substitute foods for the carbohydrate items you love.
- How to function in supermarkets and restaurants, and at dinner parties, after you've begun your new lifestyle.
- How to personalize your diet so it is uniquely suited to your tastes, lifestyle, and metabolism.
- How animal foods can suppress your craving for sweets.

PERSONAL AND FAMILY CHANGES

- How to explain your diet to family and friends.
- How to eat comfortably with them, even if their style of eating remains different from yours.

HOW TO MAINTAIN THE DIET

- What to do if you have cravings for sweets and starches.
- How to go on a maintenance diet that will already be second nature to you.
- How to follow the maintenance plan for a lifetime.
- How to break the diet and still survive.
- How to use dietary fat and enhance your health.
- How to adjust and return to your ideal weight if you gain weight at some point.
- How to never be more than five pounds above your ideal weight.

This Just Might Be the Diet for You

That's an ambitious program I've just outlined, and I have wide-eyed and romantic moments in which I almost wish I could tell you it's going to be difficult and that you'll have to summon up all your reserves of energy and courage to march in step with it. But the truth is, I can't claim anything so heroic. It's going to be surprisingly easy, and it's going to make all the difference in your life.

I've spent over thirty years in the trenches with people who didn't like what their excess weight was doing to them—young and old, some only ten pounds overweight, some two hundred. I've seen people sit down in my office and start to cry uncontrollably because they were so appalled by their repeated failures, and so despairing of help.

I hope I've finally convinced you that you're holding help in your hands right now.

3 | *Is This You?—Three Types Who Need a Ketogenic Diet*

You have a right to wonder if I'm talking about you. I've said that if you have a weight problem, there's better than a 90% chance I can help you solve it. Is that really relevant to your own particular, very individual weight situation? In order to help you understand where you do or don't fit in, I'll profile my typical obesity patient. It's not hard to do. There are several signature patterns about overweight due to disorders of carbohydrate metabolism that are instantly recognizable.

Does This Describe You?
Group A Responders

- Are you overweight despite the fact that you don't eat that much?
- Do you follow standard weight-loss diets and still make no headway losing weight or get stuck far short of your goal?
- Have you noticed that slim people definitely consume more food and more daily calories than you do?
- Are you just plain unpleasantly hungry on low-calorie diets?
- Do you find the amount of food you eat is really the least you can take in without feeling physically unsatisfied?
- Do you feel a sense of unfulfillment when you eat a normal meal?
- Do you find that when you eat the amount of food that feels just right, you don't lose—or you even gain?
- Have you often said, "I'm really very disciplined; it must be my metabolism"?

Or Is This a Better Description Of You?
Group B Responders

- Do you have an inexplicable obsession with food?
- A habit of night eating?
- A tendency to binge?
- A craving for such carbohydrate foods as sweets, pastas, and breads?
- Do you nibble all day long when food is available?
- A strong desire to eat again shortly after you've eaten to fullness?
- Do you consider yourself a compulsive eater? Have you ever said, "I only wish I could control my eating behavior?"
- Do you have specific symptoms of ill health, such as the ones I'm about to list, that lessen or vanish as soon as you eat? Do you suffer:
    - Irritability?
    - Inexplicable drops in your strength and stamina at various times throughout the day—often overwhelming bouts of fatigue, especially in the afternoon?
    - Mood swings?
    - Difficulty in concentrating?
    - Sleep difficulties—often a need for considerable quantities of sleep, sometimes a habit of waking from a sound sleep?
    - Anxiety, sadness, and depression for which there's no situational explanation?
    - Dizziness, trembling, palpitations?
    - Brain fog and loss of mental acuity?

Or Perhaps This Describes You:
Group C Responders

- Do you have a single food or beverage you feel you could not do without?
- Would you pass up an elegant meal to get your favorite food?
- Is there a specific food or beverage that makes you *feel* better as soon as you get it?
- Do you ever think, "I wonder if I could be addicted to that food/beverage?"
- Do you feel this way about a *category* of foods? (Sweets, soft drinks, dairy products, grains, etc.)

What These Answers Tell You

Now let's see what you do with this information. First of all, let me say I would find it hard to believe there could be a significantly overweight person who had no "yes" responses. If you respond in the affirmative, then this book is about you and for you, and I probably do have a solution for your problem.

If most of your "yes" responses are in group A, you have a metabolic problem, manifested either by a) a relative inability to lose weight or maintain weight loss, or by b) hunger or inability to achieve and maintain satiety.

If most of your "yes" responses were to group B questions, then you probably have glucose intolerance, commonly known as hypoglycemia.

If most of your affirmatives were to the group C statements, then you probably have an addition to the food/beverage you singled out. Other terms for the phenomenon are "food allergy" or the more accurate "individual food intolerance."

If you're a group C responder, and the food/beverage you've identified is or contains a carbohydrate, then you have a carbohydrate addiction, and this book will provide you with more answers than you've thought possible.

These Three Responders Are All Facets of the Same Problem

You A and B responders (and most of you C responders as well) have a condition that is the common denominator behind nearly all your problems, and it's called hyperinsulinism.

Before I explain the significance of hyperinsulinism and the very good news of how easily you can tame it with this diet, I want you to reflect on the significance of eating.

Stop and ask yourself, *"What else do I do in the course of a day that constitute such a dramatic and intense alteration of my body as swallowing the food I do?"*

Between the time you rise and the time you go to bed, you put pounds of organic matter into your mouth. Your body runs on it. Don't be surprised that if you make bad choices, you'll pay a price.

Now, before I explain more about the mechanism of the metabolic problems that result, let's look at the impact of sugar and carbohydrate consumption upon real people.

Life Without Control

Food-obsessive behavior is common, and some of the tougher cases can be difficult to cure even on this diet and impossible on any other. Certain writers in the diet area have spoken of carbohydrate addiction, and the term isn't a bad one. The men and women who binge and fantasize and often almost live for food are as much between a rock and a hard place as the addict of alcohol or narcotics. They desperately need a metabolic approach to their problem.

Gordon Lingard, a real estate executive, was an extreme example. He was 53 when he came to see me and was 306 pounds on a 5'10" frame. Gordon had progressed from a normal weight in college (when he was a lifeguard) to extreme obesity by his late twenties. His weight had gone as high as 450 pounds. He had no hormonal imbalances, and he had tried everything—stomach stapling, emetics, laxatives, and every diet from B to Z.

Gordon was an inexplicable to himself as to his many doctors. All he knew was that he had to eat. The cravings were indescribable. He told me he was constantly planning his next binge. Gallons of ice cream disappeared as swiftly as an ordinary carbohydrate addict downs a candy bar. Sugar was Gordon's master obsession.

> "There was never a moment I didn't desire it. Often I would shake until I could put some sugar in my mouth. The symptoms were totally physical, and they were really frightening. For me there was nothing else but food. I had an hour's drive from my office to my home, and I knew every restaurant, every dinner, every candy machine, every soft drink dispenser along the whole route."

I bet you'd be willing to bet this was almost entirely psychological—and you'd be wrong.

Gordon Lingard's case was a special one and, for a while, treating him was no cinch. In his case, some of the vita-nutrient aids I describe in Chapter 21 were an important part of the solution. But what I'd like you to realize is that Gordon's problem was only a more extreme version of the problems so many overweight people have.

His difficulties were basically metabolic difficulties, and they were solvable metabolically. Today Gordon Lingard has nearly reached his normal weight for the first time in thirty years, and he no longer feels the drive to consume sugar.

Gordon had failed repeatedly on low-fat/low-calorie diets. And why not? His problem lay in his metabolic response to carbohydrates. To solve an out-of-control situation like this by restricting calories while not restricting carbohydrates is like marching into the surf with a firm intention of turning back the ocean.

You may have picked up this book with the secret inner conviction that you're a "compulsive eater." In all probability, you're a carbohydrate addict. How many compulsive eaters of steaks have you come across? Not too many, huh? Let me tell you, it's a rare breed.

A Craving for Sweets Is Often a Sign

Many people start off when they're kids eating the so-called "balanced" diet, but by the time they're adults, it's becoming progressively less balanced. Eating didn't seem all that important to them once, but now it does. So they look at their waistlines, they look at their eating, and they realize they have a problem. Usually they notice that their taste in food has gone off in a specific direction.

Carbohydrates now form the bulk of what they eat; breads and baked goods, cakes and candies, pasta and popcorn. Surprising and illogical food cravings are typical. Do you ever have dinner with a big dessert and almost immediately afterward find that you want some candy? That's a sign, as is fatigue, that your carbohydrate metabolism is out of whack.

It's not that you eat when you're not hungry, but you seem to be *always* hungry. And yet when you eat the carbohydrate food you crave, you feel only briefly better. Your situation is the exact opposite of the one you'll experience on the Atkins diet. There, you'll find that your appetite has diminished, but your satisfaction in the food you eat has increased.

Do You Feel Like a Compulsive Eater?

Many carbohydrate addicts could no more walk past a refrigerator without opening it than Pete Sampras could let a short lob drift overhead without smashing it. I've heard many patients say, "It's irresistible, Dr. Atkins. I'm a slave. How can you possibly help me?"

I say, "That's all right—your compulsions have no terrors for me and soon they won't for you. When you pass that refrigerator, open it, have some chicken salad or sliced pot roast. If you eat the way I'm asking you to eat, you'll find that food is still delicious, but the compulsions will fade."

You see, your food compulsion isn't a character disorder, it's a chemical disorder called hyperinsulinism, and you have it simply because you've eaten the same unhealthy way that *most* people in our culture do.

The Diet That Does It

There are marked similarities in the diet eaten in all the developed, modern countries of the world, so, for now, I'll just mention the statistics for the United States. Once you understand what healthy eating can be like, you'll find them as bizarre and shocking as I do.

First, and worst, there's sugar. Let me tell you just a little bit about that. Two hundred years ago, the average person ate less than ten pounds of sugar a year. Then almost exactly a hundred years ago, the lid blew off. In the 1890s, the craze for cola beverages swept the nation—which means that when we were thirsty and craved water, we got sugar as well. The net result was that the sugar intake, which had been twelve pounds a year in 1828, was nearly ten times that in 1928. The latest Department of Agriculture statistics show that the average American consumed 118 pounds of caloric sweeteners (principally refined sugar and high fructose corn syrup) in 1975 and 152 pounds in 1996.[1] This means that sugar and corn syrup alone form a whopping percentage of the average American's diet. Those figures translate into 190 grams of sugar (and corn syrup) a day. Compare that with the 300 grams of carbohydrate the government expects us to consume each day, and we see that sugar now comprises over 60 percent of the carbohydrate total.

Sugar has no nutritional value and is directly harmful to your health. Despite vociferous attempts to defend it, there are hundreds of studies that clearly show how deadly its effects can be.[2] I won't go into them now, because I want you to learn about hyperinsulinism in the next chapter, and sugar deserves a whole book.

But I do want you to remember what the modern western diet consists of, especially in America. Remember, too, that if you don't take your sugar straight, you'll find it already inserted into a thousand different foods and beverages before they come to your table, put, for the most part, into stuff that, if it hadn't been made so sweet, you'd wrinkle your nose up at. Sugar is the American food industry's friend, and it seems to be the friend of some highly regarded medical organizations, as well. For example, some of the most sugar-laden cereals (often half their calories are sugar), with names such as Froot Loops and Pop Tarts, bear the Heart-Check seal of the American Heart Association. If you've allowed yourself to be overawed by the vast quantities of anti-fat propaganda issued forth in the guise of nutritional education during the past ten years, you may almost have forgotten what's *really* packed onto those supermarket shelves.

Let me assure you that eating meat, fish, and fowl isn't a health hardship—it's what the human carnivore has eaten for millions of years.

Look at the way people ate in the 19th century. They were liberal in the use of butter and lard, they were beef and pork eaters, and their eggs were unrestricted. Yet hardly anyone died of heart attacks. The coronary occlusion, the heart attack, was first described in a medical journal in 1912. And Dr. Paul Dudley White, who was Eisenhower's personal cardiologist, recalled that he didn't see his first heart attack until after his first year of postgraduate training in the 1920s. If you want an even more illuminating fact, chew on this one: The 20th-century Frenchman with his butter-, cheese-, and goose-liver-paté-laden diet has a heart disease rate 60% lower than his American peers.[3] (The Frenchwoman does even better—she has the lowest heart disease rate in the western world.)

So what caused the avalanche of degenerative diseases? The only thing I ask is that you observe how our diet actually changed in the last century. Not only were colas invented in the 1890s, but to make matters worse, the mills that could refine wheat into a white, nutritionally barren flour were developed in the same decade. Once that flour was put together with sweetness and saltines, we had the makings of the junk food culture of America and many of the other developed countries—but not all of them.

Let's look at the Frenchman again—the fellow with his teeth buried in the *paté de foie gras*. As anyone who's been to France or who watches *60 Minutes* knows, the French are far less afflicted by obesity and heart disease than Americans. Yet their diet is *higher* in fat. (They eat comparable amounts of meat and fish, four times as much butter, and twice as much cheese as Americans.) What does it all mean? *Could it have anything to do with the fact that the American per capital consumption of sugar is 5½ times that of the French?*

And in the crucial 60-year time span between 1910 and 1970 when coronary heart disease escalated from a yet-to-be-recognized problem to the killer of more than half of us, this is what happened to our diet: The intake of animal fat and butter dropped significantly, while the intake of cholesterol was not changed, but the intake of refined carbohydrates (mainly sugar, corn syrup and white flour) went up by 60%.[4]

Yet we all know that fat is the source of all ills. Don't we?

Keep Your Eye on Your Metabolism

Sugar, you see, activates certain metabolic processes that are both harmful to your health and folly for your waistline. Sugar is a metabolic poison.

You could, of course, ignore this fact and attempt to control your overweight by calorie counting and eating only so many pieces of this and only so many grams of that. That is, you could direct yourself to the quantity instead of the quality of your diet. Isn't that what conventional dieting advises you to do?

But I want to tell you that *the likelihood that you'll permanently lose weight by controlling your calories is almost nil.*

Bet you guessed that before now. Common sense dictates that when a lot of people try the same answer to the same problem and they all fail, there's something wrong with their solution. You may have tried a low-calorie diet. I'm sure you've seen other people try it. After a promising start, they end up as failures. Perhaps there is no sense beating your head against the wall.

Melissa Jackson, a 35-year-old insurance executive, came to me weighing 223 pounds on a 5'4" frame. She had tried literally every diet that she read about or that anyone proposed to her since she was 16. She had been fat even as a child. The situation had always tormented and obsessed her, because not only did her accumulated body fat interfere with her life, it was something she simply couldn't handle. She tried diet pills and liquid-protein diets. By the time she was in her thirties, she was used to being told after months of conscientious struggle that she was "plateauing at 200 pounds."

"The situation was out of my control and because of that I didn't like myself. It got to the point where I would be hungry all the time on low-fat or low-calorie diets, and I'd lose maybe two pounds a month. Then I couldn't even lose that. I would literally starve myself to the point of collapse, and after four or five days of eating nothing I'd find I'd lost half a pound."

Melissa Jackson went on the Atkins diet and lost 77 pounds in a year. Without hunger. She has always liked—and during a large part of her life had craved—cake, candy, soda, and pasta, and she gave those foods up. But everything else she enjoyed eating, she ate. After the first few weeks, she didn't miss what she wasn't having. She had more energy, needed less sleep, her cholesterol level went down, and her ratio of HDL to LDL cholesterol went up. She used to wear a size 20 dress, but now wears a size 8 or 10.

If all this still seems mysterious to you, I can only say, *read on.*

I said one whole large category of obesity, which we agreed to call group A, was metabolic. Let's learn in what specific way.

4 | *Insulin— The Hormone That Makes You Fat*

I'm going to talk to you about the hormone whose name you've heard many times—insulin. Even though this chapter is going to cover some technical points, I think you ought to read it carefully, because for many of you, the answers are here.

Almost everyone has heard of insulin because it's given to certain kinds of diabetics to help control their blood-sugar levels. This insulin hormone is one of the most powerful and efficient substances that the body uses to control the use, distribution, and storage of energy.

Your body is an energy machine, never resting, always metabolically active—and it powers its operations mainly through the use of glucose (a basic form of sugar) in the blood. It *must* have the glucose, and even under conditions of starvation it will continue to obtain it so long as there's anything in the body it can convert into glucose. Thus, even on a prolonged, total fast, the body can maintain its glucose level within a rather narrow normal range. As a general rule, of course, the body obtains its principal supply of fuel by eating.

Eating a Meal

Dinnertime comes. You sit down at the table and consume a three-course dinner. What does your body do? Somewhere between chewing and excreting, it absorbs certain substances from your food, mostly across the surface of your small intestine. At that moment, the food is actually entering your body for use.

From the carbohydrates you eat, your body will absorb simple sugars, all of which either are, or quickly and easily become, glucose. From fats, it absorbs glycerol and fatty acids, and from proteins it absorbs amino acids, the building blocks of protein.

Obviously, if you eat a lot of carbohydrate, you'll produce a lot of glucose in your blood. Sounds good, doesn't it? All that energy coursing through your system. Eat sugar and starches and fruits and you're going to get those blood-sugar levels up fast, aren't you?

If you love candy bars, perhaps you're saying, "That's great—the more I eat, the stronger I'll be."

Alas, a bad mistake. You see, your body was designed way back in pre-Neanderthal days when they didn't have any candy bars. Your body's capacity to deal with unrefined foods as they occur in nature is quite adequate; its capacity to deal with an excess of quick-energy, simple sugars is pretty poor, which is the true reason why our 20th-century diet gets us into trouble.

If you don't understand this yet, then let's look at what insulin and the other energy-controlling hormones do when you eat.

As Your Blood Glucose Rises

If your blood-sugar levels go sharply up, as they do soon after you eat carbohydrate, your body makes an instant decision. How much of that pure energy is it going to use for immediate needs and how much will it store for future requirements.

The instrument of its decision is insulin, because insulin governs the processing of blood sugar.

Insulin is manufactured in a part of your pancreas called the islets of Langerhans. As the sugar in your blood goes up, insulin rushes forth and converts a portion of that glucose to glycogen, a starch stored in the muscles and the liver and readily available for energy use. If all the glycogen storage areas are filled, and there is still more glucose in the blood beyond that which the body needs to function, insulin will convert the excess to fatty tissue called triglyceride, which we carry in our bodies as the main chemical constituent of adipose tissue—the stuff you're reading this book to get rid of. That's why insulin has been called "the fat-producing hormone."

Insulin is a pretty efficient worker. If it were not, your body could not process glucose, its basic fuel, and blood glucose levels would escalate while the body searched for other fuels—first your fat stores, and then your muscle tissue itself. That's what happens in insulin-deficient diabetes when no insulin is present. On the other hand, suppose insulin is too effective, or in too great a supply. It would process too much, leaving too little glucose to circulate in the blood to fuel the brain. The body attempts to adjust by liberating counterregulatory hormones—mainly glucagon, adrenocorticoids, and adrenaline to raise the glucose level, but a stiff dose of insulin can overpower the lot of them. Fortunately for most of us, this glucose balancing act takes place automatically and our blood sugar stays in a fairly narrow, normal range of between 65 and 110 mg per 100 cc of blood.

Hyperinsulinism

It's easy to see that there's a relationship between the kinds of foods you eat and the amount of insulin in your bloodstream. Carbohydrate food, especially simple carbohydrates such as sugar, honey, milk, and fruit, which contain glucose, and refined carbohydrates like flour, white rice, and potato starch, which, because they are readily absorbed through the gut, speedily convert to glucose, require a lot of insulin. Foods made of proteins and fat, on the other hand, produce almost no alteration in the insulin level. (Protein requires some insulin; fat essentially none.)

As an overweight person becomes fatter, the insulin problem expands too. Numerous studies have shown that the obese (and diabetic) individual is extremely unresponsive to the action of insulin. That's where you will see the term "insulin resistance." Carbohydrates are triggering the release of large quantities of the hormone, but the body is incapable of utilizing it efficiently. The body responds by putting out yet one more insulin. Consequently, overweight and high insulin levels are almost synonymous.*

What appears to happen is that the insulin receptors on the surfaces of the body's cells are blocked from carrying out their function, which in turn prevents insulin from stimulating the transfer of glucose to the cells for energy use. It's one reason why overweight individuals are tired much of the time. Because insulin

---

*And, to confuse the cart-before-the-horse issue a little more, it has been shown experimentally that high levels of insulin can themselves *increase* insulin resistance. This means that the high insulin levels can be the *cause* of the entire vicious carbohydrate–insulin–insulin resistance cycle.

is not effective in converting glucose into energy, it transfers more and more into stored fat. You'd like to slim down, but your body is, in fact, becoming a fat-producing machine.

Your body's hormonal system is now in desperate straits. Insulin—your fat-producing hormone—is now being secreted all the time to deal with high sugar levels, and it is doing its job less and less effectively. In time, even the insulin receptors that convert glucose to fat start getting worn out—this forecasts diabetes. In severe cases, the pancreas itself becomes exhausted by the effort required to produce so much insulin—and a high-insulin diabetes changes into the insulin-dependent type.

To have your insulin levels more or less permanently high and yet to be resistant to the effects of insulin is what's called *hyperinsulinism*.

Diabetes to Follow?

The next step in this tragic process is indeed diabetes, a disease that's *epidemic* among the overweight.[1]

In this situation, the first sign of diabetes is often that the obese person, who's never been able to lose weight, starts losing weight inexplicably. That's because blood sugar is no longer being converted into energy *or* body fat. Insulin, that crucial fat-producing hormone, has been reduced to impotence.

Diabetes is a heavy-duty illness, not only vastly increasing the risk of heart disease, but having long-term adverse effects on the eyes, kidneys, nervous system, and skin.

A Few More Insulin Problems

Not all fat people reach diabetes, but afflicted as they are with hyperinsulinism, they are in a pre-diabetic condition that may have more significant perils than diabetes itself. Those of you who responded "yes" to the B group of symptoms should recognize yourselves.

First, and most noticeable, the persistent bouts of daily fatigue that overweight people can't seem to do anything about; then shakiness and hunger often traveling in company with depression, irritability, and poor mental function. Not only are fat people tired because their cells are not effectively taking in energy, but off and on throughout the day, they are the victims of hypoglycemia, or low blood sugar, the ironical consequence of consuming too much sugar.

As a man or woman goes deeper into carbohydrate-induced metabolic disorder, hypoglycemia becomes more and more ingrained. Just a touch of glucose will send insulin pouring forth, dropping blood-sugar levels to an abnormal low. If you are a group B person, you become tired, irritable, and hungry. A midafternoon attack of hypoglycemic exhaustion is very typical. This, of course, makes you hungry, you eat more, and the whole sad process goes on. Thus you see that what you thought was compulsivity, a behavioral problem, is really a glucose-triggered mechanism, a metabolic problem. So don't feel so guilty.

There is more to say about hypoglycemia and I'll be doing that in Chapter 11, when I describe it as one of the branches of a very prevalent modern epidemic, which I call Diet-Related Disorder.

Diabetes-Related Disorder

Many academic researchers describe type II diabetes as having five stages, three of them detectable *before* diabetes, with its elevated morning blood sugar level, is diagnosed. They are:

The Five Stages of Diabetes

Stage 1—Insulin Resistance (IR) only.
Stage 2—IR, plus hyperinsulinism (HI).
Stage 3—IR, HI, plus abnormalities in a glucose tolerance test.
Stage 4—Type II diabetes, with high insulin levels.
Stage 5—Type II diabetes, with low insulin levels.

I consider that anyone in any of these stages has what I call Diabetes Related Disorder, and since 90% of these people put out too much insulin after a carbohydrate meal (stages 2, 3, and 4), that Diabetes Related Disorder is a more serious health challenge than diabetes itself.

Here are some further reasons why high insulin levels can lead to big problems.

- Insulin increases salt and water retention—a recipe for both hypertension and continued overweight.

- Insulin aggravates hypertension by increasing the responsiveness of arteries to the effects of adrenaline
- Insulin affects the body's supply of neurotransmitters and can cause sleep disorders.
- Insulin is directly involved (according to numerous animal studies) in creating atherosclerotic plaques.
- Insulin is the primary contributor both to high levels of triglycerides and low levels of the "good" HDL cholesterol.
- Insulin provokes the liver into producing more LDL cholesterol. It may be one of the most significant components in the cholesterol/heart disease connection.

Since obesity and high insulin travel in company, the latter three factors are probably the reasons why overweight is such a major risk factor for a heart attack.

This Is Why You Can't Lose Weight

The last few pages recount a horror story that might be headlined: *Innocent Possessor of Human Body Is Turned Upon by Own Hormones!* But we did it to ourselves, you know. Remember, no culture in world history has ever consumed even a fraction of the sugar we 20th-century westerners do now.

Perhaps you've been overweight for a long time. Once there was a stage in the progress of your metabolic disease when you could lose weight pretty well, if you sharply cut your caloric intake. You'd gain the pounds back, but at least at the price of hunger, you could take them off for a while, if you really needed to.

Now you may be past that stage. If you are, insulin has really closed the trap. The pancreas, faced with your abuse of simple and refined carbohydrates, has become so efficient at secreting it that just a touch of blood sugar will release a flood.

Mediated by high insulin levels, your body has become intent on saving fat. And, in so doing, group A responders will recognize the role that excess insulin plays in preventing weight loss, either directly by lowering your apparent caloric needs, or indirectly by giving you a constant sensation of hunger that can be satiated only by constant overeating.

Now that you're reached this understanding of metabolic overweight, imagine the fat person who goes into his doctor's office and is told, "Well, if you just had a little more willpower . . ." Sad, isn't it.

To lose weight, you're going to need the low-carbohydrate diet offered in this book. You may also need the two other legs of the Atkins Program triad: exercise and nutritional supplementation.

How It's Done

I know I've produced a really heart-sinking analysis of why the fat stays on your body. So, what does one do now?

One makes an end run around insulin.

One needs glucose for fuel, but one doesn't need to get it from one's diet. It's time to turn off the insulin spigot. Weight loss? The answer is in two golden words: KETOSIS/LIPOLYSIS.

5 | The Great Fat Meltdown— The Secret of a Ketogenic Diet

Once you've been fat for some time, you're in a metabolic trap, a sort of high-walled box created in large part by high insulin levels.

You may already have noticed that you're trapped. Certainly, trying diet after diet and failing on all of them is depressing. I know from personal experience and from the comments of thousands of my patients just how tightly the lid of metabolic obesity seems to press down. Ketosis—the Benign Dietary Ketosis (BDK) I'm talking about—opens the lid up.

The term "ketosis," when it applies to the benign diet-induced type we're talking about, is really a shortening of the term ketosis/lipolysis, which is enough of a tongue twister that you can see why it is commonly referred to only by the name "ketosis," and why the diet that is responsible for this remarkable (to dieters) achievement is called a "ketogenic diet."

The definition of lipolysis sounds like Nirvana to dieters and diet doctors alike. It means "the process of dissolving fat." Now, isn't that exactly why we're all gathered here today?

When your fat is used up metabolically, it break down into glycerol and free fatty acids, which in turn break down into pairings of two-carbon compounds called "ketone bodies," leaving a newer fatty acid, shorter in chain length by the two-carbon fragment that entered the metabolic pool to be used as fuel. Apparently this is the *only* metabolic pathway for fat breakdown (lipolysis).

Therefore, there is no lipolysis without ketosis, no ketosis without lipolysis. The two terms are biologically linked and, therefore, it is appropriate that they be linguistically linked.

How does the process actually work? Are there any drawbacks?

There are plenty of laypeople and even physicians who think there must be. Burning one's fat off sounds like a faddish trick. These folks give a skeptical shrug and say, "I'm sure people lose some weight on your diet, Dr. Atkins, but don't they gain it right back again?"

The interesting thing is, not many do. The Atkins weight-maintenance diet, though more indulgent, is quite similar to the Atkins weight-loss diet, and weight regain is not very common.

As for the weight-loss portion, that is simple and overwhelmingly effective. I don't see any reason why I should understate the facts. Ketosis is one of life's charmed gifts. It's as delightful as sex and sunshine, and it has fewer drawbacks than either of them. Many low-carbohydrate diets have been proposed over the years. They work with some degree of effectiveness for some people. However, many of them do not bring carbohydrates down to a level—generally less than forty grams a day—that will permit BDK. For people who are metabolically obese and have great difficulty losing that is a grave weakness.

The Atkins ketogenic diet, on the other hand, is state-of-the-art in weight loss. The safest, healthiest, most luxurious way to start the slim, second half of your life.

Going for It

You've heard me say you can burn the fat off your body. How does ketosis/lipolysis work?

Being in ketosis simply means that you're burning your fat stores and using them as the source of fuel they were meant to be.

When your body is releasing ketones—which it will do in your breath and your urine—that is a chemical proof that you're consuming your own stored fat. Once more, for emphasis: *When a person on a safe low-carbohydrate diet such as mine is releasing ketones, he or she is in the fat-dissolving state known as BDK, or ketosis/lipolysis, which is simply the most efficient path ever devised for getting you slim.*

The more ketones you release, the more fat you have dissolved.

BDK is the physiologic method of weight loss—the exact opposite of the process that got you fat to begin with. It can be your life raft, gaining you not only slimness but health, putting you at a good, healthy distance from the obese person's perils of diabetes, heart disease, and smoke.

Most of all, of course, it is the achievement of your goal—to use up the fat stored on your body.

The phenomenon of ketone formation as the major alternative fuel system is so scientifically well-studied that it is simply not disputed in academic circles. It is as agreed upon as any scientific fact can be. In fact, Dr. George Cahill, the Harvard professor considered to be the preeminent teacher of metabolic-pathway research, after noting that brain tissue utilizes ketones more readily than glucose, announced that ketone bodies were a "preferred fuel" for the brain.[1]

Why, then, are you likely to hear or read that ketosis is undesirable or in some way bad for you? My only answer can be that there are too many "experts" who don't do their homework. Making a statement that benign dietary ketosis is anything other than beneficial is like wearing a sandwich board that says "I'm an expert" on the front panel, and admits "I don't know my field" on the back.

True, there is confusion in the minds of laymen (and some ill-informed doctors) between BDK and the ketosis of diabetic ketoacidosis. The latter is the consequence of insulin-deficient subjects having their blood sugar levels out of control. The two conditions are virtually polar opposites and can always be distinguished from each other by the fact that the diabetic has been consuming carbohydrates and has a high blood sugar, in sharp contrast to the fortunate person in BDK.

Ketosis vs. Glucosis

In the previous chapter, I suggested that you need glucose for fuel: that statement is only partially true. Ketones, as I pointed out, are the fuels that energize our cells when stored fat is our fuel, just as glucose is the fuel when we are subsisting on carbohydrates. These are the only two fuels that come from food. (Alcohol is a third one.)

I find that people understand the concept when I tell them "If you're not in ketosis, you're in glucosis." "Glucosis" is a newly minted term to remind you that the two fuel sources are your body's alternative, completely parallel options for energy metabolism.

Misconceptions about BDK nonetheless abound—and by people who should know better. The authors of *The Zone*, for example, mistakenly believe that ketones represent the breakdown of protein, not fat. Unfortunately, millions of readers are being exposed to such misinformation without being aware of the lack of scientific understanding behind such statements.

Let's see just how BDK is the dieter's best friend.

Why Does Ketosis Work?

Ketosis is the reversal of the biologic pathways that are involved in obesity. You'll remember that insulin was there to convert all your excess carbohydrate into your body stores of fat. As you gained more weight, your pancreas released more insulin to carry out this process.

Most obese people become so adept at releasing insulin that their blood is never really free of it, and, even at night, when weight loss most naturally occurs, they're still not able to use up their fat stores. In a normally functioning body, fatty acids and ketones are readily liberated from adipose tissue and converted into fuel during those hours. But the overweight subject is overweight because the high insulin levels prevent this from happening to him or her—or to you.

Now, with very little carbohydrate in your diet, your insulin levels will become normal—perhaps for the first time in years or decades.

Back in 1971, Drs. Neil Grey and David Kipnis convincingly demonstrated that insulin levels drop as carbohydrate intake is lowered. When carbohydrate drops to ketogenic levels, an abnormality in insulin can no longer be detected. Numerous studies over the past two decades have reconfirmed that insulin levels drop on ketogenic diets.[2]

In ketosis, you burn the fat placed in storage by insulin when the obesity cycle began, and this fat powers your brain and your other vital organs.

The reason that BDK can take place so smoothly, if you know the "secret" to unlock its latent power, is that your body elaborates specific substances to sustain and facilitate the process. Back in 1960, three English researchers, Dr. T.M. Chalmers, Professor Alan Kekwick, and Dr. G.L.S. Pawan, whom I'll be telling you about in the next chapter, isolated the most significant of these, a Fat Mobilizing Substance (FMS), from the urine of animals and humans who went on ketogenic diets containing virtually no carbohydrates.[3] When they injected that urinary fraction into nondieting animals and humans, the recipients *lost weight without dieting*. Subsequently, other researchers discovered other substances that have similar effects, and a class of compounds called lipid mobilizers was identified.

Presumably what happens is that in the absence of carbohydrates to fuel the body, a signal is sent out to release a symphony of lipid mobilizers. The burning of stored fat in the absence of dietary carbohydrate is a *natural* mechanism of our bodies—it's what sustains hibernating animals—and our bodies provide natural messenger substances to ensure that the process of fat mobilization, heralded by ketosis, takes place smoothly and is self-sustaining. For you, this is a sort of biologic utopia. Once you reach a state where fat mobilization is supported by blood-borne enabling substances, the process of losing weight becomes as painless and hunger-free as "eating naturally" was in the days when you were gaining weight.

Yes, No Hunger

This is one of the most attractive features of any low carbohydrate, ketosis-producing diet. Frankly, it first attracted me because back in the 1960s, when I was a young doctor with an ever-increasing paunch, I wanted to diet but didn't want to be hungry. I knew very well that I couldn't stand being hungry for very long. I had too big an appetite and too little willpower, two facts which haven't much changed.

When I found out about Kekwick and Pawan's work and realized that the body could satisfy its hunger by burning its own fat as fuel, I thought I saw an escape hatch. Ketosis turned out to have certain metabolic similarities to fasting. After the first forty-eight hours on each, the body suppresses hunger and lowers appetite.

There was still another advantage. A prolonged fast can be dangerous and has one severe metabolic disadvantage: When fasting, the body not only burns fat for energy, it also burns protein. This means that it burns off some of the body's lean muscle tissue, which is clearly not desirable. Investigation has shown that on a high-protein, ketogenic diet, virtually no lean tissue is lost, only adipose tissue. And that's why I am able to put extremely overweight individuals in ketosis/lipolysis for six months to a year (and longer), knowing that they will suffer no ill effects of any kind.

These enlightened people are able to consume their own fat for energy and feel good while they're doing it.

The Message of Smooth and Happy Weight Loss

The beauty of BDK is that it bypasses the agony of low-calorie dieting, which is carried out with the help of almost no lipid mobilizer support. And ketosis is not only pleasurable, but frequently essential. People who've been fat for a long time or who've tried many diets often find it very nearly impossible to lose much weight *unless* they're in ketosis. I've treated people who, on 700 or 800 balanced calories a day, couldn't lose weight. That's less than half the normal caloric intake of an average woman. And yet they lost weight when they were placed on ketogenic diets of even more calories.

When I make this claim, that you can lose more weight on a higher number of calories, I seem to be breaking the law—one of the hallowed laws of thermodynamics. Many powers-that-be get terribly provoked when I repeal their laws. But the calorie theory is a false law that is meant to be broken, and ketosis/lipolysis is the instrument for breaking it. You'll see exactly what I mean in the next chapter.

6 | The Metabolic Advantage— Every Dieter's Dream

I can't wait to get you started on the convincer—the real clincher—the 14-day trial on the *Induction* diet. That experience will be worth a thousand chapters.

But before I do, I have something designed to increase your enthusiasm to a fever pitch. Are you ready for this?

You can lose more weight and more fat, calorie for calorie, on the Atkins diet than on any other diet you've ever tried.

In other words, this diet will give you an edge, what in scientific lingo would be called a *metabolic advantage*. That's what will enable you to lose weight on the Atkins diet eating the same number of calories you used to gain on. And, if you're eating fewer calories on this diet, as you probably will be, it will enable you to lose with considerably greater rapidity. You'll remember I pointed out that the calorie theory, as an explanation of weight gain and weight loss, has enough loopholes to render it invalid. Nothing could be more evident to anyone who has spent a long time working in this field.

But let me tell you right here and now that the enormous dietary bonus I call metabolic advantage is an area of controversy and has remained so in spite of innumerable studies affirming its reality. I began describing this surprising phenomenon long before I ever heard the expression *metabolic advantage*. In 1973, the term was thrust upon me by the American Medical Association. Annoyed by the extraordinary success that *Dr. Atkins' Diet Revolution* was having in promoting a low-carbohydrate diet at just the time that they themselves were choosing to side with the supporters of high-carbohydrate, low-fat diets, the AMA put together a council of carefully chosen nutritionists to attack low-carbohydrate dieting and, in particular, my book, as the most prominent example of that trend.

Virtually all of their criticisms were inapplicable to easily refutable merely by reviewing the scientific reports already published at that time, but one of the stray arrows they fired off is fascinating since it called *my* attention to one of the most striking pluses provided by low-carbohydrate dieting for weight loss. Their comment was, "No scientific evidence exists to suggest that the low-carbohydrate ketogenic diet has a metabolic advantage over more conventional diets for weight reduction."[1]

Since I had scoured fifty years of scientific research on ketogenic and low-carbohydrate diets and found only confirmation of the phenomenon I'm about to demonstrate to you in some detail, I must admit I was more than taken aback by their statement. Were they suggesting that none of the studies had actually been done or that none had any validity? Since the AMA has never bothered to retract the palpably erroneous statement I quoted above and since metabolic advantage remains one of the most spectacular pluses that an overweight low-carbohydrate dieter has in his favor the minute he goes on the Atkins diet, I've decided to lay out for you the actual scientific evidence that undergirds the advantage you'll be experiencing on the diet.

I know many of you are not of scientific bent and are put off by doctors talking medicalese to you. But, if you pay close attention to what follows, I promise you that you'll be privy to some of the most exciting scientific studies a person interested in weight loss ever gets to learn about. And, before the chapter's over, I'll give you a small reward by demonstrating, though one of my patients, just how the concept works in the case of a flesh and blood person and his diet.

Let me start by introducing you to the academic achievements of two brilliant, painstaking British researchers, Professor Alan Kekwick and Dr. Gaston L.S. Pawan, whose seminal experiments on mice and on obese humans provided the breakthrough concept, the mechanism and rationale, and the irrefutable experimental evidence that a low-carbohydrate—yes, even a high-fat—diet has a significant metabolic advantage over balanced or low-fat conventional diets. Let me point out that my intellectual allies in this pseudo-controversy were not mad scientists writing in the Podunk Medical Journal, but rather represented the top echelon of British obesity research, both serving as chairmen of many international conferences. Professor Kekwick was Director of the Institute of Clinical Research and Experimental Medicine at

London's prestigious Middlesex Hospital, and Dr. Pawan was the Senior Research Biochemist of that hospital's medical unit. The AMA's panel of experts could not have been unaware of their research or of its far-reaching significance.°

The Kekwick and Pawan saga began in the early 1950s when they were struck with the many studies that suggested that differently composed diets provided differing rates of weight loss. They had read the exciting clinical studies of Dr. Alfred W. Pennington on employees of the Dupont Corporation, as well as German and Scandinavian papers showing success in dieters who restricted carbohydrate. So they did a study on obese subjects and found that those on a 90% protein and (especially) on a 90% fat diet lost weight, but when they were given a diet of the same number of calories, 90% of which came from carbohydrate, the subjects *did not lose*.[2]

Kekwick and Pawan were so impressed with the potential importance of their unexpected findings that they devoted nearly two decades of their collaboration to learning why and how the theory that all calories are equal seemed to be so patently wrong. They then replicated an animal study of theirs on humans and found the same phenomenon: A low-carbohydrate diet of 1000 calories worked well for weight loss and a high-carbohydrate 1000-calorie diet took off very little weight.[3] They then showed that their subjects did not lose at all on a balanced 2000 calorie diet, but, when their diet was mainly fat, these same obese subjects could lose even when as much as 2600 calories were given. A typical example was their subject JB, who lost 9 pounds in 3 weeks on the 2600-calorie low-carbohydrate diet, yet not an ounce on the 8 days he was on the balanced 2000 calorie diet.

Skeptics with the calorie-is-a-calorie mindset were in a state of shock and set out to disprove this intellectual bombshell that Kekwick and Pawan had dropped on them.

A spate of studies followed. One, by T.R.E. Pilkington and his associates, was published in Lancet in 1960.[4] But the study dealt with the 1000-calorie level, a level at which nearly everybody loses weight, and only 3 of the subjects in the study were kept as low as 32 grams of carbohydrate, the upper limit of intake to provide a ketogenic diet. But if you look at their data, you'll see the same striking accelerated weight loss on restricted carbohydrates that Kekwick and Pawan showed, except that the Pilkingtonians blithely elimi-

---

°They did acknowledge reading one of the Kekwick/Pawan reports.

nated the first 12 days of the low-carbohydrate diet from their mathematics, which just happened to be the only way they could make their conclusion—that all low-calorie diets give the same result—fit their data. Their reasoning? They said the low-carbohydrate diet causes water loss. How did they know? Unlike Kekwick and Pawan, they did no water balance studies to prove their point. With the ivory tower complacency Galileo's contemporaries showed when they insisted the Earth could not possibly move around the sun, Pilkington and his associates concluded that their preconceived dogma must certainly be true.

I'm embarrassed for the nutritionists at the AMA who, in their desperate search for ammunition, even cited that study. If you did something like that too often, you could get a reputation as The Gang That Couldn't Think Straight.

But Kekwick and Pawan stuck by their guns. Their data had shown water loss to be only a small part of the total weight loss. For the next two years, they embarked on a study of mice in a metabolic chamber. By measuring the loss of carbon in the feces and urine, they were able to show that the mice on the high-fat diet excreted considerable unused calories in the form of our friends the ketone bodies, as well as citric, lactic, and pyruvic acids. At the end of the study period, they analyzed the fat content of the animals' bodies and found significantly less fat on the carcasses of the high-fat-diet mice. Nevertheless, the AMA's team of scholars didn't even bother to review this study, although it was published in the prestigious American journal *Metabolism.*[5]

There is more to the Kekwick and Pawan story. During the time they were providing the reality of the metabolic advantage of ultra-low-carbohydrate dieting, they detected and extracted a substance from the urine of the low-carbohydrate dieters that, when injected into mice, caused the same metabolic events they had observed in the mice on low carbohydrate, indicating that fat was melting off the body. The carcass fat decreased dramatically, the ketone and free fatty-acid levels rose, and, most significantly, the excretion of unused calories via urine and feces rose from a normal 10% to 36%! This substance was named fat-mobilizing substance (FMS). FMS is the instrument of your metabolic edge; it enables you to sneak out some unused calories from your body that you wouldn't be able to remove so easily on a low-fat diet.

Kekwick and Pawan attributed hormonal properties to FMS, and at least four other research groups coming at the subject from a variety of directions felt they had identified fat mobilizers. Thus, the idea that you have a metabolic ally in sustaining weight loss has been demonstrated by a plenitude of researchers.[6]

The Struggle Continues

There were two more studies that the AMA panel of experts reviewed on the subject of metabolic advantage. One was by Olesen and Quaade, which again showed extremely favorable weight loss on a low-carbohydrate diet.[7] Like the Pilkington study, this favorable result was attributed to water loss, and once again no attempt was made to document the water-balance dynamics. The other study by Sidney Werner simply did not apply, being a study of a 52-gm carbohydrate diet—far too much for demonstrating ketosis and lipolysis.

Now let's look at the studies that were deliberately excluded from the AMA critique. First let's look at the study done by Frederick Benoit and his associates at the Oakland Naval Hospital.[8] Impressed with the Kekwick and Pawan success, they decided to compare the 1000-calorie, 10-gm-carbohydrate, high-fat diet with fasting in seven men weighing between 230 and 290 pounds. On the 10-day fast, they lost 21 pounds on average, but most of that was lean body weight; only 7.5 pounds was body fat. But on the ketogenic diet, 14 of the 14.5 pounds lost was body fat. Think of it. By eating foods such as bacon, whipped cream, cream cheese, and mayonnaise, their subjects lost their fat stores almost twice as fast as when they ate nothing at all! Benoit's other exciting discovery was that on the ketogenic diet, the dieters maintained their potassium levels, while there were major potassium losses when fasting. You may recall that about a decade later, many dieters were to lose their lives on very-low-calorie formula diets that were very much like fasting, presumably due to potassium losses leading to heart arrhythmias. Had the medical establishment accepted the Benoit study for what it was—the needed confirmation of the Kekwick and Pawan research that should have made the ketogenic diet the treatment of choice for the overweight—these lives might have been spared.

Benoit presented his findings at the Golden Anniversary session of the American College of Physicians and his paper was published in the *Annals of Internal Medicine*, both in 1965. Hardly an obscure study. Why was it not included in the AMA's critique? I admit that trying to explain that without using the words "intellectually dishonest" is difficult.

Actually, the Benoit study set off quite a furor in the minds of establishment spokesmen such as Francisco Grande, who knew that Benoit's data had to be wrong because it contradicted the calorie theory.[9] Grande calculated that 650 gms per day (the amount of fat the ketogenic dieters actually lost), if multiplied by 9 calories a gram will equal a 5760 calorie deficit, and no one could lose that much weight. What he was saying in effect was, "Don't bother me with data, I've already calculated the results."

But this confirmation of metabolic advantage continued to be replicated, sometimes from the most unlikely sources, such as Dr. Willard Krehl, a determined opponent of low-carbohydrate dieting.

Krehl went on to study two obese women, average weight 286 pounds, for 10 weeks on a 12-gm, 1200-calorie low-carbohydrate diet and recorded weight losses averaging a half-pound *daily*.[10] He then described this as "commensurate with caloric restriction and exercise." (Three hours a day.) But is it? To lose a half pound per day, a woman would have to burn up 1750 calories a day, over and above the 1200 calories she was eating on Krehl's diet. That means that Krehl assumed these women, one of whom had a basal metabolism 18% below the norm, would normally burn up 2950 calories a day. The accepted theory, however, is that the average obese woman does *not* lose weight on 2000 calories a day. Therefore, to me, Krehl's figures conceal a metabolic advantage of 950 calories a day or more.

Still not convinced? Try this one. The AMA panel of nutrition experts, most of whom certainly read the *American Journal of Clinical Nutrition*, failed to acknowledge an important paper by Charlotte Young, professor of clinical nutrition at Cornell University, published in that journal just two years before.[11] This time, the subjects were overweight young men, and the three diets compared were of 1800 calories, all with some degree of carbohydrate restriction. The diets contained 30, 60, and 104 gms of carbohydrate and were followed for nine weeks. Young and her colleagues calculated body fat through a widely accepted technique involving immersion under water. Those on 104 gms lost slightly better than 2 pounds of fat per week, out of 2.73 pounds of total weight loss—not bad for 1800 calories. Those on 60 gms lost nearly 2.5 pounds of fat per week, out of 3 pounds of actual weight loss— better. Those on 30 gms, the only diet which produced ketosis and, presumably, FMS, lost 3.73 pounds of fat per week—approximately 100% of the weight they were losing each week.

We should forgive Dr. Young for editorially concluding that she preferred the 104-gm diet she had been working with for twenty years. After all, she had published the fourth peer-reviewed medical study demonstrating the metabolic advantage of the ketogenic diet and quantitated it rather accurately. Look at her figures. These young men, by dropping 74 gms of carbohydrate and replacing it with 300 calories of protein-based food, will lose an extra 1.7 pounds of body fat each and every week. In other words, if they were to replace their cereal, banana, and skim milk with a ham and cheese omelet every day for 30 weeks, they will lose 51 more pounds of fat than if they stayed with the cereal.°

That's the edge the frustrated, struggling dieter needs. That's what metabolic advantage provides. That's what has enabled most of my patients to succeed. That's what has made the Atkins Center a success, and that's what will make you a success.

Before we leave Charlotte Young, I've got good news for those of you who have been trying to lose weight with the major commercial plans. Most of them have been trying to get you thin with diets containing 60% or more carbohydrate. Dr. Young's *highest* diet was only 35% carbohydrate. But what I, in treating many thousands of weight-loss patients, and Charlotte Young in her meticulous research, and virtually every other scientist who has actually studied low-carbohydrate diets have discovered, is that *the more the carbohydrate, the less the body fat lost*.

Here's the part of the story that has hurt you the most. What do you think happens to exciting, breakthrough-potential medical research when it runs afoul of the medical establishment? Does the truth come out, no matter what? Can the establishment win even though truth is not their ally? The answer to that can be deduced from recent history: Power wins. Once the AMA spoke out, no further research on the question of metabolic advantage was ever done in the U.S. And that's one of the major reasons why you're struggling with your weight and getting nowhere. *The proper, easy solution is not being offered as one of your options*.

Fortunately for the world, German science is not as inhibited by AMA position statements as is American research, and on the European continent, metabolic advantage continued to be explored. One example was a study done at the University of Wurzburg on 45 patients who were studied in the hospital for 5 weeks.[12] Once again

---

°Providing the rest of the diet contained 1500 calories and 30 grams of carbohydrate.

the low-carbohydrate diet demonstrated a significant metabolic advantage, this time an extra 9.24 pounds was lost on the low-carbohydrate version of the 1000-calorie diet. Moreover, careful water-balance studies demonstrated that the proportion of those extra pounds that could be set down to water loss was not significant. Five other German studies[13] make the score:

Number of studies showing metabolic advantage—10
Number of studies showing no advantage on ketogenic diet—0

But even the successful German clinics succumbed to these powerful politico-economic deterrents and stopped writing about the success of their low-carbohydrate programs by 1981. That marked the beginning of the "Nutritional Dark Ages" in which food industry–dominated nutritionists held uncontested sway and convinced the unsuspecting public that white flour was so good for everyone that all of us should consume at least six servings each day and that meat, eggs and butter were bad for everyone. No voices pointed to the fact that meat, eggs, and butter are all produced by independent producers and cannot be sold above the fair market price, whereas food consisting mainly of cheap refined ingredients (flour, sugar, corn syrup, and corn starch) could be sold at an enormous markup. No voices questioned whether perhaps nutrition teaching is strongly influenced by economics, or whether such interests encouraged the stonewalling of information about the metabolic advantage of protein foods.

Metabolic Advantage in Action

Perhaps you will now understand how Harry Kronberg, the patient I mentioned in Chapter 2, was able to lose fifty pounds in three months on a diet containing an abundance of calorically-dense foods, even though in the previous three years all he had been able to do on a moderately-low-fat balanced diet was gain 70. This does not contradict reason, but it is an outstanding example of metabolic advantage.

Let's look at the mathematics and then you'll understand that Harry isn't losing all this weight because he's restricting his calories.

It works like this. To lose a pound a week one has to be eating 500 fewer calories a day than one burns up in energy. To gain a pound a week, one eats 500 calories a day more. Harry had been gaining half a pound a week for 35 months, which means he was taking in 250 calories a day too many. He was eating three full meals with chicken and fish for dinner and he was taking in 2129 calories a day.

Chart 6.1
Harry Kronberg's Before and After Menu
A TYPICAL PRE-ATKINS DAY

Breakfast	*Calories*
Cheese Danish	308
Coffee (decaf with half 'n' half)	2
Lunch	
French Fries (3 ½ oz.)	175
Pastrami/Corned Beef (4 oz cooked)	410
Rye bread (2 slices)	140
Pretzels (3 oz)	220
Snacks	
Nestle Crunch Bar (1 oz)	138
Orange	71
Dinner	
Herring (4 oz kippered)	217
Vegetables (1 cup cabbage)	24
Salad (lettuce/tomato/no dressing)	80
Crackers (4 rye thins)	52
Diet Soda	0
Vanilla Ice Cream (1 cup)	290
Total	2129

A TYPICAL POST-ATKINS DAY

Breakfast (Brunch)	*Calories*
Tuna Salad (1 cup)	240
½ grapefruit	41
Decaf Coffee (black)	0
Lunch	
Grilled Chicken (light meat, 6 oz)	280
Small Green & Tomato Salad	80
Salad dressing (1 oz)	170
Diet Soda	0
Dinner	
Rib Steak (6 oz)	490
Summer Squash (½ cup)	19
Small Green & Tomato Salad w/dressing	80
Salad dressing (1 oz)	170
Seltzer	0
Snacks	
Almonds (1 oz)	176
Coleslaw (with Sweet 'n' Low	174
Cucumber (½ medium)	8
Total	1928

Now on the Atkins diet, Harry was losing 3.9 pounds a week, which means that according to conventional calorie theory, he would have to be taking in 1950 fewer calories a day than he burned in energy. We already know that at 2129 calories a day, he was taking in 250 calories a day too many. Thus Harry's break-even point is 1879 calories a day. To lose 3.9 pound a week, he should be taking in 1879 calories minus 1950 calories, or −71 calories a day—clearly an impossibility since you can't eat less than nothing.

You've seen Harry's menu. In fact, that menu calculates out to 1928 calories a day. Harry is eating 49 calories a day over break-even point and therefore, according to calorie theory, he should be gaining 0.1 pound a week, and after 13 weeks on the Atkins diet he should have gained 1.3 pounds, not lost 50.°

All the calories Harry eats over and above −71 is metabolic advantage. That means he has a metabolic advantage of 1999 calories a day. Impossible? Not according to the research that's been done on low-carbohydrate dieting, and not according to the facts of Harry Kronberg's case.

The metabolic advantage is there. It can't be disguised, evaded, put down to water weight, or wished away.

I would have no difficulty going into my charts and finding hundreds of other such examples.

Back when I wrote my first book, I described a patient of mine who lost 5 pounds a week for 17 weeks, 85 pounds in all, while consuming enough meat that his documented food intake was 3000 calories per day (2 ½ pounds of red meat, plus a cheese omelet).

By not eating carbohydrate, this patient, like Harry Kronberg, had stimulated the release of FMS to sustain the breakdown of his fat stores. This lipolysis (fat dissolving) became his major metabolic event. He, too, had created a metabolic advantage.

I have followed over 25,000 patients on the program you're about to learn—better than 90% of them showed some measure of metabolic advantage. Now it's your turn.

From studying the medical literature, which, as you've seen, is in surprising agreement on this point, and from studying my own patients, I can safely say that the bonus benefit of switching from high- to ultra-low-carbohydrate diets of the same caloric content varies from one-half to three pounds per week. This may not seem

---

°Incidentally, for those of you who aren't familiar with how diet research is done, 13 weeks is a very long time to test out a diet; there's nothing short-term about such results.

like a lot, but done for a year that calculates out to from 25 to 156 pounds of extra body fat lost.

Henceforth, the AMA will never be able to say metabolic advantage doesn't exist. The strongest statement they can make in the future is: "Well, yes, there is a proven advantage, but why would you want it?"

To have an edge, a bonus, the vigorish, the odds on your side. Would you want that? You could bet the ranch on it.

May the Edge be with you.

PART TWO

How to Do Your Fortnight Diet —14 Days to Dieting Success

You have just ahead of you what I believe will be a remarkable experience. Fourteen days of healthy, hearty, hunger-free eating will rapidly begin to take your excess pounds away and will show you the first outlines of a new you. It will be a "you" that is slimmer, more energetic, less driven by cravings, and very possibly freed of innumerable minor symptoms of a nutritionally inadvisable lifestyle. It will be a you that begins to understand through your own body what I can only sketch out for you in words. The flesh teaches faster than the pen. If you are metabolically obese, if you have been driven hither and yon by the lure of carbohydrates, then I have great surprises in store for you. Welcome to a whole new world!

7 | In the Beginning— Getting Your 14-Day Diet Off on the Right Foot

I know you want to get into the 14-day *induction* diet, so I'll make this chapter fairly brief. Here are two pre-diet steps well calculated to prepare you for success. In spite of your impatience to start dieting, I believe you should consider them.

I assume your weight and your physical well-being are both extremely important to you. It follows from that you're going to make a sincere attempt to abide by the not-so-very-difficult requests that I'll be making of you. I won't be angry at you if you don't—after all, we won't have met—but if you're not willing to try, you really should be angry at yourself.

With my own patients, I'm sometimes very frank. A patient if mine named David French—a 52-year-old stockbroker—had by his own account tried 6,000 diets and failed on all of them. He came to me somewhat reluctantly, nagged by his wife and children, I think, expressed his skepticism, groaned at the thought of taking a lot of vitamins, and looked to me like someone who would never make it off the ground. He weighed 206 pounds on a 5'8" frame, and his only real symptoms were fatigue and a clearly observed tendency to have a hard time with even very mild physical exertion.

"Let's at least check your blood chemistries, Mr. French," I said, "and then we'll have some idea of whether you have anything to worry about."

Those blood tests were quite enlightening. He had a whopping cholesterol level of 284 and a nearly incredible triglyceride level of 1200. At our next meeting, I leaned forward and, coming on a lot stronger than I normally would, let him have it with both barrels: *"I'd say you're probably going to die in the next year or two, Mr. French."*

That caught his attention. In all probability, I remarked, a heart attack or a stroke would be his undoing. He also showed signs of being a borderline diabetic. His condition was completely reversible, but it was apparent he wasn't going to make the effort to reverse it.

Six months later, Dave French weighed 162 pounds, his cholesterol level was 155, and his triglycerides were 90. He had been a heavy-carbohydrate eater his whole life, someone who always hit the coffee carts for bagels and rolls, liked to stop on the way home from work for a calzone, and drank soda pop every day.

He thrived on my diet, reassured by the fact that there was no limit to the amount he could eat. "If you're hungry, eat," I said. "That's what God gave you a mouth, tongue, and lips for."

Getting into BDK was no trouble at all for Dave French. I got him to do a half hour of exercise four times a week. He found that he slept better, and he felt far less tired during the day.

Physical exertion was no longer beyond him. Of course, it shouldn't be when you're only 52. Quite simply, he became a slim and healthy man. But let's let him have the last word.

> "I have a picture that I keep on the desk in my office that shows the maximum me—I look like I'm having a baby. I keep it right there where I can see it, to remind me of what I'll never be again. Nowadays, I don't even look like the same person."

He's right, too—he doesn't look like the same person.

The Pre-Diet Steps

Now let's look at those pre-diet steps. They're both important. *You should not do the diet without considering these questions carefully.*

1. Stop taking any *unnecessary* medications.
2. Arrange to have a medical checkup, so you can determine your general state of health—and so you will be aware of your levels of cholesterol, triglyceride, glucose, insulin, and uric acid before you start the diet. These are the blood tests that often change with drastic dietary change. Since these levels are at the center of controversy about what constitutes a healthy diet, you may regret not having a "before" level to compare with the "after" level.

Medications

The list of medications that inhibit weight loss is a long one. If you are on one or more of them, you will be disappointed in your diet results. For a more extended discussion of these pharmaceutical diet impediments, please turn to Chapter 18.

But there are also some drugs that combine with this diet to produce a dangerous overdose. They are the diuretics (the diet is itself a potent diuretic) and the anti-diabetes medications, including insulin. The insulin requirements invariably change on this diet. If you fall into either of these two categories, you stand to benefit more than most people. Without knowing how much and how fast these medications can be decreased, you could get into serious trouble. You or your doctor should call, write, or e-mail the Atkins Center for Complementary Medicine for specifics.

Checks and Tests

NOW FOR THAT MEDICAL CHECKUP

My second recommendation was that you get a medical checkup.

Even if you're not on any medication, this is a wonderful opportunity for you to take a look at your overall physical condition. If you have a personal physician, then he or she will be the best guide to interpreting that condition for you.

Obviously, if you're under 35 and have no evident health problems, then you don't have to have that checkup, but I still recommend it. There's something else I recommend at the same time and that's getting your blood chemistries done.

What an advantage it is—for me and for you—to know these numbers before you begin!

If you choose to keep track of those hidden physical changes that are measured in your blood—and these numbers your doctor can best interpret for you—you'll find, after you go on the diet, that they begin improving steadily. I'm talking about the uric acid levels; cholesterol, HDL, LDL, and triglyceride levels; glucose and insulin levels.

You may be startled because there's a whole body of published literature suggesting that you ought to be terrified of a diet that allows you to eat as much eggs, meat, fish, and fowl as you desire.

The most common question I'm asked when I tell a patient what I expect him to eat is, "But won't my cholesterol go up?" I have no hesitation in answering, "No, it will go down."

A low-carbohydrate diet has a plenitude of health advantages that I'll explain in Part Three of this book. Meanwhile, if you have your blood chemistries done, you'll discover that the "experts" on low-carbohydrate dieting—those physicians who never studied a low-carbohydrate diet in their lives—will be proved wrong yet again. For them, being wrong must be habit-forming.

Here's what you should expect: Your uric acid levels will be normal, your kidney function will be excellent, your blood glucose and insulin levels will have stabilized, your triglyceride level will almost certainly have fallen sharply, and your cholesterol level will already be starting to go down.

I suggest you get these blood chemistries, and quite possibly the glucose tolerance test, measured before you start the diet, so you'll have a baseline. If you're obese, many of these measurements will not be too good before you start the diet, and, if you haven't been seeing your doctor for regular checkups, you probably don't have any idea what they are. Most of the conditions that get revealed through lab work are quite insidious—your numbers can be highly abnormal and yet you will have no symptoms referable to them.

I don't want you to do the lab work for a few weeks into your new diet, because then you may think any remaining abnormalities are the result of your dieting. I treat dozens of people every month who have high cholesterol two weeks after they start on the diet, but they had *even higher* cholesterol before they started.

While checking your lab work, get your entire state of health estimated. Make sure to have your blood pressure done. High blood pressure is known for its insidiousness, and overweight and hypertension go together like, oh, like pancakes and maple syrup. What happens to blood pressure on the diet? Just this: Nothing is more consistently and rapidly observed on the Atkins diet than normalization of blood pressure.

Certainly, you're also going to want to know about your thyroid function. A sluggish thyroid is one of the legitimate causes of metabolic obesity other than hyperinsulinism. If you are one of the approximately one in ten overweight subjects who needs thyroid, your weight problem will suddenly get very much easier, once you take it.

A Very Special Test

Let's talk about the most illuminating and specific laboratory test of all—*the five-hour glucose-tolerance test (GTT) with insulin levels*. I hope I've convinced you that the metabolic defect in obesity is hyperinsulinism and that some combination of pre-diabetes, reactive hypoglycemia, and diabetes itself are found in the *majority* of significantly overweight people. Wouldn't you want to know if that applies to you? If you're really overweight, wouldn't you want to know the *extent* to which it applies to you?

Since your reading of this book is *a priori* evidence of superior intelligence, I'm going to assume that your answer to the above question is "Yes." But you may legitimately ask, "When? Should I do it now or later?"

First, let me tell you why I drive the car consistently rated number one in consumer satisfaction. My wife and I wandered into their showroom never having heard of this make of automobile. The salesman said nothing to us except, "Here are the keys. Why don't you take it for a test drive?" Eight blocks later, I said, "Where do I sign?" You can be sure that I cannot wait to get you to test drive the 14-day *Induction* diet. I know you'll sign on immediately.

So I don't want to impose an inconvenience, or a delay in getting started on the program, which would also be a delay in getting on with the best part of the rest of your life. After all, performing a GTT properly involves having blood tests drawn seven or eight times in one morning, and you must schedule it with a doctor or a commercial medical lab. Fortunately, it is covered by most major medical insurance policies, so for most of you finance will not be a problem.

There is one point I must make. The test results are not considered accurate unless you are on full-carbohydrate intake (200 gms a day for four days), so you cannot decide in the middle of this diet that you are finally ready to take the test. This leaves you only two intelligent choices.

1. Do the test (with all the other lab parameters) *before* you begin the 14-day *Induction* diet.
2. Start the diet and promise yourself that before you commit to a lifetime on the Atkins program you will get this and the other tests done properly. That sounds like your best option, but remember once you experience how great it feels to rid

yourself of your carbohydrate addictions, you won't *want* to go off your new diet and get re-addicted again!

The other option—never getting the test done— is not intelligent unless the following conditions apply: You are young, you have less than 15 pounds to lose, you don't experience energy, mood, or concentration problems that vary from hour to hour, and you do not have a pot belly (upper body obesity connects strongly with hyperinsulinism).

Whatever you have decided to do about your GTT, this is the information you will need:

The glucose-tolerance test traces your sugar (glucose) level over the course of 5 to 6 hours after you take in a test dose of glucose with no other food or beverage. Any variation from the perfectly normal response may be viewed with suspicion. If the highest reading is over 160 mg, it may suggest pre-diabetes; a drop 25% below the baseline, or below 60 mg%, suggests reactive hypoglycemia; a delta (difference between the highest and lowest readings) over 90 points suggests an abnormality, as does any hour in which the sugar drops 60 points or more. And many other criteria exist to show deviations from normal—all of which take on more importance if the symptoms (the group B responses) are characteristic.

But to really be informative (and to make your mini-ordeal worthwhile) insulin levels should be drawn along with the glucose levels, at least for the first 2 hours. After all, it is hyperinsulinism that *is* the laboratory correlate of obesity. The fasting insulin should be below 25 units, but the level drawn two hours after the glucose drink is a very important reading. In Western cultures this number seems to go up with age. This may not be a healthy change, but it is usual. My rule of thumb is that it is significantly elevated if it is 1.5 times your age, up to the age of 50. Thus, 75 is a high reading for anyone.

Now it is obvious that doing a lab test doesn't make you any healthier, but by providing you with a *bona fide* laboratory confirmation of your medical condition, it may motivate you to a degree you just haven't reached by looking in the mirror at a gradually expanding waistline.

And now for the 14 days that will change your life.

8

The Rules of the Induction Diet— This Is Your 14-Day Test Drive

First of all, let me welcome all the new arrivals who will be trying to start the book at this point. The *Induction* diet printed here is the prelude to the Atkins diet, not the Atkins diet itself, although it will probably be analyzed and reanalyzed as if it were and as if these words were never written. My critics, who realize they can't win on a level playing field, will seize this opportunity to prove it is an unbalanced diet, as if that magic word "balanced" represented a virtue rather than a hardship.

This *Induction* diet is a corrective diet; its primary purpose is to correct, as expeditiously as possible, an unbalanced metabolism. *An imbalance cannot be corrected by adding balance; it can only be corrected by counterbalancing with an unbalanced correction.*

Let me show you my favorite diagram.

An unbalanced modern metabolism with a) an unbalanced (low-carbohydrate) diet and b) a standard balanced diet applied to it.

a)

unbalanced metabolism   **unbalanced corrective diet**   **balanced result**

b)

unbalanced metabolism   **balanced diet**   **unbalanced result**

Which looks like the better solution to you?

The diet below is called the *Induction* diet because its purpose is to induce a successful weight-loss by creating ketosis/lipolysis and thus summoning the body's own production of FMS and other fat-mobilizers.

These are the things the *Induction* diet will be doing for you:

1) Efficiently switching your body from a carbohydrate-burning to a fat-burning (your fat!) metabolism.
2) Stabilizing your blood sugar and abruptly halting a myriad of hypoglycemia symptoms that cause fatigue, mood swing, brain fog, weak spells, and the like.
3) Stopping your cravings through abstinence, rather than moderation.
4) Breaking addictive eating patterns to chocolate, sugar, wheat or corn derivatives, alcohol, caffeine, grain gluten, or whatever you may have developed an allergy/addiction to.
5) Letting you experience metabolic advantage firsthand.
6) Knocking your socks off by demonstrating how much fat you can burn off, while eating liberally, even luxuriously, off the fat of the land.

Nonetheless, attractive though it is, the *Induction* diet is not going to be your lifetime regimen. That regimen will be determined by a series of steps I will teach you to take, so that the diet is eventually geared to create the best possible balance between your metabolic responses, your food tastes and lifestyle, and your total health profile as it relates to diet, which it most often does.

In permanent dieting, once the 14-day test drive you are about to begin now is over—once, in fact, you're a dieting success and you're enjoying the even-more-luxurious, lifelong Atkins *Maintenance* diet—the *Induction* diet will still serve a purpose. It will be a start-up mechanism allowing you—when necessary—to get back in stride by resuming the diet at the level you were originally successful at. Thus, when you've broken your permanent maintenance diet for whatever good (or bad) reason, you will return to the *Induction* diet, and, like the ignition mechanism of an automobile, it will turn your engine over and start you rolling down the road again. For this latter purpose, in the fine days to come when you've reached your ideal weight and then just slipped out of it for a moment, it won't be necessary to stay at the *Induction* level for two weeks. You'll only have to do it until maximum ketosis/lipolysis takes place, as evidenced by a full measure of appetite suppression. What *that* is you'll learn this first time around.

The Rules of the Induction Diet

1. *Your diet must contain no more than 20 gms of carbohydrate a day*. For most people, induction of ketosis/lipolysis can be achieved on this intake. This allows for approximately 3 cups of salad vegetables (loosely packed) or 2 cups of salad plus ⅔ cup of cooked vegetables in the below-10%-carbohydrate category.
2. You are no loner on a quantitative diet. Therefore you should adjust the quantities to your appetite. When hungry, eat the amount that makes you feel satisfied but not stuffed. When not hungry, eat nothing or just a small protein snack to accompany your vita-nutrient supplements.
3. You are, however, on a qualitative diet. This means that if the food is not on your diet, you are to have absolutely none of it. Your "just this one taste won't hurt" rationalization is the kiss of death on this diet. Addicts will find this rule builds character in a hurry.
4. Your diet will consist of pure proteins (not many of those in nature, however), pure fats (this means butter, olive oil, and mayonnaise are permitted), and combinations of protein and fat (this is the mainstay of your diet). Foods which are protein-and-carbohydrate or fat-and-carbohydrate are *not* on this diet, because carbohydrate is *not* on this diet.
5. Using a carbohydrate gram counter, one could find other combinations totaling less than 20 gms of carbohydrate. One would be using foods like nuts, seeds, olives, avocados, cheeses, cream and sour cream, lemon and lime juices, and Atkins low-carbohydrate diet foods such as the Shake Mix, Bake Mix, and Advantage Bars.° Don't assume these foods are low, unless you absolutely know the carbohydrate content of the portion you are eating. In the Carbohydrate Gram Counter on page 327, I will include the carbohydrate content in grams of the foods you may include on this 14-day *Induction* diet as well as on more liberal levels of the diet that you will be doing as your lifetime diet plan.

°Available thorugh Atkins Nutritionals, see page 251.

FREE FOODS:

MEAT	FISH	FOWL
Beef	Tuna	Chicken
Pork	Salmon	Turkey
Lamb	Sole	Duck
Bacon	Trout	Goose
Veal	Flounder	Cornish Hen
Ham	Sardines	Quail
Venison	Herring	Pheasant
in fact, all meat	*in fact, all fish*	*in fact, all fowl*

SHELLFISH	EGGS	CHEESE
Oysters	Scrambled	Aged and fresh
Mussels	Fried	Cow and goat
Clams	Poached	Cream cheese
Squid	Soft Boiled	Cottage cheese
Shrimp	Hard Boiled	Swiss
Lobster	Deviled	Cheddar
Crabmeat	Omelets	Mozzarella
in fact, all shellfish	*in fact, all eggs*	*in fact, almost* all cheeses*

Exceptions: 1) luncheon meats with nitrates or sugar added;
2) products that are not exclusively meat, fish, or fowl,
such as imitation fish, meatloaf, and breaded foods.

OTHER INDUCTION DIET FOODS:

SALAD VEGETABLES:

Lettuce	Mache	Celery
Romaine	Bok Choy	Jicama
Escarole	Chives	Posse Pied
Arugula	Parsley	Alfalfa Sprouts
Endive	Cucumber	Mushrooms
Radicchio	Radishes	Morels
Chicory	Fennel	Olives
Sorrel	Peppers	Daikon

SALAD HERBS:

Dill	Basil	Rosemary
Thyme	Cilantro	Oregano
Pepper	Sage	Cayenne
Tarragon	Ginger	Garlic

For salad dressing use the desired oil plus vinegar or lemon juice and spices. Grated cheese, chopped eggs, bacon, or fried pork rinds may be added.

---

*All cheeses have some carbohydrate content, and quantities are governed by that. (See Carbohydrate Gram Counter.) No diet cheese, cheese spreads, or whey cheeses. Those with a known yeast infection, dairy allergy, or cheese intolerance must avoid cheese. Imitation cheese products are not allowed, except for tofu (soy cheese)—but check carbohydrate content.

VEGETABLES IN ADDITION TO SALAD VEGETABLES:
Vegetables of 10% Carbohydrate or Less

Asparagus	Scallions	Snow Pea Pods
String or Wax Beans	Leeks	Sauerkraut
Cabbage	Spinach	Collard Greens
Beet Greens	Summer Squash	Dandelion Greens
Cauliflower	Zucchini Squash	Christophene
Chard	Okra	Broccoli
Eggplant	Pumpkin	Broccoli Rabe
Kale	Turnips	Spaghetti Squash
Kohlrabi	Avocado	Celery Root (celeriac)
Tomato	Bamboo Shoots	Brussels Sprouts
Onion	Bean Sprouts	Artichoke Hearts
Rhubarb	Water Chestnuts	Hearts of Palm

SALAD GARNISHES:

Crumbled Crisp Bacon	Sour Cream
Grated Cheese	Minced Sautéed Mushrooms
Minced Hardboard Egg Yolk	

SPICES:

All spices to taste, but make sure sugar is not in the seasoning.

BEVERAGES:

Water
Spring Water
Mineral water
Club Soda
Essence flavored seltzer (must say "no calories")
Decaffeinated coffee or tea°
Herb tea (no barley, dates, figs, sugar)
Clear broth/bouillon (not all brands)
Cream (heavy or light); note carbohydrate content
Diet soda (read label) †
Iced tea with artificial sweetener†
Natural and artificial orange soda (products have some carbohydrate—they may
    be one of your options for a few grams)
Carbohydrate-free, artificially sweetened powder for making fruit-flavored
    drinks†
Lemon or lime juice (note that each contains 2.8 grams carbohydrate per ounce)

Grain beverages (i.e., imitation coffee substitutes) are not allowed.

Alcoholic beverages are not part of the *Induction* diet, but those without
carbohydrate, in moderation, are an option for other levels of the diet.

°Caffeine mimics the effect of sugar on blood glucose levels by stimulating insulin release.
It should be avoided by those who suspect they are caffeine-dependent and taken in limited
quantities by others.

†Contains aspartame (usually). Must keep quantities low. See note on following page.

FATS AND OILS:

Many fats, especially certain oils, are essential to good nutrition. Include a source of GLA (gamma-linolenic acid) and omega-3 oils (EPA, salmon oil, linseed oil). Olive oil (monounsaturated) is valuable. All vegetable oils are allowed. The best are canola, walnut, soybean, sesame, sunflower, and safflower oils, especially if they are labeled "cold pressed." Do not heat polyunsaturated oils. Butter is allowed, margarine is not. Margarine should be avoided, not because of its carbohydrate content, but because it is a potential health hazard. Mayonnaise is permitted unless you are on yeast restriction. The fat that is part of the meat or fowl you eat is permitted.

Avoid the seeming paradox provided by today's "diet foods." Understand why cream is allowed but not skim milk, why sour cream can be used but not yogurt, why low-fat chicken breading is not allowed even though chicken may be pan-fried. The answer common to all these seeming inconsistencies lies in the higher carbohydrate content of the low-fat dieter's foods.

ARTIFICIAL SWEETENERS:

Dieters must determine which artificial sweeteners agree with them, but the following are allowed: saccharine, sucralose, cyclamate, acesulfame-K. Sweeteners such as sorbitol, mannitol, and other hexitols are not allowed, nor are any natural sweeteners ending in the letters -ose, such as maltose, fructose, etc.

Aspartame (Nutra-Sweet, Equal) requires a special note of explanation. Whereas virtually all published scientific studies (many sponsored by the principals) show aspartame to be safe, there has been a great volume of word-of-mouth complaints attesting to its potential risk (headaches, irritability, seizure disorder, and vision problems, among others, have all been claimed).

My concern is its possible adverse effects on weight and sugar metabolism. I have taken scores of aspartame-users who seemed to be metabolically resistant to weight loss off this sweetener and observed weight loss to resume. Accordingly, I recommend its use only in small quantities (less than 3 packets of Equal or equivalent daily). People with known sensitivity to MSG should avoid it.

COMMON MISTAKES TO AVOID:

1. Note that the 14-day diet contains no fruit, bread, grains, starchy vegetables, or dairy products other than cheese, cream, or butter.
2. Avoid diet products unless they specifically state "No carbohydrates." Most dietetic foods are for fat-restricted, not carbohydrate-restricted, diets.
3. The word "sugarless" is not sufficient. The product must state the carbohydrate content, and that's what you go by.
4. Many products you do not normally think of as foods, such as chewing gum, cough syrups, and cough drops, are filled with sugar or other caloric sweeteners and must be avoided.

How to Fashion a Diet from the Above List

Once you know what you can have, the meal plan should leap out at you. You should instantly see that for breakfast, a ham, cheese, and mushroom omelet, or bacon and scrambled eggs, or a mixed selection of smoked fish with cream cheese would start the day off on the right note.

For lunch, the typical chef salad with ham, chicken, cheese, and hard-boiled egg on a bed of greens, covered with a creamy garlic dressing, will qualify, as will a bacon cheeseburger without the bun. Or maybe a Caesar chicken salad (no croutons) or a scoop of tuna salad with a scoop of chicken salad.

Dinners should be your favorite protein main courses—rack of lamb, poached salmon, roast chicken, filet mignon, buttered lobster tails, seafood mixed grill, or whatever you fancy, plus a salad. You might have included an appetizer such as shrimp cocktail with a mustard and mayonnaise sauce (the red sauce has carbohydrates), or pate, or steamed mussels in garlic butter. And for dessert, assorted cheeses or diet Jell-O with whipped heavy cream.

Remember, the purpose of these 14 days is to improve your health, not to win a gourmet eating contest. Of course, gourmet eating is more likely to be achieved on this diet than on the low-fat diets currently making the rounds. But, for the moment, I merely want to introduce you to the notion that gourmet dieting will be yours once you master all the possibilities offered by a diet allowing butter and cream sauces. That's a beautiful prospect of eating to come. Here and now, your attention should be totally focused on whether you feel you are in control of your eating and whether you feel healthy.

Now that you have the rules of the diet, you may benefit from some pointers. It's one thing to know the rules of chess or backgammon, but it takes some instruction to become a master player. Two of the major pointers I'm going to explain here and now as part of the diet rules: nutritional supplements and lipolysis testing strips.

The first will build up your health while you pare off your weight, and the second will make it possible for you to obtain confirmation of the fact that your fat is melting away—that is when you're in the state of ketosis/lipolysis.

Dietary Supplements

In starting people on the diet, I have found that their vitamin and mineral reserves are often so depleted that it frequently takes a week or two of supplementation with vita-nutrients to build those reserves back up again. This is one of the many reasons that by the time you complete your 14-day trial period on the diet, you're likely to experience a burst of energy.

Some critics of low-carbohydrate dieting have made the suggestion that the Atkins diet is so restrictive in certain areas that I have no choice but to advise everyone who goes on it to take vitamin and mineral supplements. There's only a smidgen of truth in this; when you go down to a very low level of vegetable consumption during the first 14 days—the strictest portion of the diet—you'll certainly be consuming inadequate portions of certain nutrients.

But the real reason you'll need vita-nutrients is likely to be the diet that you are following as you read this. If you have been on one of the low-fat diets, your need for supplementation can be profound. You will have to play catch-up with possible deficiencies of essential fatty acids and the fat-soluble vitamins A, D, and E. Several minerals are in short supply on a low-fat diet, and often B_{12} intake is quite low.

If on the other hand you've been bingeing on junk food (sugar and flour), then you've been consuming anti-nutrients, and your nutritional needs are even greater. Chromium, zinc, manganese, magnesium, B_6, and folic acid are among the nutrients used up faster than they are taken in on a thoughtless diet.

The third reason you need vita-nutrients is to maximize your body's ability to function optimally as a fat burning unit.

I Recommend Supplements for Everyone

The more I learn about nutritional supplements, the more I discover nutritional components that can help nearly everyone.

In fact, I consider the prescribing and individualizing of programs of vita-nutrients to be one of the two pillars of nutritional medicine. For the overweight, this diet, of course, is the other pillar. The key word is "individualizing," for each health problem a person might be facing requires a different roster of vita-nutrients.

I won't spend a lot of space in this book describing all the many ways vita-nutrients can help you overcome the many conditions you might have to deal with. I did that in another book, *Dr. Atkins' Vita-Nutrient Solution* (Simon & Schuster, 1998). If you ever need information on how nutrients can solve a health problem better than drugs, you'll find it in that book.

To give one example of how everyone can benefit from vita-nutrients, take the antioxidant group (vitamins A, E, C, beta-carotene, selenium, glutathione, coenzyme Q_{10}, and flavonoids), which can protect you against heart disease, cancer, and aging. Now, who wouldn't benefit from that? Add to that the vita-nutrients known to be useful for each of the myriad medical problems my patients face, and you'll see why many of them take over 30 vitamin pills each day.

In this chapter, however, all I want to do is provide adequate nutritional support for a 14-day diet, not the lifetime program my face-to-face patients get after a two-hour evaluation. When you opt to become a lifetime Atkins dieter (notice, I didn't say "if"), you will have to familiarize yourself with Chapter 22.

So for now, this is what you do:

1. Find a very broad multiple vitamin, a model for which you can find in Chapter 22, "Nutritional Supplements," where I gave the breakdown of my Dieter's Formula, Basic #3. Such a formula should contain considerably more than the RDA of B complex factors and of vitamin C and should contain at least 40 different nutrients. Don't expect to take fewer than four pills a day. Ideally, chromium picolinate, 200–600 mcg, should be included.

2. Part of a basic formulation for anyone, including non-dieters, is an oil-containing capsule providing Essential Fatty Acids. (That formula, too, is found in Chapter 22.) Essential Fatty Acid deficiency may be the most prevalent dietary shortage in our culture.

3. If you have sugar cravings, you should include L-Glutamine 500–1000 mg before each meal.

4. If you are concerned about the possibility of an elevated cholesterol level from the very beginning, you should be sure to include 2 tablespoons of lecithin granules per day, plus pantethine 300 mg before each meal, and inositol hexanicotinate, 300 mg before each meal. The formula I give my patients for cholesterol control is also shown in Chapter 22.

Lipolysis Testing Strips
How to Get and Use LTS

Using lipolysis testing strips, which hereinafter will be referred to by the acronym LTS, to measure your degree of ketosis/lipolysis is another category from nutritional supplementation.* You don't

---

*"Lipolysis testing strips" is a generic term for a variety of products available for determining, some quantitatively, the presense of ketone bodies in the urine, thus healding fat breakdown. They are available under the names of Lipostix, designed for low-carbohydrate dieters, or Ketostix, designed to warn of ketoacidosis in diabetics. However, both are quite serviceable as lipolysis testing strips.

necessarily have to do it, but it can be an extremely convenient aid to doing the diet. And, if you're not getting the results you expect, then they will surely help you to clear up the mystery of why that's so.

After all, the clear basis for going into the strict *Induction* phase of the diet, the first 14 days, is that you be in ketosis. I'm going to allow you one medium-sized tossed salad a day to start. After you've used up your 48-hour supply of stored carbohydrate—it's called glycogen—you'll almost certainly enter ketosis.

Your LTS will help to measure how deeply you've done so. After the first two weeks, as you increase your carbohydrate, your LTS will help to ensure that you don't increase them too much and fall out of the effective state of ketosis/lipolysis.

What Are Lipolysis Testing Strips?

Lipolysis Testing Strips are urine test sticks that when placed in your urine change color depending on what they find there. If you're excreting ketones in your urine, then the LTS will turn purple. The more ketones excreted, the darker the purple.

LTS are moderately inexpensive, and you can find them in your local drug store or you can ask your druggist to order them or you may contact the Atkins Center. My patients often tell me that LTS are psychologically supporting. To see them go from beige to purple is to receive in chemical code the message *I'm losing weight*.

What If They Don't Turn?

Well, basically, they must, unless you're not doing the diet correctly or you have very severe metabolic resistance. First, make sure that none of your foods—except the salad—have carbohydrate. No hidden sugars, no breading, etc. Then follow the diet for five days, using the LTS each day. If they still haven't even changed to at least the color of lavender, then cut out that one salad. It's the only significant source of carbohydrate that you're consuming. As soon as the LTS turn purple, put the salad back in the diet again.

Do your LTS testing at the same hour each day. Usually the evening works best, because that's when you generally get the deepest reaction.

For the vast majority of you, there will be no difficulty getting your LTS purple at this stage. You'll have more interesting variations as you go up the carbohydrate scale later in the diet. At that point, in the *Ongoing Weight-Loss* phase, you'll be testing out where your Critical Carbohydrate Level lies.

However, should your LTS not turn purple, yet you are doing everything correctly, you may still show a decrease in appetite, an improvement in well-being, and a steady weight loss. This simply means that you are producing enough ketones to succeed, even though not enough to register on the LTS.

Critical Carbohydrate Levels?

This is an interesting aspect of the diet, because this is where the individualization process begins. The diet aspect of the Atkins program has four stages. First, there is this, the 14-day *Induction* diet for fast weight loss. Next, there will be the stage of *Ongoing Weight Loss* (OWL). Then, there will be the *Pre-Maintenance* diet, a stage of transition to your lifetime diet, which will take place while you're losing your last few pounds. Finally, there will be the lifetime *Maintenance* diet.

For each of these levels of the diet, there is a critical Carbohydrate Level that pertains to you. Your individual metabolism has a certain quantity of carbohydrate beyond which it will cease to lose weight, or—after you've reached your ideal weight—beyond which you will begin to gain it back. Therefore, in Part Four, I'll tell you all about those very critical levels.

What Does This All Mean Metabolically?

Principally, of course, your purple LTS and your capacity to stay below your Critical Carbohydrate Level for Losing will mean that you've found the easiest method of losing pounds and inches.

Your LTS are evidence for the fact that you've carved out a different metabolic pathway. On all other eating patterns, the first fuel your body burns for energy comes from the carbohydrates you eat and drink. Now that you've lowered your carbohydrate consumption to a level that can't finance your energy expenditures, you must burn your stored fat. Easily, if you're metabolically average, reluctantly, if you're metabolically resistant, your body draws upon those stores of fat. A new metabolic pathway for supplying energy has been successfully taken. And, at that moment, your body converts from being a carbohydrate-burning engine into being a fat-burning engine.

You really are doing the diet now. I'm very happy for you. This should be the last diet you'll have ever to do.

9 | *Doing the Strict Level of the Atkins Diet at Home and at Work*

The 14-day *Induction* diet is primarily about losing eight and feeling good. You now know how to do it, but let me add one necessary caution before you begin: If you have serious health problems, seeing your doctor is *essential*.

The Atkins diet has a strongly positive effect on virtually all conditions, but it *is* a major lifestyle change, and, if you have a serious medical problem, you should monitor your changing metabolism with a physician's aid and counsel. Enough said. But please don't forget.

Also, I must insert a crucial warning: *this phase of the diet is* not *appropriate for pregnant women and people with severe kidney disease.*

Now, how about my other suggestions?

Have you laid in your stock of vitamin supplements and lipolysis testing strips as suggested in Chapter 7?

What about those blood tests I spent so much time urging on you? Have you had them? I hope so, but, if you're young and healthy, and you just haven't' been able to get your act together and do them, so be it. It's a pity to remain uninformed, but it would be a far greater pity to remain fat.

But don't think I'm letting you off the hook here. I do strongly, intensely, urge you to do them. If money is a problem, then be aware that the federal government conducts cholesterol screening programs that you can participate in and that will give you at least your cholesterol and triglyceride levels.

Dieter's Morale

Psychologically, have you made a firm commitment? Don't start something this important with the shallow notion that "Oh, well, I'll give it a whirl." At the least, you should have decided that you'll give two weeks of your life without deviation and without compromise to this diet.

If you can commit yourself to that, then quite frankly I expect great things for you. By the end of your 14 days, you'll be walking with new energy, getting out of bed in the morning with new zest, and joyously anticipating your every encounter with the bathroom scale.

Blast Off! You've Begun—Munch Away

Naturally, you begin by eating—something you've always done with some degree of guilt. But don't hesitate as you plow into the spare ribs or the roast duckling. If you're an experienced dieter, you may have to suppress an involuntary shudder as you begin downing high-calorie food you always thought would make you fat.

Once again have faith. In the absence of carbohydrates, the body has no choice but to burn its own fat. Moreover, at this stage of your dieting, eating the rich, fatty foods your last dietitian advised you to flee from can only be advantageous.

You're starting off at the most extreme low-carbohydrate end of the diet, and I'm encouraging you to eat as much as you like.

I want you to be totally, shockingly unafraid of fat during these two weeks. Fat is much more ketosis-inducing than protein. After all, 58% of protein will become glucogenic amino acids, i.e., convertible to glucose, but only 10% of fat will become its glycerol portion, which is similarly convertible. The ease of getting into deep ketosis/lipolysis is based on the ratio of fat to carbohydrate. The higher that number, the more ketosis. Thus, you should strive for the maximum amount of fat during this initial period, and in doing so, you will almost certainly find yourself experiencing the deepest, sharpest, most appetite-suppressing aspects of the diet.

As an overweight person, you're very likely to be resistant to ketosis, since ketosis means parting with your fat, and that's just what your body has obviously been reluctant to do. During your fortnight trial diet, we're taking no chances. We're going to make sure those LTS turn purple.

Have the Food on Hand

Stock the refrigerator and the cupboard with the food you're going to eat. Go to the supermarket and check out the protein goodies you're fond of. Naturally, avoid the aisles where the carbohydrate temptations are found. I had a nineteen-year-old patient named John Connors who, standing 6'4", dropped his weight from 290 to 209 in six months. He used to tell me how he'd go to the supermarket on some legitimate food errand, get sucked into one of the sugar aisles, and end up walking out of the store with a package of candy bars. In the course of his journey home, self-control would reassert itself, and he'd lower the car window and throw it into the street!

What permitted foods do you like to have in front of you when you open the refrigerator door? Deviled eggs, turkey, chicken, shrimp salad, your favorite cheese?

If you live alone, don't keep the things you won't be eating. Invite some friends over to finish off the ice cream. Have a final party. Give away all your forbidden foods to a neighbor or an in-law. (Blood relatives may share your inherited metabolic disorder.) Or just throw them away. Alter your mental picture—for you, that food doesn't exist.

If you don't live alone, then it almost always makes sense to prepare your significant others for the "shock" of your new diet. Unless you come from a family of vegetarians, it actually shouldn't be too shocking. You're planning to eat things you've always eaten.

If you do the cooking, unless you can convince your household to share the Atkins diet experience, you'll have to cook for yourself and make additions for them. They may want bread, potatoes, and dessert. There's a little problem with temptation here, but if you really want to lose weight I think you'll bite the bullet and not the breadstick or the banana. You have this comfort: Human beings are remarkably adaptable, and, in as little as a week, your tastes will start to change. Soon you'll find that sugar and refined carbohydrates don't tempt as much as they did. And the appetite suppression I've told you so much about will be your constant ally.

If, for the first few days, you find it a bit of a downer watching other folks eating foods that you're fond of and can't touch, then comfort yourself in your own way. Take a double portion of what's permitted. Remember, weight loss is now your destiny; these moments of temptation are just momentary afflictions. Make sure you tell family members that you need a strong show of support and understanding. You certainly don't want them tempting you with illicit food and saying vile and inappropriate things like, "Don't worry, this tiny piece of cake won't harm you." *It will!*

Tell people in advance that you take your diet seriously, and you'd appreciate their doing the same. The Atkins diet is a breeze, the most luxurious diet you'll ever be on (and the last), but we all know what a tricky, emotion-laden, family-connected, downright passionate business food is.

I understand that the other people in your house may not automatically be entranced with your new diet. In the nicest possible way, tell them it's your diet, not theirs, and they don't need to be entranced. All they need to do is show respect for the major decision you've made. You're about to lose a lot of weight and gain a lot of health. After you've done the diet, you won't need to request respect for it; the results will speak for themselves.

But above all, remember: If other people are going to be impressed with your resolve, then you yourself must take your diet seriously. Do so! Go at it, as if it were a life-and-death matter. For overweight people, over the course of years, that's exactly what it is.

What's the First Thing You Notice?

You're not hungry.

Indeed, how could you be? Ketosis, just like a fast, always induces appetite suppression once a body's two-day supply of glycogen is burnt off.

Two days are past. Your glycogen is gone. You're solidly into ketosis/lipolysis. At this point, you're finding out that this appetite suppression is the *most striking thing* that has ever happened to your appetite in your entire life.

Suddenly, you find yourself eating quite moderate quantities of food and feeling no hunger pangs.

You certainly know you're in ketosis, when you find yourself saying: "You mean lunchtime was an hour ago?"

You may be a person for whom incessant, almost hourly food cravings have been a way of life. I'm sure you remember Gordon Lingard, the patient who came to see me at 306 pounds. He used to say, "I'd always be planning the next binge. I'd be in a business meeting, very serious, a lot of money at stake, and one-half of my brain would be figuring out what I would eat, how much I would eat, when and where I would eat. Food seized my brain."

Now that's enslavement to food. Yet in the end, Gordon succeeded, and if he could do it, almost any one of you can, too.

Willpower is not required on the Atkins diet, only the wisdom to put yourself into a position where you won't be needing it.

What's the Second Thing You Notice?

Unless you have an exceedingly high energy level, the next thing that will strike most of you is a feeling that you've latched onto some misplaced, long-lost energy. Typically, this feeling arrives around about the third or fourth day. Some people experience a slight euphoria. Most simply find that those dreary, weary hours that used to hit them two or three times a day have been reduced to mere occasional moments.

Conversely, there are people who experience fatigue during their first week on the diet. Most often this means that the diet is going too fast for their particular metabolism—they're losing weight too fast, losing water and minerals too fast, and their bodies aren't adjusting to these quick changes very readily. Usually, I advise patients who have these problems to back off and slow down. I suggest they add a second salad or a helping of vegetables with their evening meal. Though their bodies would almost certainly adjust during the second week, there isn't any good reason for feeling washed out and sickly for five or six days.

There is a second mechanism providing adverse reactions you should all know about—withdrawal symptoms. Quite a few people get addicted to foods they consume every day. Common offenders are caffeine, sugar, wheat, and other foods capable of quickly changing blood sugar levels. Withdrawal symptoms are quite variable—ranging from fatigue, faintness, and palpitations to headache and cold sweats. Bad as that seems, it is really good news. The withdrawal process is usually completed within 3 days, and when accomplished, you are finished with the problem (unless you re-addict yourself) and feel better than ever. If you cannot "stay the course" and progress through withdrawal, then do it gradually by consuming progressively smaller amounts of addictive foods (you'll know what they are) until you get to zero.

I'm happy to say that with most people it's the energy lift they experience. It tends to send them roaring on through the diet because it's such clear evidence of the satisfying influence their dietary change is having on their metabolism.

This Is Your Diet Wherever You Go

It's true I began by talking about eating at home, and for a reason. The person in his or her own habitat, living with the refrigerator, is the basic prototype. This is the world in which food is always there for the asking, this is the land of temptations, and often gluttony. Sitting at the kitchen table and wondering, *What shall I eat*?

The answer is always the same: Eat as much as you want of the *permitted* foods. If you've spent a whole lifetime plagued by food cravings—usually, I know, straightforward carbohydrate cravings—then the pleasant truth is that hunger isn't going to occupy as much of your time and thought. Oh, yes, you'll still have an appetite, and you'll still eat with pleasure and delight, but the days of obsession are on the way to being past. What a joy not to always be hungry and always be tired and always be searching for some satisfying physical solution that you've never been quite able to reach. That's the lifestyle of the carbohydrate addict, which so many of you are, and it's a profoundly exhausting and irritating lifestyle that you'll be eternally happy to be rid of.

But what about when you're not sitting at the kitchen table? Well, I hope it's clear to you just how easy this diet is to follow in all the circumstances of life. On weekends, in restaurants, on the job, when you travel a lot—unless someone imprisons you in a candy store, you really have nothing to worry about. Of course, the diet is not completely adaptable to dinner parties given by hostesses with fixed ideas about what everyone should eat. You'll need a little ingenious diplomacy to get you out of that one.

Of course, there are also the airlines—the Last Final Frontier of Junk Food. I'll have some further remarks on airlines in my chapter on eating in the Real World, but for the moment, I have a suggestions to make that applies just to your 14 days on the *Induction* diet. I think you should try to choose a two-week stretch in which you're not traveling, not vacationing, and not attending other people's dinner parties. These first two weeks are important, so why make them difficult?

Outside Eating

Let us consider eating outside the home. If you eat five lunches a week at work or in a restaurant, that's no problem at all. And certainly the Atkins diet is wonderfully accommodating to the needs of those of you who like as many weekly occasions of restaurant dining as you can manage.

If you eat out a lot at restaurants, or at your office cafeteria, then you must become familiar with the possibilities of the menu, and you must be alert for hidden pitfalls. If the eating establishment is one you go to often, talk to the waiter or the maitre d' and be quite clear about the fact that you're on a diet that doesn't permit you to eat sugar in any manner, shape, or form. A surprising problem can be sugar in salads. Sometimes fruit juices are used as a sugar substitute. For your diet, this is absolutely not permissible.

Go right down the list and make sure that your appetizer, main course, and salad all qualify for the diet. Avoid sauces, breading on your meat, bread crumbs, flour as thickener. Such carbohydrates ingredients can be hidden in surprising places. There may be flour or grain in your hamburgers, or bread crumbs in your crab cakes.

Eating out requires alertness. Otherwise, one meal can destroy your weight-loss program for the day and set it back for the week. Your first week's results won't look so good, if, instead of losing three-quarters of a pound on Wednesday, you gained half a pound that day.

If the choices are really limited at the cafeteria or luncheonette where you dine, then you may prefer to pack a lunch. Bring along some finger food—chicken drumsticks, hard-boiled or deviled eggs, slices of ham, cheese, and chicken roll.

At this point in the diet, you're simply looking to have what it takes to stabilize your blood sugar and avoid hunger. Make sure, if you're bringing your own food, you have enough food with you. Don't allow for even the slim chance that you might be hungry enough to turn to the carbohydrates.

More information about doing the diet with your family and in the outside world can be found in Chapter 23.

Special Situations

Once the diet begins to become a habit, you won't have to think about eating the right foods, because you really won't think about eating any other way.

Cynthia Marlborough, who for many years was executive secretary to one of the top corporate chairmen in New York, had battled mood swings and fatigue for years when she first came to see me. Cynthia, a chocoholic, had recently quit smoking.

"I had been overweight since I was a child; I can remember dieting when I was twelve but this was different. The weight was really piling on. And worse yet, it was a tense, stressed-out time at work. It got so I didn't know how I could handle the pressure and my poor physical state simultaneously. This actually began to depress me to a degree that people noticed. After lunch, I could have slept for hours. Instead I had to work through the fatigue. My job, which is one of the central things in my life, was just becoming torture."

Yet Cynthia Marlborough easily lost weight, cured her sugar cravings (it was a lot easier than quitting smoking), and went from a size 16 dress to a size 6 in less than six months. She also acquired an uncanny sensitivity to the foods she was eating. Two weeks into the diet, she had dinner at a girlfriend's house. She found herself eating some sliced filet mignon, a green salad, and a helping of horseradish.

"As soon as I ate the horseradish, I knew something was wrong, and I stopped and asked my friend if there was sugar in it. She said there was, and, of course, I didn't eat another bite of that. By that time I had a lot more energy, and I'd lost seven pounds, and I'd already become very careful what I put into my mouth."

This sensitivity to the taste of sweets is not uncommon among people who are curing themselves of sugar addictions. It's a good, protective sensitivity that will help you out in some of the situations I described above. Sugars and refined carbohydrates have gotten you into a bad physical pickle, so be wary of them.

A New You

This introduces us to an idea I want to emphasize right here at the end of this *Induction* diet chapter. *It's a lot easier to change diets than you imagine.*

I know that some of you are still hesitating about doing the Atkins diet because you're thinking, This isn't really the way I eat—how will I live without my favorite foods? Psychological attachment is more important here than physical. We're attached to ourselves, our habits, the customs of our lives, our cultural and culinary traditions. Sharp changes are like the rending of old attachments, the breaking of friendships.

All I can tell you is that it must be done. You'll find after you change the way you eat that the essential you is still intact. And since that will be true, what you must look to is the salvation of the physical you.

You *can't* afford to be fat and unhealthy—it's as simple as that. This is a path that will cure you; for many of you, it will be the only path. You may imagine that your tastes won't change, but you're wrong. The body, faced with the necessity of eating, the passage of days, the inevitable renunciation of old habits, adapts. This is it, simple, almost humiliatingly basic: *The body adapts.* The body learns new tastes and forgets old ones. And since much of the desire for carbohydrate food is metabolic addiction, once the path of renunciation is completed, the desire for the old goodies is really very small.

Look at Ernie Kingman, who came to me for the oddest of reasons. At 55 years old, Ernie felt pretty healthy, but he had one problem: He was carrying 290 pounds on his 6' 1¾" frame. He had tried a liquid-protein diet in the '80s and gotten a temporary weight loss of no long-term significance, except, after the lost pounds came back, he found it was even harder to lose again.

Ernie didn't know what to do because he had developed a weight-related lifestyle problem. His children rode horses, and three years before, he'd taken it up to have something to do with them and found he loved it. He felt he needed to be agile and limber for horseback riding, and, as he put it, "At my weight, it isn't fair to the horse and it's dangerous for me."

His best friend, who's fair comment had been, "All you can do is get on and pray," was a patient of mine and urged Ernie to come, too. "Another diet doc," Ernie said. "Oh, I don't know."

Soon after, Ernie was taking a business trip to Florida and while he was waiting in the airport, the public address system paged him to a phone. It was his friend, and what he had to say was, "You have an appointment with Atkins next Thursday at nine o'clock."

My patients aren't usually sent to me as forcibly as that, but I was glad to have Ernie, who is a charming guy, and who was definitely in need of a little lifestyle improvement.

I looked at his diet, which had more than its share of cakes, cookies, ice cream, and sweet goodies, and which, amazingly, nobody had attempted to change in the direction of carbohydrate limitation, not even his previous doctor, who had told him, "You're an accident waiting to happen."

You won't be surprised to hear Ernie was a resounding success. He got his weight down below 240 in eight months and his pounds are still falling off, slowly now, but steadily.

Where he used to have cake and coffee in the middle of the afternoon, he now has a slice of turkey on Swiss cheese. Ernie had been so afraid he wouldn't be able to bear life without his sugar-loaded carbohydrate diet that I made him promise he'd call me up if he felt he was going to quit.

It never came to that. Ernie got used to his change, he adapted, and moreover he noticed that "I feel better when I have protein, lots of protein on my diet. I'm really glad that I don't want to go back to eating the way I ate before." Ernie was an overweight person with typical glucose intolerance and an addiction to the very carbohydrates that made his condition worse. A couple of weeks eating the Atkins way pretty well took away the urge to eat the sweets and starches that were at the root of his weight problem. Ernie admits that now and then in a restaurant he'd like to reach for a roll or order up a gushy dessert, but the urge is hardly irresistible.

Some people go even further and simply find their former urges aren't there at all. Marjorie Burke, an excellent chef and a woman who had craved starches her whole life long, found after a month on the diet that starches no longer filled a spot in her imagination. She could cook delicious breads for other people without so much as a desire to taste them.

Such a complete conversion is rare, and I don't recommend that any Atkins dieter become a baker. Nor do I recommend going back at some later stage to eating those white flour foods or those dreadful sugars, especially if you were addicted to them. But if you weren't addicted, it is possible to enjoy an occasional indulgence, as you'll see in the *Maintenance* chapter.

10 | *Time to Review Your 14-Day Results*

You've gone through 14 days on the Atkins diet. For approximately 90% of you this will have been a highly satisfying experience. You're taking stock of the successful loss of considerable girth. How did you do it? By eating luxuriously and without stint! You'll remember I promised you a diet fit for royalty? That's what you've been eating.

At the same time, you probably noticed that though self-indulgence reigned supreme, you weren't eating as much as you had expected to. Your metabolism changed markedly after the first few days. *Your appetite became controllable, and, for some of you, that will have been a new experience.*

Now you're at the end of your diet fortnight, and you have choices ahead.

Do I Go On?

This is the logical time for you to make a decision, and I hope you will join the vast majority of dieters who choose to go on with the Atkins diet. They do this for a number of reasons. First, they're losing weight easily. Second, in direct contrast to the experiences they've had on so many other diets, they're not only feeling no pain, they're also feeling more vigorous and energetic than they did before they began. Third, a significant percentage of dieters, especially those who are over forty, have discovered that a variety of nagging minor physical ills, from headaches to body aches, have completely vanished.

Those are impressive general results. But as an individual, you may want more information to help you in making your choice. I suggest you get a second round of lab tests done at the 14-day break point. In just two weeks, blood chemistries can change a lot.

I think it's important for you to realize that not only do you feel good but good things are happening inside you. This is especially important because *high*-carbohydrate dieting has been elevated to the status of a religion during the last two decades, and you're bound to feel a slight uneasiness over going against the grain—and against the potatoes, for that matter.

Your real decision ought to be not whether or not to have repeat blood tests done, but whether to continue with the diet while you're waiting for results or go off the diet and see what those results are first. If you haven't done your initial blood tests, particularly your glucose/insulin blood tests, you certainly should go off the diet, spend at least four days on your previous eating pattern, and then have the tests done.

Most people go right on to the next level of the diet, a vote of confidence I'm vain enough to appreciate, but, in all honesty, each of these decisions has its advantages. You have a whole lifetime in which to take the weight off and keep it off, and a week or two of reflection will do you no harm.

Some Questions to Ask

- Did you experience any hunger
- Did you have any problems with constipation?
- Did you like the food?

If you were hungry, then you weren't following my counsel to eat as much as you wanted. If you were constipated, then you'll do better as you progress to an easier phase of the diet, as your body learns to adjust, and as you accustom yourself to eating some of the low-carbohydrate bulking agents or bowel-stimulating vita-nutrients we'll discuss in Chapter 22. A certain amount of constipation is common during the first week, but it almost always gets solved a lot more quickly and easily than your weight problem.

As for liking the food, that's a classic difficulty of any major dietary change. Fortunately, most people enjoy protein food. If your tastes run to the vegetarian line, you can still do the diet but not without major efforts. The lack of selection on a diet that's low in carbohydrate and simultaneously excludes animal food is a serious taste difficulty. It's theoretically possible to construct a healthy low-carbohydrate vegetarian diet, but there aren't a lot of foods on it. In general, I've found that a person who will not eat any animal food at all will not stay on the Atkins diet indefinitely. The narrow range of selections is too boring.

The rest of you can enjoy a very delicious diet. What you'll chiefly regret is the loss of some favorite carbohydrate foods. Pasta and bread, as well as fruit and juice, are very often missed in the first few weeks.

So why do bread lovers continue on the diet? Simply this: The upside is much larger than the downside. Weight loss, of course, but feeling physically better and in control of your eating are paramount issues, too. I've told you about these improvements so many times that I hope you're beginning to understand I'm not talking through my hat. Feeling good is a major part of the Atkins diet.

At this point, I'd like to take inventory of your 14-day experience. You may well start with the quiz below. If you feel better in a number of these areas, that should provide strong support for the idea of going on with the diet.

14-Day Quiz

Problem	Worse	Same	Better	Much Better
Energy Level	___	___	___	___
Anxiety	___	___	___	___
Depression	___	___	___	___
Headaches	___	___	___	___
Premenstrual Symptoms	___	___	___	___
Sleep Function	___	___	___	___
Comfort with Appetite	___	___	___	___
Concentration	___	___	___	___
Willpower	___	___	___	___
Mastery of Eating Behavior	___	___	___	___

Other Symptoms:

1. _____

2. _____

3. _____

Scoring Your Quiz:

SCORE:
−1 for worse
−1 for a new negative symptom
 0 for same or does not apply (you didn't start with the symptom)
+1 for better
+2 for much better

A score of +4 should encourage you to stay on the diet.
A score of +8 should mandate you to.

Medical Indicators

Now, assuming you've taken my advice let's look at the results of your blood tests.

First, let's look at the cholesterol reading. Lipolytic low-carbohydrate diets have been well studied in this regard, and even the extreme high-fat version of such a diet generally drops the total cholesterol level a little bit in the group starting with readings over 200. But this process may take up to 4 to 8 weeks. During the first week the cholesterol may be elevated, a phenomenon reported on all diets that act quickly in using up fat stores. Even zero food, i.e., fasting, has that effect.°

Now, since you will be doing this test after only two weeks, you may get unpredictable results. Unless the cholesterol has shot up considerably (over 20 points), it may be assumed that it would be lower by the time another reading is taken after 3 to 4 more weeks. If the cholesterol has not gone to a healthy level, yet you were satisfied with the diet's advantages, you should make it a point to remain on the diet, take the cholesterol-lowering nutritional supplements outlined on pages 147–149 and repeat the test within a month.

On the other hand, if your triglyceride level was elevated, or even high normal (anything over 100 increases the risk of heart disease), it will plummet down dramatically. Drops of 40–80 percent are

---

°The biphasic cholesterol response is so well known that one has to take notice of the study by Rickman purporting to show that a low-fat and low-carbonate diet such as the one proposed by Stillman is a cholesterol, elevating diet, even though Rickman's study covered less than two weeks on the Stillman diet. That study, which has been quoted many times because it served the purposes of those who wish to critize low-carbohydrate diets, must be classified as either an incompetent and poorly thought out investigation, or as an intellectually dishonest hatchet job.

commonplace. If you don't get such a response, make sure you followed the diet correctly; or else, repeat the test making sure you wait 14 hours after your last meal before the blood is drawn.

Make sure you look at your HDL and LDL cholesterol levels. Your heart risk is dramatically decreased whenever the "good" cholesterol (HDL) is at least half as high as the "bad" cholesterol (LDL). If the after-the-diet readings are better than the pre-diet ones in this regard (as it usually will be), then you will have gone a long way toward reducing your heart risk factors.*

The other lab parameters should remain as good as before, except that there may be an elevated uric acid level. Should this happen, know that you can control it by going to a higher level of the diet and slowing your weight loss to less than two pounds per week.

Practical Problem Solving

If, however, you simply don't seem to be losing much weight on the diet, then you need to turn immediately to Chapter 18, "Metabolic Resistance." Sometimes, some very simple problems can give adverse results. Simple problems usually mean simple solutions. When I say that only 2% of dieters are unable to succeed on the Atkins diet, I mean precisely that—2%—one dieter out of fifty. I think that means the odds are good that Chapter 18 will correct your difficulty.

On the other hand—I suppose there always is another hand—too much success can sometimes masquerade as failure. When the diet works too well, and the weight loss is too rapid, there can be weakness or other slightly debilitating symptoms, presumably caused by sodium or potassium shifts, that can be corrected by the simple measure of tripling or quadrupling the vegetable intake and slowing the weight loss down. Whenever weight loss exceeds 1 pound per day, you should suspect that you may experience some symptoms. Another problem that people occasionally experience is leg cramps at night. This is due to a rapid excretion of calcium, magnesium, or potassium, and almost invariably indicates that the

---

*You should be aware that elevated triglyceride levels, espeically when combined with low levels of HDL cholesterol, have been shown by a multitude of well-conducted studies to be the most important combination of heart risk factors ever discovered. (Gaziano, J. M., *Circulation* 1997; 96(8):2520–2525) And you should know that these two abnormalities are caused primarily from the consumption of carbohydrates by persons who are high-insulin responders.

dieter has not followed my recommendations on vitamin and mineral supplementation. See Chapter 22.

Success and Long-Term Satisfaction

The Atkins low-carbohydrate diet has many levels, and is made for many different types of people. The high-fat, deep-ketosis form of it that you've just experienced is not *the diet* but an extreme variation of it. And the fact is most of the time spent on the Atkins diet is not spent on this level. This first level, the *Induction* level, is to be used whenever ketosis/lipolysis must be induced, but I do not advise staying on this level for any length of time, unless it is the only level that works.

Instead, I want you next to find the level of carbohydrate restriction that works best for you as you're making your passage through the pleasant waters of long-term weight loss, whether that passage is 6 weeks to lose twenty pounds or 10 months to lose a hundred. Later on, you'll go one step further and find the level of carbohydrate restriction that works best in sustaining you at your ideal weight level once you've attained it.

All you gung-ho types may think the ideal level is simply that which takes the pounds off fastest, i.e., the diet you've just been on for the first 14 days. But why, in heaven's name, should that be true? Fast weight loss isn't a very important consideration when you're going to be solving your weight problem for the rest of your life. What *is* an important consideration is being comfortable, contented, and healthy. I want you to feel at ease on the Atkins diet. Physically well, satiated, pleased with your daily menu, confident in your body. The vast majority of you will find that the level of carbohydrate consumption that achieves that best is *not* the first level.

In Part Four of the book, I'll show you how you go on through the four Atkins diets, passing from the *Induction* diet, to the *Ongoing Weight Loss* diet, and then to the *Pre-Maintenance* and *Maintenance* diets. On the last of those diets, you'll learn how to find and work with the lifetime carbohydrate level that's right for you.

Now it's time to look at some of the health advantages of the diet you've already discovered has the capacity to take weight off more efficiently than any diet you've ever been on before.

PART THREE

Why the Diet Makes You Healthy

11 | *Diet-Related Disorders and You*

Now that many of you have experienced the remarkable improvements in well-being that accompanied your 14-day diet experience, I will assume that I got your attention. I promised you weight loss while taking in lots of food, and since I prepared you for it, you're probably not surprised. But I'll wager that many of you were quite surprised to see that symptoms you have never connected to weight loss cleared up too.

Over thirty years ago, I reasoned that if a diet could predictably clear up a cluster of symptoms, then that symptom cluster must have been partly caused by whatever diet my patients had previously been on. I was convinced I was seeing hypoglycemia, and I so stated.

But over the next few decades I witnessed thousands of patients whose symptoms promptly cleared up on their new diet, but who were not hypoglycemic. I classified the whole lot of them—patients whose symptoms came and went *according to whether they were consuming carbohydrates*—as people with Diet-Related Disorder. And, over time, I realized that was a category of illness in its own right. Besides unstable blood glucose, the two other principal carbohydrate-based conditions that are part of the Diet-Related Disorder syndrome—DRD—are a) individual food intolerances, and b) the yeast syndrome, the condition caused when the organism *Candida albicans* gets numerically out-of-control in your intestinal tract. Less commonly, we found nutritional deficiencies or addictions to certain foods as other contributing causes of the disordered body harmony that clears up when carbohydrate is sharply restricted. These are the elements of Diet-Related Disorder.

A pretty intelligent question, and the one you are probably asking, is: "Why did you feel you had to invent a disease you call Diet-Related Disorder? Why couldn't you just identify who has hypoglycemia, who has yeast overgrowth, and who has specific food intolerances?

The basic answer to that question is that there is considerable confusion among those doctors clinically expert in these conditions as to which symptoms should be attributed to which conditions. For example, when the hypoglycemic complains of abdominal bloating is it not his/her yeast syndrome? If a chemically sensitive individual craves sweets, is it not his/her hypoglycemia? When a yeast patient reacts to dairy products, is it not his/her food intolerance? More and more doctors have come to recognize that they must deal with all of these problems in a single individual because they are so frequently found together in individuals.

Interestingly enough, the majority of people on the ketogenic/lipolytic diet feel better even before weight loss mounts up to more than a handful of pounds. That's one of the reasons why this section will be important to you. It's going to have a major positive impact on your lifelong commitment to the diet. After all, if you know that the diet corrects a specific condition or conditions that you have that will inevitably motivate you to stay on it. All diets are not alike, and all do not correct Diet-Related Disorder.

In these next five chapters, let's see how much you can learn about yourself.

12 | The Sorrows of Hypoglycemia and the Perils of Diabetes

I assume you recall that in Chapter 3 I talked about hypoglycemia as the symptomatic aspect of the hyperinsulinism that correlates so strongly with the presence of obesity. Now here I am talking about it as the cornerstone of DRD.

I won't be repetitive, but I do want you to know the vast extent of the scientific discoveries that justify your considering the real probability you may have or may eventually develop disturbances of your glucose and insulin metabolism.

A brief review is in order:

1. If you are, or have been, significantly overweight, or if you have an eating (behavior) disorder, chances are much greater than 50/50 that you have insulin resistance and hyperinsulinism.
2. Insulin resistance and excess are the first abnormalities on the way to developing glucose disorders (glycopathy).
3. Hypoglycemia, pre-diabetes, and type II diabetes are stages of the same disease—glycopathy. The denominators common to all of these conditions are insulin resistance and excess.
4. Insulin and glucose disorders accelerate the development of atherosclerosis, the mechanism leading to heart attacks.
5. In fact, insulin has been shown to be a more probable cause of atherosclerosis than is glucose.
6. This means that people with pre-diabetic glycopathy share with full-fledged diabetics the biochemical mechanism leading to heart disease.
7. Therefore, stop the insulin-based chain of events, and you can protect your heart and extend your life.

First, I'd like to stress the symptoms you may be experiencing right now. Let's look at hypoglycemia first.

Why Do People Feel So Much Better So Fast on the Atkins Diet?

The correct answer certainly is (most of the time) that the diet deals with the unstable levels of blood sugar that we speak of, somewhat loosely, as reactive hypoglycemia.

This instability produces symptoms, such as:

- Frequent bouts of fatigue—sometimes overwhelming—often in the afternoon.
- Sleep difficulties, usually combined with a need for considerable amounts of sleep. Awakening from a sound sleep is a specific example.
- Emotional instability, mood swings, sadness, and weepiness for which there's no explanation or cause. Inability to concentrate, irritability, anxiety, brain fog, and confusion. Becoming easily obsessed with annoyances.

This list of symptoms, some of which obviously share common ground with mental disorders, could be expanded. My patients often don't want to talk about them. They think it's their fault, just like being fat. I hear them make remarks like this:

Maybe I should be seeing a psychiatrist.
I just don't seem to care anymore. Life can do what it wants with me.
I don't have any control over my life.
I'm so weak-willed that I don't know why I even try.
Sometimes I feel suicidal.

These remarks, coming from people who quite clearly have nutritional disorders, arouse my suspicion that a fair percentage of the "mental illness" that doctors diagnose would vanish if only people would eat right.

I'm sure you'd like to avoid these symptoms as well as the physical ones, but following a low-fat diet isn't necessarily going to do that for you. I've seen many people who go on a current low-fat fad diet and feel worse because they're consuming more fruit, fruit juices, frozen yogurt, and Gatorade. The knee-jerk reaction in favor of low-fat dieting simply doesn't address many of the actual diet-related problems of body and mind that a sizable percentage, perhaps even a majority, of human beings have.

Coming Alive Again

Let's look at the physical first. I'm sure you remember what it was like being a kid, bouncy with energy and sure of your physical capacity to meet any challenge. Well, how would you like to have part of that back again?

Changes come quickly once you alter your blood glucose dynamics, and those changes are one of the reasons people stay on the diet. There's no doubt that feel-good changes can make their appearance in Atkins dieters long before there is significant weight loss. Over the years, I've seen thousands of people come into my office with expressions of lethargic weariness and plop themselves down in chairs in a manner that makes me wonder if a crane and derrick will be required to lift them out again.

Yet when I see them next, two or three weeks later, the change is generally remarkable. They have pep, and the air of helplessness I noticed at the first visit is gone. I had a patient, whose story I recounted at length in a previous book, who had been suffering from fatigue for the previous twenty years, had gotten no help from a half dozen doctors, and had then come to me and cleared up all his symptoms in less than a week on the low-carbohydrate diet. A few weeks later, as he recounted at an office visit, he went out to dinner at an Italian restaurant with a client, ate a lot of pasta and bread, and afterward, driving home alone, stopped for a red light. The next thing he knew a policeman was waking him up. The fatigue induced by his meal had put him to sleep right there in the middle of traffic.

And What If the Problem Seems More Than Physical

Direct physical results are most common, but the complexity of human beings can produce more complex and serious problems than fatigue. For instance, Phillip Rossi, a 35-year-old wrestling promoter, came to me because for years he had been the victim of extreme panic attacks. Various doctors blamed it on "nerves" and some of them helpfully prescribed Valium, which Phil dutifully took, occasionally supplementing their soothing effects with self-prescribed marijuana joints.

Naturally, drugs, whether prescribed or recreational, were no cure, though there were times when they toned down the situation. Yet, Phil still had panic attacks, which were so frightening and upsetting that, as he put it, "My whole day consisted of trying to stay calm."

Many of us when confronted with a grown man who has attacks of trembling, cold sweats, heart palpitations, and absurd over-whelming fear—and has these grim things inexplicably and repeatedly—are perhaps tempted to dismiss these problems as simply too bizarre and irrational to understand. Yet they are utterly real and overwhelming. Phil's anxiety was so great that "Big things scared me and little things scared me. Driving scared me and being in the dark scared me."

By 1988, Phillip Rossi had become so dependent on his drugs and so disgusted with himself that he decided to go "cold turkey." He went off everything, and the result was an anxiety attack so severe that he didn't leave his house for three months. "Even the sound of the phone ringing terrified me."

I know you're thinking, "Are you really going to tell me this is *all* hypoglycemia, Dr. Atkins?" My answer is, no, I wouldn't necessarily say that. But I treated it as if it were! And with success!

Though I suspected what the major diagnosis would be, the GTT was, of course, the giveaway. His fasting glucose was 122, going up to 166 in a half hour and plummeting to a low of 45 after three. The difference between the high and the low is called the delta, and a delta of 121 is a definite indication of blood sugar abnormality.

The results of treating Phil's panic attacks with a low-carbohydrate diet were very satisfactory. It's true he had to dump his Oreos and his banana barges, but in compensation, within two weeks, his anxiety became manageable and his panic attacks were very, very rare. He says he has about four a year now.

And since this is a weight-loss book, I may as well mention that when Phillip Rossi came to see me he weighed 224 pounds, and, after four months on the diet, he weighed 180, which is a region he's remained in ever since.

Phillip Rossi's comment? "My life has changed; now I feel up to manufacturer's standard."

Enormous Effects

So you see that when we talk about blood sugar disorders, we have a condition that can radically effect an individual's physical and mental states. Women with severe premenstrual syndrome often find, for instance, that a change of diet will correct the underlying hypoglycemia that can fiercely exacerbate this hormonal condition. When their next menstrual period comes around, they often find they've dramatically improved.

But let's look at hypoglycemia and its frequent follow-up disease, diabetes, in some sort of logical order and try to understand their mechanics.

First There's "Low Blood" Sugar

As I mentioned earlier, your blood glucose powers most of what your body does, as well as fueling your brain. Anytime you're feeling good, you can take it as given that your body is working off of optimal quantities of glucose (or ketone bodies, if you're in ketosis).

Hypoglycemia (low blood sugar) is not a good thing, but what is hypoglycemia? The word itself is Greek, derived from *hypo* meaning "under," *glykis*, meaning "sweet," and *emia* meaning "in the blood." *Too little sugar in the blood.* That sounds clear, but what it demonstrates is that the word "hypoglycemia" is actually a misnomer.

Stick with this literal translation, and you will assume it's the opposite of diabetes, which you probably remember involves too *much* sugar in the blood. You may have heard it said of a diabetic that he's "spilling sugar in his urine." That is indeed the product of excess—and yet the fact is that, far from being opposites, hypoglycemia and diabetes are actually successive stages of the same disease.

The proper term for describing the hypoglycemic's real problem is "unstable blood sugar," for it is the overreaction of the glucose mechanism (going up too high and then dropping too far and too fast) that explains the hypoglycemic's problems.

One of the most intriguing evidences for the hypoglycemia-diabetes connection was found by scientists in the 1960s.[1] These researchers studied the offspring of *two* diabetic parents—people who were almost, by definition, prediabetic. They found a classic series of abnormalities in these patients. First came hypoglycemia—

a sharp drop on the glucose tolerance curve I showed you in Chapter 4. Years would pass. Then these subjects, still hypoglycemic, showed elevations of their blood sugar readings within an hour after glucose was administered. These elevations lasted 2 hours, then 3 hours. Finally, the very high blood-sugar readings of early diabetes occurred throughout the test and throughout the day.

What happened was this: In the early stages, these individuals, genetically sensitive to any abnormalities of blood glucose, were reacting to the high levels of serum glucose that their diet produced by manufacturing large quantities of insulin and forcing the glucose down. This led to the typical hypoglycemic curve in which blood sugar rises fairly quickly after eating and then falls in the third, fourth, or fifth hour to an unpleasantly low level. It's this *full*, too rapid and to somewhat too low a level that constitutes hypo-glycemia, rather than a low level of blood sugar, *per se.*°

This early stage is typical of people with insulin resistance—the very people who tend to become fat. People of normal insulin sensitivity tend to stay thin, because just a touch of the "fat-producing hormone" is enough to lower their blood glucose to a normal level and more insulin need not be released.

If you're insulin resistant—and you probably are, if you're reading this book to lose weight—then your body at some fairly early stage in your life lost the capacity to respond quickly to insulin. It "resisted" the insulin, and so the pancreas had to secrete more. The metabolic dynamics of glucose and insulin are thrown awry by this abnormal effort, and the body generally loses it capacity for fine tuning in this essential area. Consequently, too much insulin is secreted, and the blood-glucose level is temporarily knocked down to an undesirable low level. The unpleasant symptoms I mentioned at the outset of this chapter are either caused by the fact that the glucose level is too low to supply the brain's needs, or by the adrenaline-like activity initiated to counter-regulate the precipitously falling sugar level.

This is a first step in an unhealthy metabolic path. Eventually, the body can absolutely lose its capacity to produce insulin in the quantities required or its capacity to employ the insulin that's being produced, so that high blood-sugar levels result, and the early stages of diabetes are reached.

°I make this point because critics of hypoglycemia have attempted to obfuscate the issue by suggesting that something called *low blood sugar* is really very rare. As a permanent state of affairs, of course, it is. It's a response to glucose rather than a constant deficiency such as you have when your potassium or iron levels are too low.

Lifelong students of diabetes have suggested that the potential for the disease exists in 20% of the population.[2] Keep in mind that most of that 20% is found among the overweight, since, when the final tally is made, 80% of all diabetic are obese. Some studies have suggested that, *if you're significantly overweight*, your chances of becoming diabetic will be one in two.

In fact, the progression to type II diabetes has been described by some important diabetologists as having 5 stages (see page 41) and the first three stages—those of (1) insulin resistance, (2) hyperinsulinism, and (3) abnormal glucose tolerance—were all present before the elevated fasting blood sugar that allows for an official diagnosis of diabetes.[3] It is abundantly clear that much of the harm wrought by diabetes comes from the unattended insulin disorder present in people not classified as diabetics.

And After Hypoglycemia, Diabetes?

Amazingly enough, many specialists have managed to suggest precisely the wrong diet for their hypoglycemics, pre-diabetics, and diabetics. I have treated hundreds of patients with Type II diabetes who were put on low-fat, high-carbohydrate diets and consequently had to be on insulin—sometimes as much as a hundred units a day—to cope with the unnecessary and *avoidably* high glucose levels that resulted. Of that fact, I am certain, because the majority of these insulin-taking type II diabetics, with the help of a low-carbohydrate diet and vita-nutrients targeted to overcome insulin resistance, *were*, in fact, able to get completely off insulin.

I hate to be so cynical as to suggest that proper diet might adversely affect the thoroughly profitable administration of insulin and oral diabetic drugs, but I will certainly say that if sugar and high-carbohydrate diets were denounced from the scientific pulpits as if they were sin, it would seriously compromise a mutually supportive food and pharmaceutical industrial cartel.

It is difficult to avoid the damning implications of a high-carbohydrate diet, especially with regard to hypoglycemia and diabetes. As far back as 1970, Muller, Faloona, and Unger wrote in *The New England Journal of Medicine* of the effectiveness of a low-carbohydrate diet in preventing excess insulin production.[4] Four years later, two German doctors, E.F. Pfeiffer and H. Laube, at an

International Symposium on Lipid Metabolism, Obesity, and Diabetes Mellitus presented the result of research indicating that diabetes might not occur at all, if it were not for the effects of sugars and starches on insulin levels. (And for T.L. Cleave's brilliant work on the relation between refined carbohydrates and diabetes, see Chapter 16 in this book.)

In 1972, in an intriguing study, A.M. Cohen described in the prestigious American journal *Metabolism* how he and his associates had been able to create an entire strain of diabetic rats by feeding them sugar and selectively breeding the most sugar-susceptible rats.[5] Is this not what is effectively happening to a significant percentage of our 20th-century human population? I do not know if any studies indicate overweight people tend to marry other overweight people, but if that were the case, then they would be selectively breeding for a susceptibility to diabetes provoked by our culture of refined carbohydrates.

Other studies, especially a number carried out on rats from 1964 to 1982, have demonstrated, almost beyond the possibility of contradiction, how the whole process begins with a deterioration of glucose tolerance generally compensated for by hyperinsulinism and continues grimly on toward diabetes.[6]

But for You, That Will Be the Road Not Taken

This process, which may already have begun in you, must be counteracted and put to rest. Let's get practical and see how it's done.

Suppose you know from your symptoms, confirmed by your GTT, that you are a reactive hypoglycemic. Suppose you know from your medical experience that you are diabetic. Suppose you are even on medication or insulin. What is the complete how-to for you?

You must have gathered by now which diet will be best for you. My experience numbers 15,000 patients with documented abnormalities of GTT (hypoglycemics and diabetics) and over 99% showed improvement ascribed to the Atkins diet.

There's a good deal more you must know, but before I tell you about it, let me discuss a patient who went from eating the wrong foods to eating the right foods.

John Parlone, a 58-year-old real estate consultant, is a good example of what the program can do for a Type II diabetic in the early stages. John had already been diagnosed before he came to see us (his fasting blood sugar was 315) and put on glipizide, an oral diabetic medication.

Treating John wasn't difficult. Look at how across-the-board his improvements were! He started the Atkins diet two months before he came to the Center for a checkup, and by then his blood pressure, which had been dangerously high for nearly a decade, had already fallen to 140/80. We eventually got it down to 116/70. In the two months before John came to the Center, he had also gotten his weight down from 225 to 204 using the low-carbohydrate diet. (John is 5'8".) In the next six months, we took it down from there to 169. John's cholesterol was 296 when he came to the Center; in five months we took it to 251. His triglycerides were 187; they fell to 77.

As for his diabetes, it proved to be eminently controllable. By his third month on the diet, John Parlone's blood sugar had fallen to 80, and we were able to take him off his medication.

John had been a big sweets eater with a passion for cake. He adjusted very well to his new diet and adjusted even better to the fact that his pants size went from a 40 to a 34. He felt better than he had in years and looked a heck of a lot better. What you see in John Parlone's results is a reflection of the fact that diabetes is a disease of carbohydrate metabolism completely bypassed by a low-carbohydrate diet. You may think I chose to write about John because he improved so rapidly and so thoroughly, but in reality, he's just a typical case.

Start with the GTT

Let's see how one diagnoses blood glucose problems and the possibility of eventually developing diabetes.

I told you on page 67 that you must demand a 5-hour test and that drawing insulin levels is imperative if you are 15% above your ideal weight. But how does the test get interpreted?

Your doctor will tell you if you are abnormal, right? Maybe right and maybe wrong. The prejudice against the diagnosis and management of reactive hypoglycemia by the medical establishment represents one of its most prolonged failures to practice good, responsive medicine. For the past forty or more years, the majority of physicians have taken a hypoglycemia-doesn't-exist attitude and, for them, presenting grossly abnormal results done at a proper medical lab will get you nowhere. It will get you angry denials, sometimes replete with expletives.

Who Are These Doctors?

By and large, these doctors represent the mega-orthodoxy within the profession—doctors who worship medicine with religious fervor, but not the process of medicine, rather the conclusions of its Holy Synod, the amorphous but all-powerful medical consensus.°

It is consensus medicine that denied the existence of reactive hypoglycemia even though GTT testing has always revealed deviations from the normal, or ideal, picture in the majority of obese subjects. The scientific rationale for their position is a series of studies on so-called "healthy normals," many of whom showed abnormalities that fulfilled most criteria for the diagnosis of reactive hypoglycemia. Their conclusion: If healthy normals show it, then the lab test has no meaning. But these healthy normals were not screened for family histories of diabetes, obesity, or heart disease, nor for symptoms like sugar craving, food addiction, or academic underachievement. Just how normal were the ones with the abnormal lab findings? Suppose someone had studied the same subjects for their cholesterol level? Would all of them have been below 200 mg%? I doubt it. Yet, if someone had concluded that those healthy normals with cholesterol elevations were to be treated without concern, he would have been drummed out of the corps.

How to Measure a Normal Glucose Tolerance Test

Use this as unequivocally normal:

Fasting 70–100 mg%
Peak (30–60 minutes) 120–160 mg%
Nadir (2–4 hours) 60–90 mg%
Delta (difference between the lowest and highest reading) 30–80 mg%

Without going into all the criteria for ferreting out abnormal values that I published in 1977 *(Superenergy Diet),* let me call your attention to one criterion—the delta.

If the delta is over 80 points, and you are overweight, you most probably have hyperinsulinism.

If the delta exceeds 100 points, you have fulfilled *my* official criterion for abnormality.

If it exceeds 125 points, you've got it, baby.†

°I have discussed the matter at length in my second book, *Dt. Atkins' Superenergy Diet*, and those of you running into difficulties with physician close-mindedness will find it of value.

†Remember that during glucose tolerance testing, when hyperinsulinism is present, there is usually a "free fall" of the glucose just before it hits its low, at which time adrenaline release raises it very quickly. It only stays at its real nadir for two or three minutes. Therefore, the lab's chance of drawing blood (on a once-an-hour basis) that reflects that real low is about 1 in 20. Consequently, the *rate* of fall in any given internal is an important criterion.

The real diagnosis of reactive hypoglycemia is based more on symptoms than on the GTT results. The bottom line for the diagnosis is the correction of the symptoms by a diet known to stabilize hypoglycemia. And for overweight, symptomatic people, that's this one.

What About the Diagnosis of Diabetes?

Here you can get help from your personal physician. The medical profession does recognize diabetes. For cases in the gray area, the criteria given in the box on this page have been agreed upon.

The Glucose Tolerance Sum System:

Add the first four numbers in your GTT together. This means the numbers at fasting, 30 minutes, 1 hour, and 2 hours.

If the total (in mg%) is below 500, that is considered normal.
If the total (in mg%) is above 800, that is considered diabetic.

The gray area, between 500 and 800, is called impaired glucose tolerance, and nearly half of the significantly obese fall into that area. So you see, there's a very good chance I'm talking about you. The closer your total approaches the 800 mark, the more probable it is that you will eventually be classified as a true Type II diabetic. But there is still some good news for you. Even if you are considerably into the diabetic range and are obese, the normalization of your weight by the lifelong curtailment of carbohydrate can get you to, and keep you in, the normal range for life.

Special Nutrients for Glycopaths

If you do have one of these glucose/insulin disorders, there is a great deal that can be done *in addition to going on the diet*. First and foremost is the use of chromium supplementation.

Chromium is an essential part of the Glucose Tolerance Factor (GTF), and GTF has such a profound effect on facilitating sugar metabolism that several researchers suggested it be elevated to vitamin status, meaning that it is *essential* to health. I certainly believe it to be an essential nutrient for those with overweight tendencies.[7]

The problem was finding a source that the body assimilated well. For years the only effective source was brewer's yeast, which posed problems for the many people with the yeast syndrome that you'll be learning more about in the next chapter. But in the nearly twenty years that chromium picolinate, and later polynicotinate, have become available, I have seen a definite further benefit in the glucose metabolism of patients with both hypoglycemia and diabetes. Even more striking is the benefit of lowering the cholesterol and raising the HDL levels, a fact that strongly points to the value of controlling cholesterol by way of controlling carbohydrate metabolism.

The effective dose range of chromium (as picolinate) is 200–700 mcg per day.

Beyond Chromium, What?

The second most important mineral for diabetic/hypoglycemic individuals would now have to be vanadium. Most research, done with vanadyl sulfate, showed benefits for combating both insulin resistance and the lack of insulin.[8] The dose range of vanadyl sulfate is 20–100 mg daily; however, two newer vanadium compounds, BMOV and BGOV (both organic) may prove more reliable. Their dosage range is smaller, 10–20 mg daily.

I have long opposed the use of drugs such as insulin and the insulin-mimicking sulfonylurea type of oral anti-diabetes medications on the grounds that obesity generally is the result of too much insulin in the first place. My patients benefit dramatically from lowering the dosage or getting off these medications. However, in recent years, two drugs have reached the market that work on the very pertinent insulin resistance problem, thus lowering both the blood sugar *and* the insulin levels. One of these, troglitazone (Rezulin) can cause severe liver disease, and tends to lead to weight gain, so it, too, is not a good choice. The other, metformin (Glucophage) helps lower the body weight, lipids, and insulin level and is one of the few drugs worth using.

If the Atkins diet and the full roster of vita-nutrients targeted for diabetes fail to keep your blood sugar close to normal, you may want to ask your doctor to consider the pros and cons of starting or switching to this drug. I have prescribed it to several hundred of my patients and have found it helpful in selected cases.

The third most important mineral is zinc.[9] Perhaps the best of readily available forms of zinc is the monomethionate, and other minerals probably advantageous for diabetics are magnesium, manganese, and selenium.

Vitamins, especially vitamin C and the B complex, facilitate most of the metabolic pathways that diabetic subjects use and must be a liberal part of any nutritional supplement. A single paper on one B complex constituent, biotin, in doses 100 times greater than you get in a good multivitamin pill, looked very promising.[10]

Other promising nutrients to help the diabetic are coenzyme Q_{10}, alpha lipoic acid, and the essential fatty acids GLA and EPA. (You can learn more about these and other diabetic control supplements in *Dr. Atkins' Vita-Nutrient Solution*.)

What About Hypoglycemic Symptoms?

Suppose the symptoms of hypoglycemia, the ones you've been treating all your life with a "fix" of sugar or other carbohydrate, won't respond to abstinence and instead are worse than ever. How do you rectify that?

Fortunately, abstinence almost invariably does work, but there can be a time when the symptoms seem to become a hurdle impossible to scale.

There is a nutrient almost *designed* to get you "over the hump" of symptoms so severe it seems only a direct dose of glucose will make your life bearable. The nutrient is one of our natural amino acids, L-Glutamine, the one amino acid that can directly serve as fuel for the brain. Doses of 500 to 1500 mg, four to five times a day, may be necessary until the cravings and related symptoms abate. Chromium and the other glucose-modulating nutrients I just mentioned are an integral part of the solution, as well.

Another nutrient you can call upon here is glycerol, sold as Glycerine, U.S.P. A tablespoon taken along with glutamine when the cravings are at their worst will surely help. I rarely have to prescribe other remedies beyond a few days when a person remains carbohydrate abstinent. The FMS-induced ketosis/lipolysis will take over in just a few days.

However, many dieters experience minor degrees of hypoglycemia, appearing most often as hunger developing *before* mealtime. I have made a delicious, very low-carbohydrate, high-protein energy bar available to my patients and the public. Called the Atkins Diet Advantage Bar™, it contains a small amount of glycerine, which makes it ideal for getting people "over the hump" when the blood sugar needs to be stabilized.

How Do I Know Your System Works, Dr. Atkins?

I wish I could invite you all to study the case records of the Atkins Center. Here you would see 15,000 examples of people with the combinations of glucose disturbances and overweight. In many ways, it's what the Center treats best. You would see, to cite but one example, that over 50% of the group taking insulin is able to get off insulin completely and 98% on the oral anti-diabetic medications can be successfully weaned from them.

Now, having covered the various manifestations of glycopathy, let's look at DRD from a new perspective.

13 | *The World of Yeast Infections*

What could turn out to produce a metabolic slowdown hazardous to your weight-reduction program might exacerbate hypoglycemic symptoms, if you have them, and might require you, in the end, to drop cheese, mushrooms, vinegar and other fermented condiments from the Atkins diet? The answer is yeast.

"Yeast?" Now, I know, Dr. Atkins, that you just get off on being perverse. First you recommend a diet that the AMA criticized, then you find fault with the diet that doctors all agree is good for everyone, then you make sure everyone takes vitamins, which doctors know are all worthless, then you try to get people off their prescribed medications. You go on to tell people that their problem is insulin, when the profession tells us it's cholesterol, then you try to tell us we have hypoglycemia, which the AMA has pronounced to be nonexistent, and now you want to tell us we have another nonexistent condition—the yeast syndrome."

To this irate and not too hypothetical critic, I can only answer, "When you're right, you're right." And, if you've been on the 14-day Atkins *Induction* diet, you already *know* who's right.

What you are in the process of learning is that the official consensus of the medical establishment, those same folks who brought you a national health-care price tag of one trillion dollars for 1998, can be that wrong. There are thousands of physicians in this country who treat yeast infections, but there is still an entrenched core of conservative doctors who deny they exist, except in the limited form of vaginal infections.

Why Yeast in a Diet Book?

This may be the first diet book dealing with yeast, and you may be wondering why it is necessary to do so. One reason is that yeast overgrowth is an integral part of DRD, producing many of the symptoms attributed to hypoglycemia and contributing to much of the food intolerance you'll read about in the next chapter.

Another reason is that a yeast infection affects the metabolism in many often-unpredictable ways, but by and large, those ways tend toward the addition of weight rather than its reduction. The reason for this effect is still highly speculative; the fact that it exists is well-known to any physician who treats the disorder.

So Why Is a Yeast Epidemic Denied?

Just as 60% of my overweight patients have abnormal GTTs, so different from the criteria for normalcy that it would make any impartial observer at least wonder whether some truth might be lurking in the figures, so, too, do 30% of my patients (of all kinds) have *Candida albicans* overgrowth diagnosed by direct microscopic visualization or orthodox immunologic blood tests. Yet the prejudice against recognizing this illness is so great that in New Jersey, doctors can lose their license for diagnosing it, and in all states, insurance carriers will delay or avoid payment to patients for whom candidiasis is the primary diagnosis.

Why the intense hatred of what seems to be a legitimate, rather prevalent medical problem?

Just look at the contributing causes of candidiasis and you will see an epidemic actually caused by the actions of health professionals.

Candida outgrows its boundaries (the *Candida albicans* yeast is a normal inhabitant of our bodies, generally comprising 10% of the microorganism profile of the intestinal tract) when a subject is exposed to:

1. A diet high in sugar and refined carbohydrates.
2. Antibiotics (more than 20 weeks in a lifetime would make *Candida* overgrowth a probability).
3. The mercury in silver dental fillings.
4. Birth control pills, prednisone, and other steroids.

Since everything on this list is iatrogenic—meaning caused by the medical care we receive—or diet-related and either recommended or condoned by establishment medicine, to admit that yeast is epidemic—which I believe it is—is to admit that medicine and dentistry share guilt in its causation.

First, consider antibiotics, which are capable of destroying or inhibiting the growth of germs such as the *Pneumococci* bacteria, which cause pneumonia. Unfortunately, they will also kill the friendly *Lacotbacilli* that live in your intestines and keep *Candida* from spreading.[1]

There's nothing wrong with antibiotics when you use them to save your life, but unfortunately, in our pill-popping society, they're taken for a variety of inappropriate reasons. Doctors will prescribe them to snuff out a bad cold, or to treat acne, or to prevent a nearly nonexistent complication of mitral valve prolapse.

Antibiotics are probably the main unleasher of yeast infections, but birth control pills have also been implicated, and, finally, there's the poison that almost all of us carry around in our mouths twenty-four hours a day—mercury. The silver/mercury filling that dentists still put in the mouths of their patients is approximately 50% mercury, and mercury just happens to be the most poisonous free element our bodies get exposed to. Dentists have always believed that in amalgams it was stable and would not contaminate its host.

This simply isn't true. Mercury vapor tests in the mouths of real people have made that unambiguously clear.[2]

Mercury figures into this chapter because it's a sure-fire way to weaken your immune system in just such a way that yeast infections flourish. Now let's look at diet.

What You Eat

I don't believe that your diet necessarily causes candidiasis, but my clinical practice has taught me that the wrong foods will definitely encourage a yeast infection once it has begun and will make it almost impossible to clear up.

The worst offender is sugar. Indeed, nothing is more usual than to find that the victim of a yeast infection has sugar cravings. Sugar is the major growth factor for yeast. *Candida* patients are warned to stay away from ice cream, candies, cakes, corn syrup, fructose, maple syrup, molasses, etc., etc. It is no coincidence that Atkins weight-loss dieters won't be eating any of those foods, either. You'll also be avoiding the natural sugar in fruit juice, the lactose in milk, and all those refined carbohydrates like starches, white flour, and white rice that easily turn to sugar in the body.

All of this is very critical for those of you who are going on the Atkins diet to lose weight. A yeast infection can prevent that from happening even though everything else is in your favor.

A good example is Stella Rudman, a 55-year-old woman I first saw in the late 1980s. Stella was 20 pounds overweight, but that was a minor part of her reason for coming to me. Since menopause, she had had a very hard time with both physical and mental symptoms that were beyond her control. Her weight was going up, she had extreme cravings for sweets, she had numerous gastrointestinal problems from virtually non-stop gas and bloating to extreme rectal itching, and, worst of all, she was frequently and severely depressed. Her doctors initially gave her estrogen to help her get through menopause, but she only got worse. They then turned to the psychotropic drugs to control her depression, and when she came to us she was on a formidable anti-depressant cocktail consisting of lithium, pamelor, and imipramine.

Many of you who are not familiar with yeast infections, including indeed many doctors who have never treated them, will be amazed to discover that we were able to pretty easily settle all these problems by treating Stella for her yeast infection, which we confirmed with a blood test. Put on a low-carbohydrate diet, within a week she was over her food cravings. Within two weeks her rectal itching and bloating had subsided almost to vanishing points. As her yeast cleared up, so did her depressions, and we began to wean her off her medication. We suspected that the estrogen she had been given several years before had been one of the major stimulators of her problems, since estrogen stimulates the overgrowth of *Candida albicans*.

In addition to the diet, we treated Stella by giving her forms of acidophilus to help rebalance the bacterial flora in her gut and then by giving her caprylic acid, a short-chain fatty acid that helps kill yeast in the bowel.

Stella started losing weight, and once off her medications she found herself for the first time in years free of such distressing side effects as mental sluggishness and slurred speech.

Typically, Stella's weight loss was only able to really get moving a month after she came to us, because she first had to get her yeast infection under control. Once that was done, the path was clear, and two months later her weight had dropped to 124. Three years have passed, and it remains in that range. Two or three times over the years, she's given way to temptation and started to binge on carbohydrates. Within days the symptoms of her yeast infection began to return, and she began to gain weight. Once we had to put her back on caprylic acid. But Stella Rudman understands her problem now, and, with her cooperation, these relapses quickly settled down.

She is a very good example of what a yeast infection can do and how essential it is to solve it if one wishes to solve a weight problem too. Slowly but steadily, the medical world is beginning to learn about and accept what we call systemic yeast infections. But they have been slow to do it. Very slow.

This Disorder Is Politically Incorrect

Is this because *Candida* is rare? Not at all. I'm willing to bet that there have been countless people in your life who had yeast infections—friends, acquaintances, probably relatives. One out of every three of my patients has *Candida* diagnosable by irrefutable laboratory tests. Yet comparatively little attention has been paid to it. Why? I think because—though the disease exists—it doesn't fit into the solutions that our society wants to deliver to sick people.

Candida albicans infections, though tricky to treat, are treatable. *Candida* is a yeast, a single cell fungus, and we all have a bit of it in our bodies. Indeed, there are hundreds of species of indigenous biologic forms resident in the human intestinal tract, and *Candida albicans* is just one of them. It is, therefore, a normal part of us, and, in healthy competition with our other intestinal flora, it serves us well, performing yeasty missions in our gut.

The condition called *candidiasis* begins when, through some disturbance in our body's balance, the bacterial equilibrium is upset, causing an overgrowth of yeast organisms. Most commonly, *Candida albicans* is the yeast that overgrows, colonizing areas that were formerly alien to it and suppressing less aggressive bacteria. Having, by conquest, acquired this new position in the body, *Candida* generally shows no inclination to return to its former humble role.

As you only partially saw in Stella Rudman's case, the range of problems that *Candida* can cause is so wide ranging as to verge on the fantastic—and, of course, that's part of the problem. A short list includes lethargy, fatigue, depression, inability to concentrate, headaches, gastrointestinal disorders including constipation, abdominal pain, diarrhea, gas and bloating, respiratory ailments and disorders of the urinary tract and reproductive organs. The most specific symptom is bloating—gas in the lower abdomen. *Candida* patients often have a tell-tale lower abdominal pot belly that seems forever filled with gas. If this describes you, and you have had exposure to one of the risk factors, such as oral antibiotics, do yourself a big favor and see a doctor who claims to be proficient at finding and treating *Candida*.

There is a very pragmatic reason why a yeast problem should be identified. If you have it, there must be dietary restrictions beyond those involving carbohydrates. If you don't do that, you'll wonder why everybody else got better on the Atkins diet and you didn't.

One out of three of you will find that it's necessary to avoid "yeasty" foods, some of which you might otherwise be eating on an Atkins diet. These include cheeses, vinegar and other fermented condiments, mushrooms, yeast-containing vitamins, wine, and beer. Brad and baked goods, which are not allowed on pre-maintenance levels, would be totally disallowed. In general, most people with *Candida* are allergic to yeasts and get symptomatic when fermented food items are consumed.

Will This Cure Candida?

Sometimes it does. However, it is more likely that the elimination of inappropriate foods will be only partly effective. Therefore, when yeast is identified, you'll probably find it necessary to proceed to a more aggressive solution.

The bolder treatment traditionally centers around the anti-*Candida* drug nystatin, which is effective taken by mouth. Nystatin has become the gold standard in *Candida* therapy. However, it is not my first choice of specific therapy.

I am just as interested in strengthening the immune system, cleansing the bowel, which has usually been attacked by protozoal parasites that are found in association with *Candida*, and treating for the allergy to yeast and molds most of these patients have

My choice of therapies that do attack the yeast itself include two short chain fatty acids—caprylic and undecenylic acids. I will also use ozone, hydrogen peroxide, or chlorine dioxide, which liberate nascent oxygen. All forms of free oxygen are fungicidal. Garlic is also an effective oral treatment. Like nystatin, all of the above can kill vast quantities of yeast and should be administered carefully because the dead yeast can produce a "die-off" reaction and make the patient feel even worse for a few days than he or she felt better.

Presently, my treatment of choice for making certain that *Candida* is brought under control is oil of oregano. I will build the dosage up to 15–25 drops daily in divided doses (building up is to avoid the "die-off"). A second treatment choice that also can cause the "die-off" is olive leaf extract.°

Certain treatments to improve the yeast sufferer's condition are employed simultaneously with an attack on the yeast. The care of the bowel is very important and psyllium and bentonite are often prescribed. People with *Candida* often suffer from constipation, and these agents improve that, as well as help remove the putrefying substances and toxins that have gathered in the bowel.

As you can see, *Candida* is complicated, and it sometimes requires the sort of complicated attack I've just outlined for you. But the good news for many of you will be that the Atkins diet is, by itself, so effective against *Candida* that you can have a *Candida*-complicated case of overweight and clear it up without even knowing you had it.

But that is not necessarily the end of the story, for my experience has been that yeast infections coexist with food intolerance in almost 75% of the patients who have them. Therefore, in the next chapter we will investigate that problem.

°I am concerned that not all products labeled oregano and olive leaf may be equally effective. If you believe you need such a product, here at the Atkins Center we use a brand called Prolive from Allergy Research Group in California.

14 Food Intolerances— Why We Each Require a Unique Diet

The third part of DRD is intolerance by specific people to specific foods. This is something that could affect your diet and make further restrictions necessary. Virtually everyone who has difficulty with simple across-the-board carbohydrate restriction will have to consider the possibility of specific food reactions.

This cautionary note to all of you is based on a simple, self-evident truth: *Everybody is different.*

Everyone Must Be Treated as an Individual

To the heretofore unsuccessful dieter this means: If you get into trouble or you can't achieve the results this book promises you, then recognize your individual food intolerances and eliminate them. The diet may be more stringent, but the success is just about guaranteed.

A good diet can't be bought off the rack; it's custom fitted, made for an individual. Eating a healthy low-carbohydrate diet will do a lot for your body. Finding out what foods you can't handle is what makes the diet a more perfect fit for you.

Happily, the most common sources of food intolerance are generally found in foods I recommend you either avoid entirely or approach very cautiously. The foods to which people most commonly prove intolerant are grains (such as corn, wheat, rye, and oats), soy, milk, cheese, brewer's and baker's yeast, and eggs. The only three you might be eating on an Atkins weight-loss regimen are eggs, cheese, and tofu.

But those foods are hardly the end of the story. There are many other allergy-producing foods. Strictly speaking, you *could* be allergic to *any* food you eat—and a very small number of people seem to be universal reactors, which means, as you may have guessed, reactive to all of them.

Alas, the Foods You Love

Perhaps the first and most basic principle of food allergy is this: The foods you eat and love the most will usually be part of your problem. In fact, it has been observed that many Orientals are allergic to rice, and many Mexicans are allergic to corn. Consequently, you carbohydrate addicts will often find that on an Atkins diet you do more than just lose weight and feel more energetic. You may also clear up nagging physical ills, from headaches to diarrhea, that you never did understand the source of.

The trouble with food intolerances is that we actually become addicted to the very foods we're intolerant to. The term you will see often repeated in the writings of specialists in environmental medicine is allergy/addiction. It works something like this: Those foods that make us ill actually make us feel better for a short time after we eat them. It's a classic addiction pattern, isn't it? The sugar addict, the drug addict, the alcoholic, all feel better when the fix is in. But they all feel worse later.

For each and every addicted person, there's the difficult process of withdrawal. If you're allergic to a food that has become the mainstay of your diet, then you will suffer unpleasant withdrawal symptoms when you quit. The worse these symptoms are, the happier I, as a doctor, am. That's because the greater your addiction is, the greater your physical improvement will be once you scale the withdrawal hurdle. So put up with feeling worse for a few days, because after you give up the food "you can't live without," you're almost certainly going to feel better. The general rule is that after two to five days, the withdrawal symptoms cease.

A few of the other very common allergic foods are the nightshade family (potato, tomato, eggplant, paprika, tobacco), sulfites, coffee, chocolate, citrus fruits, and—among the foods permitted on my diet—shellfish, beef, chicken, onions, mushrooms, pepper and other spices, and artificial sweeteners.

This Could Happen to You, Too

As you might imagine, going on a low-carbohydrate diet will clear up a large percentage of food intolerance. When we treat for food intolerance using the cytotoxic blood test, we find that the majority test positive for problems with one or more carbohydrates and most often show no reaction to the animal-based, low-carbohydrate foods. The conclusion is warranted that some of the minor physical miseries of your life will clear up on the basis of avoiding food-intolerant items.

But if you've been on the Atkins diet for some weeks and you do not feel considerably better than when you began, then your next move should be to look into possible food intolerances to some items you are still eating.

What Causes Food Intolerances?

No one knows for sure, but I believe many food intolerances are related to the weakening of the immune system, secondary to problems like yeast infections. It is rare to find a person with a yeast infection who doesn't have some food intolerances.

Food intolerances are implicated in scores of health disorders. One of my favorite medical studies was done in 1983 by five physicians at the Hospital for Sick Children in London.[1] The researchers took 88 children, all of whom had been having migraine headaches at least once a week for the previous six months, and put them on a rotation diet that strictly excluded many varieties of food for weeks at a time. To the doctors' admitted astonishment, 93% of the children became headache-free once their food intolerances were discovered and the foods were taken out of their diet. One child had reacted to 24 foods and was symptom-free when all those foods were withdrawn. Cow's milk, eggs, wheat, chocolate, and oranges were all foods to which more than twenty children responded. Of equal importance was the fact that the change of diet corrected such other disorders as abdominal pains, behavior disorder, epileptic fits, asthma, and eczema in a number of the children.

How Do I Discover My Food Intolerances?

The range of techniques is wide. You'll notice I haven't mentioned conventional allergists, who look for a substance in the body called immunoglobulin E, or IgE, for short. Most practicing allergists have the strange conceit that only "their" allergy—the kind caused by IgE—is a real allergy. That's why I try to use the term "food intolerance" as much as possible, so as not to get into a battle over language.

Probably less than 50% of food intolerances are related to high levels of IgE produced in the body when the antigen, as any allergy-producing substance is called, is eaten. These can be detected, therefore, by the skin tests that allergists use, though the principal test, called a RAST test, is by no means free of false positives and negative. For non-IgE food intolerances there are a variety of techniques of discovery. I prefer those systems based on the dissolution of the granules of the white blood cells (granulocytes). This is called cytotoxic testing. In cytotoxic testing, a blood test is performed in which a technician notes the degree to which granules have dissolved. Presumably this correlates with the degree of food intolerance that the patient has at that moment to each of the foods tested. Though not perfectly accurate, it is a very good test when done by skilled hands, and is quite reasonable in price.*

But even without lab tests, there is a very successful system of avoiding food intolerances that people have used with great success and that I would like to introduce to you here. The basic principle is to go on a rotation diet in which you avoid the repeated consumption of anything.

Generally, on this sort of diet, all the foods you are to eat are arbitrarily divided into four different groupings. They are assigned to Days 1, 2, 3, and 4. On Day 1 only foods from the Day 1 group are eaten; and then three days must pass before foods from that group are eaten again (i.e., on Day 5). Similarly the Day 2 menu must be avoided until it is repeated on Day 6. And so on. Thus you take advantage of a "loophole" in the production of symptoms from most food intolerances, which is that most people can ingest an "untolerated" food if the time that passes before they repeat the action is at least three days.

With this system, you may never learn what your food intolerances are, but you avoid the symptoms anyway. The disadvantage is that the choice of foods you may select on any given

---

*Unfortunately, mainly because cytotoxic testing is rarely reimbursable, many doctors have stopped doing the test. But they use other systems that may be worth doing.

day is only 25% of what it would be on your already restricted diet. This makes it a tough diet, but to the person with persistent symptoms it can be worth the extra effort.

Whatever technique is used to determine food intolerances, I employ the following system for reintroducing foods.

The first project is to eradicate the symptoms, even if it means using a diet of total austerity. This is best accomplished by using any and all systems of avoiding intolerances (cytotoxic testing, avoidance of known and suspected food intolerances, yeast restriction, removal of caffeine and, of course, sugars). Once that is accomplished, you may *then* reintroduce the foods that you hope will prove acceptable. These you replace, one food at a time. Those that bring on your symptoms upon being reintroduced are the ones you're going to have to eliminate permanently, because bringing on symptoms is the proof of food intolerance. Those that you tolerate, happily, can be restored to your permanent diet.

15 | *Good Protection for Your Heart*

One of the reasons this book is being written is that I have interviewed hundreds of my old, previously successful patients, and, although most are prospering healthwise, a certain percentage of them are now overweight, not in the best condition, and, although still aware of the need to diet, are no longer using the low-carbohydrate diet they did so well on.

Since recidivism is not a problem one often has to deal with once a person has made a low-carbohydrate lifetime commitment, I went into great detail to find out why they weren't using the Metabolic Advantage techniques I'd taught them.

I asked, "Was the Atkins diet experience a bad one?"

"Not in the least," they would answer, "best diet I've ever been on."

"Did you like the food?"

"Can't recall a diet where I ate so luxuriously."

"Well, how did you feel on the diet?"

"You know, now that you ask, that was the best I've felt in my adult life."

I then proceeded to review the old medical records and noted that their lab values improved considerably on the regimen, as they usually do. Whereupon, I inquired: "Okay, then explain to me why you don't eat that way today?"

Then the inevitable answer: "I heard (or read) that the diet isn't good for you."

Think of it! A large group of individuals absolutely turning their backs on common sense, defeating themselves by rejecting the very program that, by their own recollection, suited them best—and all because they were snookered by the prevailing winds of propaganda. Rather than choosing to repeat their previous success, they became enthralled with the naked emperor's clothes.

At first I was angry with my former patients, but now that I've observed this reaction a number of times, I'm angry with the society that creates this No Win Situation.

What I've just told you about is cognitive dissonance—the inability to believe what you've been programmed not to believe, however compelling the evidence. I imagine many of you have it, too, so I must deal with it before it defeats you.

Let us start with the main area of cognitive dissonance. People believe that the Atkins diet is bad for the heart. They believe it with such certainty that any attempt to demonstrate that the facts show otherwise is met with a smile of incredulity.

And Yet, With a Low-Carbohydrate Diet, I Found the Beginning of an Answer

I'm a cardiologist by training, and I've spent a lot of my life treating cardiac patients. Naturally, it has always been deeply satisfying to me that the Atkins diet is so remarkably heart-healthy. Almost from the first moment that I began using it more than twenty-five years ago, I saw the good effects it had on my patients.

Patients with chest pain found their angina clearing up, often within days of going on the diet. Patients with episodes of cardiac arrhythmias maintained a normal rhythm as long as they kept to the diet. Patients with hypertension lowered their blood pressure—and fast.

I'll bet that's not what you've heard. You've had the opposite message drummed into your head so repetitively that I'm afraid you think I'm lying to you. You know with more certainty than you know the sun rises in the east and sets in the west that a diet allowing cream and butter and red meat *causes* heart attacks and that it'll make your heart symptoms worse.

So let's talk about the preconceptions you may have formed, ideas that could quite possibly lead to your being touted off a diet that may fit you as well as Cinderella's slipper fit her.

I'll start with a rhetorical question: How could the Atkins Center have shown a steady 25-year growth pattern into the significant clinical facility it now is, if I had treated my patients with a diet that in any way jeopardized their health? How indeed could this very book have been a number one bestseller six years after it first came out, despite a paucity of advertising or media appearances? How could it have surpassed the 5 million books-in-print mark and its predecessor of the previous generation, the 10-million mark? How, in fact, could the only other diet books on the bestseller list have been "me-too" versions of the low-carbohydrate message? I submit that such success could only have been achieved from word-of-mouth reports to the effect that "the diet not only works but it made me healthier."

No, the facts are quite the opposite, and what may come as a surprise to many of you, the rationale and the all-important bottom-line observations are all documented in the doctor's ongoing bibles, the widely disseminated medical journals, which we in the field refer to as "peer-reviewed medical literature." As we review it together, you may then see why I have spent much of my career developing and utilizing a diet that superficial observers persist in criticizing for its hypothetical effects on the heart, and why I actually treat *cardiac patients* with probably more success on this diet as Dr. Dean Ornish claims (I'm sure truthfully) for the patients whom he treats on a wildly different diet, an extreme low-fat, vegetarian diet.

I can only applaud Ornish's achievement—he is not an ivory-tower, academic theorizer; he's shown the results on his patients. But then, so have I.

Misled by Words

The faulty preconception that a low-carbohydrate diet should, by rights, be heart hazardous is based on a knee-jerk linguistic reaction to the words "fat" and "cholesterol." There is a fixation on the idea that, if fat and cholesterol are eaten, cholesterol levels will surely go up.

In fact, criticizing my diet, the AMA said they were "deeply concerned about any diet that advocates the unlimited intake of saturated fats and cholesterol-rich foods."[1] Then they scrutinized all the medical literature they could bring to bear and came up with *a single case described in 1929.*°

°This was the study of the Arctic explorer Vilhjalmur Stefansson, who, impressed with the health of the native Eskimos he observed, volunteered with an associate to be observed for a year on an all-animal-food diet. In this study, the cholesterol levels of one of the two subjects did go up but the other's dropped. The AMA inaccurately reported that both men had cholesterol increases.[2]

Let's look at their language: "Individuals responding to such a diet with a rise in blood fat will have an increased risk of coronary artery disease." Absolutely. All I can say is: "I agree, and individuals who jump off a curb with a parachute and are thereupon attacked by an enraged bull will have an increased risk of torn garments."

The AMA's *ad hoc* nutrition panel had to phrase it that way, because they knew, of course, that they could not find any evidence that would have allowed them to make a stronger indictment.

I think it is clear from their circumspect language that the AMA was aware of the difference between the results when fat and cholesterol are added to a high-carbohydrate diet and the results that occur when they are added to a low-carbohydrate lipolytic diet. In the usual scenario, *when carbohydrates are a large part of the diet*, the undesirable lipid readings *may* get worse if there is an increased intake of fat as well; on the Atkins diet, such a result is rare indeed.

What studies were available to the AMA certainly supported my contention.

In 1979, I had occasion to review all of the published literature on the effect of low-carbohydrate diet programs on cholesterol and triglyceride levels. I was able to find ten that showed a lowering of the mean cholesterol level, and a single one covering, on average, only one week of low-carbohydrate dieting, showing an unfavorable result.

Looking in the Literature

One study was published in 1966 by P.K. Reissell and his Harvard/Massachusetts General Hospital associates.[3] They studied eight patients with both high cholesterol and triglycerides, before and after a 1500-calorie, 26-gm-carbohydrate diet. The lowering of lipid elevations was every bit as dramatic for those subjects as what I see in my office today. The average triglyceride level dropped from 1628 to 232, while the cholesterol fell from 470 to 278, with one subject dropping from 610 to 186.

Then there was the study done by Dr. Willard Krehl and his associates at the University of Iowa, which I told you about in Chapter 6.[4] Krehl was no friend of low-carbohydrate dieting, yet when he put two older women on the 1200-calorie low-carbohydrate (only 12 gms daily) diet he was testing, he found no change in their cholesterol after two and one-half months, and their triglycerides were significantly lower. In addition, the five obese teenage girls he studied dropped their cholesterol levels an average of 20 points.

In Germany, where low-carbohydrate dieting is much more enthusiastically accepted and studied, many confirmations were published. The importance of the German studies is that they were done on sizable groups of patients. Dr. U. Rabast's many studies included a group of 104 clinic patients who followed a diet of 40 gms of carbohydrate for three to four months.[5] The group's cholesterol average fell from 239 to 220, the triglycerides from 159 to 118. A subgroup with higher starting readings did better, their cholesterol dropping from 314 to 259.

Dr. Ewald Riegler confirmed the same phenomenon on a group of 128 patients.[6] The most dramatic improvements once again came when the cholesterol was very high, one group dropping the cholesterol from 465 to 216 after six months.

This painstaking review of the medical literature leaves us with a paradox that may be unequaled in the annals of medicine That ketogenic levels of carbohydrate restriction will lower a normal cholesterol level slightly, an elevated cholesterol level moderately, a midrange triglyceride level impressively, and a high triglyceride level dramatically has been demonstrated, confirmed, and reconfirmed. And with the exception of a brief study of one week's duration, there is not a scintilla of published data to refute it.[7]

By all the usual standards of medical proof, the benefit of carbohydrate-restricted diets on serum lipid levels is an established medical fact.

But the paradox is this: Because American medicine is more responsive to the dogmatic pronouncements of academicians appointed to consensus panels than it is to scientific research, it is not an *accepted* fact.

The irony is further compounded by the fact that the diets recommended by these folks have an inconsistent cholesterol-lowering effect.

In fact, we can just about throw out half a century of research on the effect of diet upon cholesterol levels now that Stephen D. Phinney, M.D., a well-respected researcher from the University of California at Davis, has tracked cholesterol levels over time in a group of patients following an extremely low-fat formula diet.[8]

These obese subjects started with a mean cholesterol reading of 211 and successfully brought it down to 139 after one or two months of austerity dieting. Nice going. But his team continued observing their patients for another six months, *while on the diet.* Their group cholesterol had risen to 234! It wasn't until they went onto their maintenance diet that the cholesterol fell to 189. Since the observation of such a biphasic cholesterol response was reported in three other studies, we can only conclude that all studies not measuring cholesterol responses *over time* are of only limited value, and, in fact, the vast majority of studies on cholesterol as it relates to diet are of that nature.

The only published study of the low-carbohydrate diet over time that I could locate was the one by Riegler, who clearly showed that the six-month cholesterol level was as low or lower than the one-month level on a low-carbohydrate diet. This correlates closely with my own clinical findings where my patients' lipid levels stay down as long as they follow the program.

But there is more good news for all of you who want to lower your risk factors and reverse heart disease. There are dozens of vita-nutrients that, by themselves, can lower your cholesterol or your triglycerides or your LDL, or raise your extremely valuable HDL. Or all four, as is the case with pantethine and inositol hexanicotinate (a niacin compound). And others will normalize your homocysteine or your lipoprotein(a). I've discussed all of them at length in *Vita-Nutrient Solution,* and for those of you who are interested in heart-protection, it will prove to be "must" reading.

Add the nutritional supplements useful for lipid-lowering to the already potent lipid control effects of the ketogenic/lipolytic diet and you see why we have collected so many examples of patients with dramatic cholesterol/triglyceride lowerings. These lowerings are of the order of magnitude found in patients who demonstrate *reversal of heart disease.*

Reversal of Heart Disease?

Some of you may not know that heart disease, once thought to pursue an inexorable downhill course, has been shown in recent years to be reversible by serious lifestyle changes. This has great significance for those for whom a coronary bypass or angioplasty has been suggested. Surgeons tend not to inform you that you can improve the circulation of your heart and cheat them out of their day in the operating room if you are willing to make lifestyle changes.

Since I am not willing to ask my patients to undergo the risk of angiography even once, let alone twice, I have not been able to *prove* reversal of heart disease on our program (as manifested by improved patency of coronary blood vessels). However, we have demonstrated reversal of the *symptoms* of heart disease in over 85% of Atkins Center overweight coronary patients who have diligently followed our program consisting of the lipolytic diet, nutritional supplements, and chelation therapy.

The combination of a high-fat, low-carbohydrate diet and nutritional supplements has been reported on in the *Southern Medical Journal* of January 1988 by Dr. H.L. Newbold.[9] During the 3 to 18 months of follow-up, his seven patients dropped their mean cholesterol levels from 263 to 189.

At the Atkins Center we tabulate our results every few years. The latest was published in my book *Dr. Atkins' Health Revolution* and we reported a drop in cholesterol from 256.4 to 217.6 and of triglycerides from 166.5 to 97.2. But only half those patients were on the weight-loss diet, which has consistently produced more spectacular results.

So you can clearly see that, if the Atkins diet is a heart-attack diet,

a) It certainly is not mediated by any worsening of the serum lipids.
b) It would contrast sharply with the usual result wherein my heart patients almost always show a dramatic improvement, as manifested by their ability to exercise longer and more vigorously without symptoms and to discontinue medications that were previously necessary.

You certainly should know *why* the ketogenic/lipolytic diet is so beneficial to the heart. The scientific literature of the past fifteen years goes a long way toward explaining it.

Gerald Reaven, Norman Kaplan, and Others

What is gradually being unveiled is an association not so much between fat consumption and heart disease (remember the French with their high-fat diets and 50% fewer heart attacks than we have), but between cardiovascular risk and four consequences brought about by a single metabolic cause.

Dubbed the "Deadly Quartet" by Dr. Norman Kaplan from the University of Texas's Southwestern Medical Center, these four consequences are upper-body obesity, glucose intolerance, high triglyceride levels, and hypertension.[10] Kaplan asserted that these problems were found together because there was a common causative element in all of them, and that element was our old friend hyperinsulinism, the very thing that, back in Chapter 4, I showed you was part and parcel of metabolic obesity. What Kaplan's article, published in the *Archives of Internal Medicine*, in fact ended up saying was that high insulin levels might, in truth, be one of the chief determining factors in heart disease. As you'll soon see, he is not alone in this conjecture. The 76 bibliographical references in his article gives you some idea of how *many* scientists' research has contributed to his conclusions.

I'll come back to the reasoning behind this, but first let me demonstrate what sort of statistical evidence there is for insulin's role in heart disease. Everyone knows that the famous Framingham study begun in Massachusetts in 1948 found a positive correlation between serum cholesterol levels and heart attacks.* Has anything of this kind been found relative to insulin levels? Just listen.

The three most significant studies were done in Wales, France, and Finland, and were published and widely discussed in the major medical journals of the world.

The Caerphilly, Wales, heart disease study observed 2,512 men aged 45 to 59 years and demonstrated a connection between fasting plasma insulin levels and heart disease that existed independently of other confirmed risk factors. In the Finnish study—known as the Helsinki Policeman Study—1,059 men from 30 to 59 years of age were initially followed for five years. The data revealed that fatal (and nonfatal) heart attacks were more common in those who had the highest insulin levels (both fasting and in response to glucose). Finally, the Paris prospective study followed 7,246 men for an average of 63 months. Again coronary heart disease was found proportionate to the insulin levels, and the relationship was greater when the subjects were obese.[11]

Somewhat more recently, a study published in *Circulation* by

---

*When considering cholesterol levels and diet, it is important to keep in mind that the Framingham study *did not* show that there was a relation between the cholesterol or the fat *in people's diets* and their rate of heart disease. The study only demonstrated that there was a direct statistical relation between the level of cholesterol *circulating in the blood* and the risk of heart disease.

the team in Helsinki showed that those with high triglycerides plus an unfavorable LDL/HDL cholesterol ratio could lower their heart attack risk rate by 71% when those problems were corrected.[12]

That study corroborated the dramatic findings of a series of papers coming out of Muenster, Germany, in which it was discovered that men who had the combination of high triglycerides and low HDL were six times more likely to get heart attacks than the rest of the subjects.[13]

The culmination of this breakthrough information about what *really* causes heart disease was a 1997 Harvard study led by Dr. Michael Gaziano. He investigated the heretofore ignored ratio of triglyceride to HDL and found it significant at all levels. The people whose ratio was in the upper 25% were *sixteen times more likely* to have coronary trouble than those in the lowest 25%. This makes the TG/HDL ratio the most predictive one, by far, in all of cardiology.

As I mentioned before, and as you will see when you review your own before-and-after lab tests, high triglycerides and low HDL are the very findings seen when high insulin is the problem *and* when carbohydrates are consumed.

These very large studies have set many of our leading medical scientists on a course of rethinking. More and more of them are beginning to question whether the high-carbohydrate diets recommended for heart patients may not be so ideal as has been supposed.

Framingham director William Castelli, M.D., commented: "The findings swing the pendulum and show that high triglycerides can be a significant risk factor for some patients."[14]

It has, after all, been consistently shown that triglycerides parallel the insulin level and that the control of insulin levels can be done with supreme effectiveness on a *low*-carbohydrate diet. Grey and Kipnis demonstrated this in the early '70s. In 1979, Dr. Sheldon Reiser did a study with human volunteers demonstrating that a diet providing 18% of its calories from sugar—and this is now less than the U.S. national average—produced significantly higher lipid and insulin concentrations than did a diet with 5% of its calories derived from sugar.[15]

Among the many scientists who have begun to respond to this really formidable array of evidence, I would first like to mention the distinguished Stanford professor Dr. Gerald Reaven and his associate, dietetics expert Ann Coulston. Reaven has been pursuing the close connection between hyperinsulinism, hypertension, and cardiovascular risk factors with indefatigable zeal for over twenty years now.[16]

He was the pioneer, but since 1985 dozens of major articles in the leading medical journals have followed his lead.[17] One piece of the puzzle that Reaven showed was that hypertension—which no serious medical theorist has ever questioned as a risk factor for both stroke and heart disease—is intimately related to hyperinsulinism. In 1989, in a major article in *The American Journal of Medicine* titled "Hypertension as a Disease of Carbohydrate and Lipoprotein Metabolism," he wrote, "Patients with untreated hypertension have been shown to be resistant to insulin-stimulated glucose uptake and both hyperinsulinemic and hypertriglyceridemic . . ."[18]

In 1988, giving the Banting lecture at Stanford, he noted a clustering of risk factors for coronary artery disease, all of which were associated with high insulin level and increased insulin resistance.[19] These included hypertension, high triglyceride levels, and decreased HDL cholesterol—the kind of cholesterol that has been found to be heart protective.

Other researchers have noted that insulin increases levels of LDL cholesterol—the kind of cholesterol that promotes heart disease. The mechanism by which this takes place was already clear. The Belfast scientist R.W. Stout had written in 1985 that: "The arterial wall is an insulin-sensitive tissue. Insulin promotes proliferation of arterial smooth muscle cells and enhances lipid synthesis and low-density lipoprotein (LDL) receptor activity. *Insulin also promotes experimental atherosclerosis in a number of species.*"[20]

The circle has begun to close, and, I must admit to my great satisfaction, the reasons why a low-carbohydrate is so heart-protective are becoming clearly visible. It is no accident that I have been able to use a low-carbohydrate diet to treat cardiovascular disease with ever-mounting success. Why should we be surprised? You remember I remarked that this was the natural diet of the human omnivore. People are well-fitted to eat fresh meat, fish, fowl, berries, nuts, seeds, vegetables, and, in moderation, fruits. Nature is not trifled with, and this was our diet for millions of years, long before the bizarre dietary habits of the 20th century were unleashed to plague us.

Vegetarians have suggested that the natural human diet is based on grain since that is what most civilizations have been growing in the form of wheat, rice, or corn for the past 5,000 years. Yes, but what about the hundreds of thousands of years that preceded that?

What are all those bones doing around the campfires of primeval man and what were they doing with all those hunting tools we've discovered? Using them for letter openers?

Let's return once again to Norman Kaplan's intriguing article on the "Deadly Quartet." Look at the diagram below.

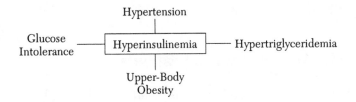

Kaplan has had the good sense needed to notice the obvious. All these conditions characteristically occur in subjects with high insulin levels, and, moreover, these conditions are very likely to coexist in the same person. Thirty-five million people in the United States are obese (20% over ideal body weight), and 40 million people are hypertensive. Among the obese, hypertension is three times more common than among the non-obese. High triglyceride levels are twice as common among the obese as among the non-obese. The association is even stronger if one measures patients with upper-body obesity. The paunch so characteristic of the middle-aged man is closely related to metabolic factors that put him at risk for a heart attack.

If you still wonder just how strong these associations are, listen to a statement made by Dr. Albert Rocchini, a medical scientist at the University of Minnesota. He writes: "It has been estimated that by the fifth decade of life, 85% of diabetic individuals are hypertensive and obese, 80% of obese subjects have abnormal glucose tolerance and are hypertensive, and 67% of hypertensive subjects are both diabetic and obese."[21]

It is now known that in all these conditions, hyperinsulinism is generally found. In fact, when I first meet an overweight patient, I expect to learn from blood chemistries that the patient has high triglycerides, glucose intolerance, and high insulin levels, and my misgivings are seldom disappointed. Of course, I am more pleased by the fact that these cardiovascular risk factors go down together, once a correct dietary approach is instituted.

And what is that approach? Well, to quote Norman Kaplan one more time: "Weight loss, however it can be accomplished, is then the obvious way to correct obesity and its attendant hyperinsulinism and hypertension. . . . However, *the use of a low-fat/high-carbohydrate diet, as usually recommended for weight reduction* [my italics] *has been found to accentuate both the hyperglycemia and hyperinsulinemia . . .*"

The alternative is, of course, a low-carbohydrate diet. And the heart-health advantage of my recommended alternative are correspondingly immense.

Special Advice for Heart Patients

Most of you are candidates for heart disease; simply having a weight problem puts you in that category. Therefore, all of you are understandably concerned with preventing heart disease, and you are certainly not interested in doing anything that would increase your risk. I hope the preceding discussion convinced you that your heart-disease risk will be considerably lessened on our program.

But for many of you, prevention comes a little late in the game because you may have learned that you already have some cardio-vascular problem. Some of you may already be taking prescribed medications.

There is good news for over 90% of those who fall into this latter group, for that is the percentage of our patients who have been able to discontinue, or at least reduce, their medication burden at the Atkins Center. The nutritional pharmacology is part of the reason behind our patients' success, as is chelation therapy. Both are outside the scope of this book, but they are very much in the scope of my most recent book, *Dr. Atkins' Vita-Nutrient Solution.* You really owe it to yourself to get it and study it as though your life depended on it. The predictable improvement of overweight heart patients on the total regimen is the closest thing to a "sure thing" in my entire medical practice.

But I do want to give some specifics for those who love to see their cholesterol levels plummet to new lows, a quest that has become sort of a national pastime.

First, let's talk about the diet strategy. Bear in mind that a low-carbohydrate diet can be relatively high in fat or low in fat, and that the fats may come in a variety of forms. You've heard the terms saturated, monounsaturated, polyunsaturated; consider, too, that each individual fat or oil has its effect on your serum lipids, both good and bad. The stearic acid component of red meat just happens to have a good effect, to give but a single example.

To perfect your lipid levels you have to be willing to have the blood tests analyzed frequently; otherwise, you are as guilty as those consensus-formers, always assuming everybody's metabolic response is the same. The strategy is to systematically test our various hypotheses and then look at blood test results to see if they are operative for you.

Testing for Fat Sensitivity

I admit that there are individuals who are fat-sensitive and will develop a less favorable cholesterol level on a high-fat diet than on a low-fat diet. Intensive study of medical reports strongly suggests that fewer than one person in three falls into this category. (Although we find the number to be smaller than that.) But you don't know if you are in that subgroup, so let me show you how to find out if you are.

Stay on the *Induction* diet and the first several levels of the OWL as long as you want, taking the supplements I will be outlining. Then draw a complete lipid profile involving cholesterol, triglycerides, HDL, LDL, etc., *to compare with your baseline levels*. All should show improvement. You should particularly note the ratio of LDL and HDL, which the Helsinki study demonstrated to be important, and the ratio of triglyceride to HDL, which the Harvard group found so important. If you (and your doctor) are satisfied with your progress, there is, of course, no need to change.

If the results are not to your liking, you may be a person who is fat-sensitive. So for the next interval, eat only the lean proteins—turkey roll, skinless chicken breast, fish, farmer cheese, lean cuts of meat, and so on—but do not increase your carbohydrate intake more than 5 grams. However, if you're not happy on the low-fat version of the diet or get hungry or don't feel as well on it, then don't bother with it; go back to the regular Atkins diet that you enjoyed more. Since there can be so much benefit from the vita-nutrient supplements, it may be better to give them a chance so that you will not have to abandon your successful diet for the sake of a cholesterol reading. But if you are happy with the new lower-fat version of the diet, still losing at a comfortable rate, and feeling just as well, stay with it and have another lipid profile drawn. If the results are better, good, but you still have one more task to perform. Go back to the original free-use-of-fat system long enough to have another profile. If it bounced back up from the previous one, *then you are fat-sensitive and should follow the fat-restricted variation of the diet.* Our studies have shown that there is generally a steady improvement on the regimen, and therefore a falling cholesterol level is expected. A cholesterol elevation runs counter to the anticipated trend and would be significant. Don't ever draw bloods if you have not been faithful to the diet, because carbohydrate deviations can raise the cholesterol much more readily than can high fat intake.

A similar experiment can be done with regard to the kind of fat. Check out the effect of switching from saturated (meat) fat to monosaturated oils, as in olive oil, canola oil, avocados, and macadamia nuts. The monosaturates may be your best ally. Another concept is the use of medium chain triglycerides (MCT), shown in research to be an aid to energy metabolism, weight loss, and cholesterol reduction. An appropriate dose of MCT is 2 to 3 tablespoons a day as a substitute for other dietary oil. You can use it in your frying pan. More MCT can be used if you're careful to avoid the diarrhea that can result in sensitive individuals. Finally, if you are curious about the effect of egg yolks (one of nature's most perfect foods), check out that hypothesis; don't assume they're bad without proving it to yourself.

And Now for Nutrients

All of the above discussion should prove academic if you find the effective nutritional supplements in the right quantity to be effective in lowering your cholesterol and triglycerides. In my private practice, I find that those patients who need still further reductions in their levels can achieve results satisfactory enough that I never have to prescribe cholesterol-lowering medications.

The following is your lipid/nutrient check list.

- Chromium picolinate. The dieter's best friend. Helps in controlling diabetes and hypoglycemia, and contributes greatly to cholesterol control. As the critics say, a must! Adults use 200–600 mcg.[22]
- Pantethine. A derivative of pantothenic acid, the precursor of coenzyme A, pantethine plays a pivotal role in cholesterol metabolism. Lowers cholesterol, LDL, and triglycerides by

25% and raises HDL similarly. Would be the "drug of choice" in cholesterol control if it were a drug. I usually provide 900–1800 mg when the lipid picture is not favorable.[23]

- Niacin. This is the nutrient that most doctors know about. Used as a drug, it can worsen diabetes and cause liver abnormalities. Used as a nutrient (i.e., with the rest of the B complex, and in lower doses), it is simply a contributor to cholesterol and LDL control. Rather than experience the unpleasant flush that niacin produces, I, and many other nutritionally-oriented doctors, prescribe the niacin compound inositol hexanicotinate, in doses of 500–1500 mg daily. The latter compound has benefits similar to pantethine; used together, the results are even better.

- Lecithin granules (much better than the capsules) two or three tablespoons daily. Can and should be sprinkled on food; goes well on salad or vegetables or mixed in with scrambled eggs.[24]

- Lots of GLA. I frequently use borage oil, 2–3 capsules daily. If you use primrose oil, you have to use more than a dozen to match the GLA content of borage oil.[25]

- Omega-3 oils. Fish oil containing EPA, DHA. I use 1500–2000 mg of the EPA on many patients. It is particularly valuable in those who have triglyceride elevations. Some studies have described a cholesterol elevation in some people taking EPA, but I'm not convinced I see that response. I think it's very valuable. Alternately, flax (linseed) oil contains a different Omega-3 oil and may be of great value to certain individuals.[26]

- Garlic. Well-documented cholesterol-lowering effect, to say nothing of its other cardiovascular and blood pressure benefits. Also great for knocking out acute infections and controlling *Candida*. I like it better on rack of lamb or scampi, but, if you like pills, consider 6 to 12 of them a day.[27]

- Carnitine. A nutrient essential for transport of fatty acids, it is valuable to heart patients with angina, cardiomyopathy and heart rhythm disorders. I use it when I want to help lower triglycerides or raise the HDL cholesterol, and I use 1000–2000 mg daily.[28]

- Fiber sources. Psyllium, glucomannan, carageenan, pectin, guar gum. All have a documented cholesterol-lowering effect, probably by binding cholesterol in the gut and decreasing its absorption. This may be less desirable than it sounds, because the body very much *needs* cholesterol. I believe it is better to present the body with all the cholesterol it needs and then still the signals in the body demanding that the liver produce more cholesterol by enhancing all nutritional enabling systems in the body.[29]

- Antioxidant nutrients. In line with the previous paragraph, you should know that many nutritionally-oriented doctors believe that cholesterol is manufactured in the body because it serves as an antioxidant (as does uric acid) and therefore will be synthesized to excess when the body is being bombarded by free radicals.°

  Providing the nutritional antioxidants seems to help with cholesterol control, and it certainly is a good idea to protect against all degenerative diseases such as cancer, arthritis, and even aging. Vitamins A, E, C, glutathione, selenium, cysteine, and bioflavonoids are the major nutritional antioxidants. Three to six capsules of a good antioxidant formula are worth everyone's consideration.

- Vitamin C. Recent research is confirming the long-term lipid benefit of using this nutrient. You may have assumed by now that I concur that vitamin C is a cornerstone of preventive medicine. Dose ranges for my patients begin with 500 mg, and many people thrive on doses 30 times that much.

- Many, but not all, of these nutrients are in my own Dr. Atkins "Cholesterol" Vita-Nutrient™ Supplement Formula, plus the Essential Oils Formula.

Cholesterophobia seems to be an American epidemic. I've already met 200 terminal cancer patients who were more concerned with their cholesterol levels than with their immune systems. I don't encourage cholesterophobia; it's as irrational as any other phobia. But it does provide one hidden advantage; it would probably impel you to use a generous assortment of the above-mentioned nutritional agents.

Combined with the dramatic lipid-lowering effects of the Atkins diet, these nutrients make you a heavy favorite to improve your cholesterol readings. In fact, with all of the above in proper dose, your chances of getting a bad result is about the same as is mine of being selected president of the United States. It is only fair to point

---

°See *Dr. Atkins' Health Revolution*, page 218, pages 225–228.

out, however, that I am over 35 and an American citizen, and would run if drafted. And I would like to clean up a few things in Washington—especially the FDA.

Just Another Cardiac Patient

I have so many cardiac patients with good results, and, alas, I only have room to tell you about one of them. But every one makes the same basic point—the Atkins diet and its adjuvant therapies are solid gold when it comes to dealing with cardiovascular disease.

Patrick McCarthy is a 55-year-old teacher who first felt the indications of his heart disease when he was tramping up and down the hills of Ireland during summer vacation four years ago. A tightness in his chest, a pain in his left arm. The alarm bells began to ring. He got back to the States and went to the HMO that handled his health care. An echocardiogram and a thallium stress test were quite clear: he had obstruction in some of his major arteries.

He was reluctant to consider a bypass, and his doctor put him on propranolol. The result was total exhaustion. Climbing a flight of stairs was a challenge, and he found he was too weak to talk to his class. Later he was put on verapamil, and when further testing revealed no improvement in his condition, the medication dose was doubled. Patrick could see in front of him nothing but risky surgery or life as an invalid. In the fall of 1989, he came to the Atkins Center.

We put him on the Atkins diet, gave him the nutrients you've just been reading about, gave him chelation therapy, and within four months he was off his medication because he didn't need it anymore. A recent stress test has shown indications of reversal of the ischemia in his major arteries. His chest pain has not returned, and all of his risk factors for heart disease have turned around.

His cholesterol level had been 199 and is now 174. More significantly, his level of good HDL cholesterol has gone up from 35 to 56. His triglycerides—now increasingly recognized as major risk factors for heart disease—have done what triglycerides always do on low-carbohydrate diets: They've sunk like a leaky rowboat in a tropical hurricane. A triglyceride level that was 341 before the diet is now 58.

His weight (Patrick is 5'9"), which was in the mid-190s when he started the diet a few weeks before he came to the center, is now 157 and has been in that region for almost two years. Best of all,

Patrick McCarthy's energy level for work and play has zoomed back up to better than normal. No more panting at the top of stairs. Patrick now takes a brisk three to four mile walk twice a week, and he's just started a course in ballroom dancing with his wife.

Is this man on an austere diet? Listen. Patrick has a two-egg cheese omelet for breakfast each morning, sometimes supplemented by some slices of filet mignon. He has chicken, beef, or fish with a salad or vegetables at lunch, and his portions are large. Patrick has always had a *big* appetite. At our last meeting, he told me he had had 9 pieces of chicken at lunch that day.

At dinner he'll have a large steak or lamb chops or a pot roast, or a beef stew with plenty of vegetables. He likes broccoli with cheese and salads with blue cheese dressing. For dessert he'll have diet Jell-O or some of the treats you'll find in our recipe section. When snacking, macadamia nuts are his favorite. Such austerity! Such suffering! Although, it's true he *has* had to give up the cakes and donuts he used to nosh on in the bad old days before he went on the Atkins diet.

I suppose his case speaks for itself. It does for me, because I have seen so many thousands of people like Patrick eating the way he eats and reversing their heart disease. And that's why I *know* that cheese omelets and steaks are heart-healthy in the context of a low-carbohydrate diet.

Those Who Have Tried the Diet Already Know the Answers

The irony is that every working day I encounter two or three others with stories similar to Patrick's. You cannot imagine the incredulity (and occasional hot indignation) these successful dieters engender when they go back to visit their previous cardiologists, who had been intent on convincing them that the best treatment they were going to get was the high-carbohydrate, high-pharmaceutical program they had prescribed for them—sometimes with a bypass to follow. My patients' resentment becomes supercharged when they actually hear criticisms of the diet that relieved their heart symptoms, their high blood pressure, their serum lipids, their excess weight, and allowed them to be free of their need for medicines. And more often than not, they were going to good, dedicated physicians who just didn't know any better.

I don't know whether I have convinced most of you of who's right in this controversy about the heart healthiness of low-carbohydrate diets. In my mind, it's not a legitimate controversy, since the scientific support for carbohydrate restriction is unequivocal, but rather a deliberate attempt by people whose ideology overrides their common sense to push a one-sided and misleading interpretation of the facts.

I do know that virtually all of you who have already completed the 14-day diet are already on the road to conviction. A successful experience is worth a thousand words.

For the remaining doubters—those who won't try the diet until they finish the book—I've written a follow-up chapter on fat. I mean the kind you put in your mouth and that advertisers of nutritionally horrific cereals and other garbage foods boast of excluding. Fat has been getting a bum rap. Let's see what we can do about it.

16 | *Dietary Fat: Real Offender or Innocent Scapegoat?*

Fat is finished, right? The United States government and perhaps a dozen medical societies have sounded the official death knell. Their consensus panels, academic medical authorities all, have unanimously concluded that we as a nation should each and every one of us reduce our fat intake to 30% of our total calories. Rich or poor, fat or thin, well or infirm, young or old, there can be no exceptions to this edict. Both Jack Sprat and his pleasingly plump wife must now heed the official dictum. The *real* scientists have spoken and those who feel we should consider biologic individuality and who would tailor diets to an individual's metabolic profile are wrong, because scientists who hold such heretical opinions are simply not worthy of being appointed to consensus panels.

These consensus panels are now in total agreement: All fat, any fat, even essential fatty acids, must not amount to more than 30% of our total intake. If our most eminent scientists appear to be in accord, then we ordinary people must conclude that there is incontrovertible evidence that eating the amount of fat we as a nation do is proven to be harmful to our health. We cannot but accept the dogma that *low-fat* diet and *healthy* diet are equivalents. But are they? The answers might surprise you.

We know that *low-fat* and *satisfying* diet aren't equivalents. Just consider the expression "He eats like a king." Was the mental picture it produced of a rather dry-skinned, austere-looking fellow wearing a crown and munching on a carrot? I doubt it.

Fat has earned its high place in the cuisines of the world because of its luxurious, satisfying taste, its richness, and its capacity to satiate appetite. Fat is *par excellence* the food of feasts. If they were of a tougher material consistency, butter and cream would undoubtedly be referred to as the backbone of fine cuisine. But you know what I mean. And so do the heart-healthy French, who put one or both of those fatty delights into as many dishes as will take them.

Fat is what makes flesh food tender and delectable. The great steak houses, now somewhat diminished by the low-fat craze (although making a comeback as more of us are enlightened), have thrived on offering their customers "select" cuts of beef that they couldn't even get in their supermarkets. What that "select" meant was that the beef had a higher percentage of fat. When you eat an absolutely mouthwatering ribeye steak, it's the fat that makes the mouth water. (Glance into the recipe section, and you'll see what master chef Graham Newbould, whom we recruited to do recipes for this book, offers in the way of delicious eating with the liberal use of cream and butter.)

Well, now, it's rather sad that we have to give all that up, isn't it? Apparently, if we don't, fat will be our executioner. The evidence is overwhelming, right?

The curious fact, however, is that the evidence is rather underwhelming! The assertion that eating a significant percentage of fat in your diet will bring you briskly down the road to heart disease and cancer is startlingly simplistic. Major studies in medical literature cast serious doubt upon these claims. Before we look at the evidence, let's see what else fat can contribute to your diet besides sumptuousness.

First, however, let's consider if I'm not beginning to sound like the fat-pusher I have been accused of being. You might think so, yet I always maintained, as the work of Yudkin and Stock illustrated, that, as a rule, people eat considerably less fat on a ketogenic/lipolytic diet than they do on their usual diet.

That's a direct result of one of fat's greatest virtues, namely that, when carbohydrates are restricted, fat causes a profound induction of satiety. Every researcher comparing diets of the same number of calories has noted that the one higher in fat produced less hunger and was considerably easier to follow.

And then there is the matter of your physical appearance. This point is a little more subtle, and no one has yet set out to prove or disprove it; yet, to me, it is as obvious as the head on your shoulders.

Did you ever study the features of one of today's "successful" low-fat dieters? It is true that their bodies look great, especially when they have worked hard at the exercise and physical-fitness aspects of their health. But study well their faces. Do you see the dryness of the skin, the pastiness of the complexion, and most specifically, do you see the deep furrows in the facial lines that extend from the side of the nose to the side of the mouth and below, called the nasolabial folds? Somehow they seem to look older than their age. You may not be as struck with this as I am, since it comes as a visual shock to me, because Atkins dieters don't get that look.

That look, the look that most people just pass off as the look of someone on a diet, is really a characteristic of a low-fat intake, and can also be seen on those who restrict fat but have not lost weight. So those of you who are dieting to enhance your physical beauty may want to prove to yourself that one advantage of a fat-containing reducing diet by studying your appearance in a mirror after a stint on both types of diet.

Now, why am I, by allowing fats and oils, so much at odds with nearly all consensus panelists, who seem to feel that the inescapable conclusion is that fat restriction is the only acceptable path to fat loss? Upon what cogent arguments do they base their end-of-discussion victory-is-ours conclusion?

Their arguments have been:

a) Fat contributes too many calories, and we will eat fewer calories if we eat low-calorie foods.
b) High-fat diets must be low in carbohydrates to work, and we will never be willing to live permanently without some carbohydrates.
c) Man is by nature primarily a vegetarian.
d) Animal foods are polluted with hazardous quantities of growth hormones and antibiotics, which we should all wish to avoid.
e) High-fat diets cause or contribute to heart disease.
f) High-fat diets cause or contribute to certain types of cancer.

A Crop of Refutations

Let's quickly dismiss the first three arguments, all of which seem to me to be rather spurious.

That we eat fewer calories when the fat is removed may be true when carbohydrate intake is high, but it certain is not true on low-carbohydrate diets. Two recent studies by Angelo Tremblay and his associates at Laval University in Quebec demonstrate that.[1] In these studies, fat was added to a high-carbohydrate diet, and it was found that the subjects of the study increased their intake of calories, but when added to a low-carbohydrate diet, there was a decrease in calories because the subjects sharply curtailed their choice of carbohydrate foods. Satiety, after all, is not a matter of fooling your stomach, it is a matter of humoral (blood constituent) factors. You eat *less* on a low-carbohydrate diet than you do on a low-fat diet. If you're not convinced, try them both.

In response to the idea that we won't be happy without carbohydrates, I can only submit that more people are happy on the luxurious butter-and-cream-containing Atkins diet than are happy on less luxurious fare.

That man developed on a low-fat or vegetarian diet is simply not true. It's even more significant that until six generations ago, man's consumption of *refined* carbohydrates was nearly zilch.

To objection d) I readily concede. We have certainly polluted our supply of animal foods with hormones and antibiotics. Unfortunately, critics of fat who mention that don't always go on and mention the next fact: We have also polluted our supply of plant foods with pesticide residues and inorganically treated soil. The situation is something of a stalemate, and it's not an argument for eating one kind of food over another, but for cleaning up our entire act. Ever since the 19th-century German scientist Baron Justus von Liebig invented inorganic chemical fertilizers, we have been doing things to our soil and the food that grows in it, the hazardous consequences of which we hardly yet know.

My recommendation to you is that when you eat animal food, just as when you eat plant food, you should go out of your way and even pay the extra few cents to get unpolluted, organic food if at all possible. Frequent health food stores. Buy free-range chickens and their eggs. Get your hands on some Coleman's beef. Mel Coleman, a rancher in Colorado, is now making major waves in the cattle industry by marketing beef free of any taint or hormone or antibiotic, and, if you'll believe me, you can also taste the difference. We can expect more and more companies like Coleman's to carve out a niche for themselves. Bother your supermarket, and let them know what you would like. You'll be surprised how response they are to their customers' desires. You're their livelihood, after all.

Now let's look at the evidence behind the heart disease and cancer claims, and, as we do, let's keep in mind that there is no good direct evidence to show that a low-carbohydrate diet leads to these health hazards. *What evidence there is in population studies showing an association between high fat and heart disease are actually simultaneously studies showing that diets high in* refined carbohydrates *are associated with heart disease. And the same is true for cancer.*

I'd like to talk to you about heart disease first.

Heart Attacks and Us

The very plausible assertion has been made that the modern diet is responsible for the extraordinary prevalence of heart disease in the 20th-century industrial societies. I'm inclined to think that's true. The further claim has been made that our rich, high-fat diet is the culprit. Long ago, I imagined this was true, too, until I began to look at the historical evidence.

You may wonder what history has to do with it. Actually quite a lot. You see, the main focus of intellectual attention with regard to the overall prevalence of heart disease has been directed to what medicine calls epidemiological studies. These are studies of the statistical breakdown of illness in various population groups. This is a crude and speculative way of studying illness but also a very intriguing one.

Let's suppose a researcher is struck by the fact that nomadic desert Bedouin don't get any heart disease but that New York City pastrami slicers do. He could scrutinize the differences between the two groups, note that the deli workers ate considerably more corned beef fat and conclude on the basis of this correlation that fat is the cause of their heart disease. Of course, if he did that, he would have overlooked the fact that heart disease *also* correlated with the consumption of rye bread and mustard and the use of subway tokens, TV sets, and meat slicers. Or that the absence of heart disease correlated with riding camelback.

More seriously, for epidemiology really isn't ludicrous, he might have concluded that the pastrami slicers get less exercise than the Bedouin or that they smoke more cigarettes or that they eat more sugar, or that they lead more driven, stressful lives. If he were interested in environmental factors, he might cast an evaluating eye over the quantities of lead, ozone, and other chemicals that the unfortunate countermen daily absorb.

But, for the most part, if our epidemiologist is a typical epidemiologist and wants to be chief of epidemiology one day, he will do what's expected of him and conclude that dietary fat did it. (As Claude Rains put it in *Casablanca*, "Round up the usual suspects.") That he jumps to this conclusion is part of the paradigm conformed to by a medical statistician at a modern American medical school, but it is easy to show that it is not a necessary conclusion from the evidence.

In virtually all the societies in which it is suggested that high fat causes heart disease, the main dietary modification in this century has been an increase in the consumption of sugar, high-fructose corn syrup, and white flour—all refined carbohydrates. Surgeon Captain T.L. Cleave, who wrote the classic study *The Saccharine Disease*, argued convincingly that increases in coronary artery disease could be traced to increases in refined carbohydrate intake.[2] He noted that diabetes, hypertension, ulcers, gall-bladder disease, varicose veins, colitis, and heart disease, to name a few, are all virtually nonexistent in primitive cultures until refined carbohydrates are introduced into the culture. *And there were no exceptions*. The process took twenty years to develop and so Cleave proposed the Rule of 20 Years—that's how long after sugar or other refined carbohydrates are added to a culture before diabetes and heart disease begin to appear in that group of people.

The epidemiologic truth is that virtually all poor, nonindustrial societies have very low rates of heart disease. Most of them also have very low rates of sugar consumption, very low rates of fat consumption, fairly low rates of urbanization, and many other differences from us modern people who live in Europe and North America. How do we tell what causes the heart disease?

A generation ago, the dean of British nutritionists, Dr. John Yudkin, and Dr. Ancel Keys, mentor for a large number of American nutritionists, conducted a running intellectual battle over epidemiology. Keys would study nations and cultures with varying degrees of heart disease and show how profoundly heart disease correlated with fat intake. Yudkin would look at the same statistics and find an almost identical correlation with sugar intake. The fact is that in over 90% of cultures there is a strong correlation between fat intake and sugar intake. Thus, to choose between the two theories, we must look at the exceptions. Let's do that.[3]

The first thing we can notice is that in two primitive cultures, the Eskimos of North America and the Masai of East Africa, a high-fat diet correlates not with heart disease but with virtually the complete absence of heart disease.[4]

Let's look at a couple of atypical Western countries. In Iceland, heart disease (and diabetes) was almost unheard of until the 1930s, although the Icelanders ate a diet tremendously high in fat. In the early 1920s, however, refined carbohydrates and sugar arrived in the Icelandic diet, and true to Cleave's Rule of 20 Years, the modern degenerative diseases arrived on schedule. Finally in Yugoslavia and Poland, the development of high heart-disease rates in the middle of this century *was concomitant with a quadrupling of the sugar intake and occurred despite a fall in animal-fat intake.*[5]

These studies prove nothing. In general, epidemiological studies never do, but they do cast serious doubt, just as an examination from history does, on the theory that high-fat diets are the main cause of the epidemic of 20th-century heart disease.

Even more serious doubt was cast by the eminent Vanderbilt scientist Dr. George V. Mann, who, in chairing a meeting on the cause of heart disease held by a distinguished group called Veritas (Latin for "truth"), pointed out that Ancel Keys had actually received data on some twenty nations showing a less than impressive relationship between dietary fat and heart disease and that he culled from that group the seven nations which best demonstrated his hypothesis. What this means, according to Dr. Mann, is that the entire Diet-Heart Hypothesis (the theory that fat causes heart disease) is in reality based on some very questionable figure-fudging.

And What About History?

Why didn't they have heart disease in previous centuries? Because they didn't eat our diet, you say. Exactly right: They didn't eat the diet high in sugar and white flour that we eat. Oh, you didn't mean that? You mean you meant they didn't eat a high-fat diet? But they did! Certainly a significant percentage of them did. Everyone who was well off, and by the late 19th century that included a minimum of several million people in America alone, ate a diet that was very high in meat, fish, fowl, eggs, butter, and lard. There was no margarine—lucky people.

These folks ate, as well-to-do people had always done, enormous quantities of animal food—their dinners were feasts, with the roast chicken followed by the fresh trout and preceded by the pork roast. Read 19th-century novels, and you'll get the picture. I know you've all seen westerns. Those giant cattle drives that began in the 1860s were aimed at getting the herds up to Chicago from whence the red meat of America was distributed.

Did they suffer from heart disease the way we did? The truth is they didn't suffer from it at all. All through the second half of the 19th century, research was being done and medical journals were being published, and yet coronary artery disease was so insignificant that the first study of it—examining four cases—was done in 1912.[6] Those several million examples of meat-eating, lard-consuming, well-to-do Americans went merrily along eating like kings and queens off the *fat* of the land, and they never paid the coronary price, apparently because there was no coronary price to be paid. In fact, the late 19th century was the great era of pathologists, and a coronary occlusion, visible even to the naked eye, was never reported.

Paul Dudley White, later to be Eisenhower's personal cardiologist, remembered that in a single year (early 1920s) in his residency training at Massachusetts General Hospital, he didn't see a single example of a myocardial infarction (heart attack).

The inescapable conclusion is that coronary artery disease was a rare illness in the 19th century. But why was it beginning around 1912? Remembering Cleave's Rule of 20 Years, I can't help wondering if it didn't date from the cola revolution of the early 1890s, which coincided with the introduction of flour mills that produced a much more refined flour.

After twenty-five years of treating heart patients who showed consistent improvement from the diet I prescribed for them, just as did Patrick McCarthy—with unrestricted meat, fish, and fowl—and who had shown every sort of ill effect while on high-carbohydrate diets, I feel there is a very strong case for the *unique* characteristics of the 20th-century diet being precisely what's wrong with people. Those unique characteristics are not fat but refined carbohydrates—the plague of our time.

I rest my case. Now, let's take a quick look at cancer.

Cancer

The same flawed epidemiology we saw with heart disease applies to cancer. No one really knows what it is in our highly complex environment—including our nutritional environment—that is most directly contributing to our explosive cancer rates. But there is good evidence that it may not be fat.

To understand that, let's first understand case-control studies. In these, we might study only the New York pastrami slicers and observe them over a period of years, noting who came down with what condition. If we decide to learn about diet and cancer from them, we collect the names of all of them who developed the disease and painstakingly question them about their diet. We then compare the food and beverage profile of those who got the illness and those who did not. Studies like this are, in fact, done all the time, but some are more important than others. And some are better because they gather the dietary data *in advance* of the illness's development.

Well, the Harvard Nurses Study was one of these, and it could always make headlines. After all, this enormous enterprise had been observing nearly 90,000 American nurses for more than four years and since *most* case-control studies have less than a thousand subjects, you can be sure that the media hung on every word issued by the head of the study, Walter Willett, M.D., and his colleagues.

That's why, at the end of 1990, every newspaper carried on its front page the story that animal fat causes colon cancer. In the interviews, Dr. Willett indicated that, if we had any sense at all, we would all restrict our consumption of animal fat. You could bet that the Nurses Study uncovered powerful, conclusive evidence that animal fat is a killer. But who would win that bet?

Let's study their study.[7] They divided every factor they looked at into quintiles, meaning five groups of equal size; thus, the 20% of the nurses with the highest intake of a nutritional element, let's say red meat, would be in the fifth quintile, and the 20% with the lowest intake in the first quintile. This was done for all the nutritional categories the researchers chose to study. In that way, they could look at each dietary variable to see whether they could identify elements where the amount of cancer in the fifth quintile was much higher than in the first.

In their study, published in *The New England Journal of Medicine*, they found 150 cases of colon cancer, which conveniently meant that if there were absolutely no effect of any given factor, each quintile could expect 30 cases (150 divided by 5). So how many cases occurred in the quintile with the highest intake of animal fat? Thirty-eight cases. Statistically significant, yes, but so minor in magnitude that it's definitely not worth abandoning a diet that controls your blood pressure and your weight, supports your well-being, and keeps down your blood-lipid levels.

Remember, this portion of the Nurses Study didn't talk about all kinds of cancer, just colon cancer. Some of you will remember that breast cancer is supposed to be another one that comes from animal fat. Official government agencies say it's so. What did the Nurses Study say about that?[8]

In the Willett breast cancer study, it was the *low-fat* quintile that stood out from all the rest. Every woman whose total dietary fat intake was 33% or *more* developed breast cancer at a rate of 114 cases per quintile (636 per 100,000), but the one quintile whose total fat intake was below 33% of the diet, just the way official government bodies suggest it should be, had a whopping 145 cases in their quintile, which comes to 813 cases per 100,000.

Willett's team denied that this finding was statistically significant, but my statistical analyst says it certainly is. In fact, there is only 1 chance in 100 that these figures, suggestive of *low*-fat intake as a contributing factor in breast cancer, could have been achieved by chance and what this really adds up to is the most significant diet/cancer connection yet discovered epidemiologically.

To return for a moment to the colon-cancer study, the underwhelming evidence that the Harvard researchers accumulated could have been predicted from some of the smaller yet well-performed case-control studies done before. Studies in Marseilles, Paris, Japan, and Belgium *all failed to show any correlation between fat intake and colon cancer*.[9] The 1989 Belgian study was even able to "finger" what I think is the real criminal—oligosaccharides, better known as the simple sugars.

What if Surgeon-Captain Cleave was right, and Professor John Yudkin was right? I think the evidence is surprisingly strong. After all, people at more fat, *because* they eat more sugar: That's because sugar leads to increased calorie intake and obesity. And *sugar is the Western world's most frequently consumed carcinogen.*

I'm sure you want to know why. The great Nobel prize–winning scientist, Otto Warburg, could have told you. Cancer cells feed on glucose, rather than on oxygen as do normal cells. Sugar intake raises the glucose and provides fuel selectively usable by cancer cells.[10]

Internationally acclaimed Russian scientist Dr. Vladimir M. Dilman, writing in the *Annals of the New York Academy of Science*, provides even more convincing evidence to support the carbohydrate-causes-cancer theory.[11] He was able to show that breast-cancer patients put out 22% more insulin than healthy controls; that colon-cancer patients had 29% more triglycerides in their blood; and that colon, rectal, and endometrial cancer patients had over twice the likelihood of giving birth to high-birth-weight babies. *The latter, plus high insulin and triglyceride levels, are all signs of disturbed sugar metabolism.*

So you plainly see that sugar has been shown epidemiologically and just-plain-logically to be a strong candidate to be the principal dietary cause of cancer, perhaps a much stronger candidate than fat.

But, you say, these Harvard scientists must have been unimpressed with what their data showed them about the correlation between cancer and the intake of sugar.

Fair enough, I asked one of my colleagues to call them and ask, "Doctors, what were you findings regarding breast and colon cancer and sugar intake?"

Answer: "We didn't look at that; we didn't consider it would have any relevance."

Ninety thousand nurses under scrutiny, zillions of taxpayers' dollars being spent via the National Institutes of Health, and they didn't look at sugar! They failed to because they were wearing blinders on which were written in indelible ink, "Faithful followers focus fixedly on fat." This is a good way to prove the conclusion you're already arrived at (although it didn't do them much good in the breast cancer study), but it's a poor way to do science. Are the endocrine mechanisms linking sugar to cancer and described in the medical journals really to be that easily bypassed?

My colleagues and I were concerned. Knowing that the *excess* breast cancer cases on *low fat* outnumbered the colon cancer excess on high fat by four to one, an that sugar-linked endometrial cancer was not included in any paper from the Nurses Study, we were legitimately concerned with the *real* bottom line of the Nurses Study—across-the-board cancer incidence.

So we asked: "What data do you have about dietary fat and *total* cases of cancer?"

Strange enough, the reply was: "We don't have that data; it's not really useful information."

Can you imagine? I can't help but imagine Peter Falk as Detective Columbo standing in the doorway in his crumpled raincoat, about to exit, and turning back to ask one last question. With fingers touching his furrowed brow, he says, "Just one more thing, Professor. I don't know much about computers, and I know you're going to think me a pest, but I just gotta ask you this. In a study this big, with all that data on 90,000 nurses and what they ate and what diseases they got, and who lived and who died, and all the rest of it, there's just one little thing that puzzles me. How do you program your computer so you *don't* get the total cases of cancer?"

Our self-effacing detective shares with me the suspicion that the overall incidence of cancer data failed to support the fat-fighters' preconceived notion and was simply no longer talked about. Had the data shown a correlation between dietary fat and all cases of cancer, you can bet anything it would have been reported and covered by every wire service in the Western world.

What looks to the paranoid among us to be a cover-up is most certainly nothing more than overzealousness, a pervasive quality indeed among dedicated scientists. To stress this point, let us consider a recent hearing on the subject of dietary fat and cancer held by the FDA and printed in the Federal Register.[12] They concluded:

> *"All of the publicly available evidence supports the conclusion that diets high in fat increase the risk of cancer, and more importantly that diets low in fat are associated with the reduced risk of cancer."*

There is only one catch. The literature cited in this major federal health publication contained the Harvard Nurses Study on colon cancer but *not* the study about breast cancer I just told you about in which 31 *more* cases were found in the 20% of nurses with the lowest consumption of animal fat. Naturally, I checked and double-checked. Could this really be true? Indeed, it was.

The studies cited in the cancer section contained many very small and necessarily tenuous reports on 200 or 300 subjects but not the largest study on breast cancer ever conducted, a study on *90,000 subjects* by the same investigators in the Harvard Department of Epidemiology, using the same nurses and published by the same *New England Journal of Medicine* as the colon-cancer study that received such headlines. (*Other* studies showing no relation between breast cancer and dietary fat were also missing.) I am more than curious about these omissions; I hope we will soon be given an explanation. I do know that consensus experts diligently study the data offered to them by the consensus panel staff. It's a shame that national-health policy can be so greatly influenced by research assistants so overworked that they miss little details like the most significant study on breast cancer ever reported.

And yet I haven't written this chapter to focus your attention upon possible discrepancies between scientific *findings* and the beliefs of certain scientists but to reassure you that the next time you confront a bacon-and-cheese omelet that you hotly desire but are afraid to approach, you needn't be afraid. The evidence that you're going to get heart disease or cancer from the fat in your diet isn't strong, it's weak; it isn't persuasive, it's remarkably unpersuasive. False accusations are being passed off as scientific gospel simply because those upon whom our political leaders rely for scientific insight have long ago become devotees of the low-fat cause and don't scruple to slant the evidence, although they may imagine that in doing so they perform a public service.

I hope the foregoing discussion has at least awakened you to the realization that there is not scientific unanimity on those points, either. As with so many other considerations involving your health, you can survive best by becoming critical enough to make your own decisions.

PART FOUR

How to Do the Diet for Life

Here you are returning to the diet once again. Some of you, of course, will never have gone off it since the day you began your original 14-day sprint. The rest of you will have taken a reflective pause to consider the significance of your initial results. Clearly you liked them. Now you are about to begin the most important part of the program. You are about to create a diet for yourself—a diet that suits your lifestyle, your taste preferences, your food intolerances, your metabolism, your medical problem areas, and even your ability to deal with temptation. The hunt for health and slimness is on. I dare to say that your prospects for success have never been better.

17 | *Ongoing Weight Loss— The Basic Reduction Diet*

If you've done the two week *Induction* level of the diet, and you're ready to go on, then you're about to become a serious dieter in the best possible sense. We continue with what I call the *Ongoing Weight-Loss* diet (OWL), and OWL, though more lenient than your original 14-day diet, will certainly show you what being on a fat-mobilizing, fat-dissolving—yet fat-containing—diet can do for you. After OWL, having become almost as wise as that dignified night-roaming bird, you'll move up to the important, though relatively brief, stage of *Pre-Maintenance* dieting, and then to your lifetime *Maintenance* diet. You're going to find that every one of those stages is a comfortable fit.

I'm never going to leave you in the lurch, with your pounds lost and nothing to do but gain them back again. And I'm never going to introduce you to a stage that's hard to do, or that makes you feel bad.

What positive changes you have already begun to enjoy! What a pleasure to lose weight, but I think, even more significantly, what a pleasure to enhance the quality of your life through painless, hungerless, healthy eating.

Let me also say appetizing. Perhaps spareribs or bacon and eggs were among the luxuries that on a low-fat diet you had to do without. Now you're on a diet that's as healthy as the most rigorous low-fat diet could possibly aspire to be, and consequently, these luxuries, as well as many others, can be yours again.

Juicy broiled New York strip sirloin steak? English cut roast prime rib of beef? Poached salmon with béarnaise sauce? Crispy duck in a Chinese restaurant? Pan fried chicken? Dig in.

But I know that you don't forget (and neither will I) that what initially brought you to this book was probably your overweight.

Let's look at the big weight loss picture, and, as the chapter unfolds, you'll see why you need never be fat again.

First of all, consider that it really helps to know how many pounds you want to lose. It focuses you. It keeps you disciplined in a psychologically pleasing way, since week after week you *do* get to see the pounds vanishing. After so many years as an enemy, the bathroom scale is about to become one of your best friends.

I'd like to remind you yet again that there are people who still can't accustom themselves to this diet because they can't get past the primitive, popular notion that a diet is something you get on and then get off, as you would a bus. But a diet is *not* an excursion, and such dieters—the uncommitted ones—are often the very individuals who need to lose forty pounds but lose interest when they reach twenty-eight. Then they go back to eating their old diet and four or five months later they're back where they were to begin with.

You can be sure that such a person will do that on the Atkins diet as well. Any diet will "fail," if you simply misuse it as a tool for some quick and easy weight loss and don't adapt it to your own tastes as a lifetime diet plan.

Your goal—for a large percentage of you, it will be your destiny—of reaching your desired weight and staying there for life is best met by realistically considering which levels of carbohydrate intake apply to you. While you're losing weight, you want to find a level of carbohydrate restriction that sustains ketosis/lipolysis. Thus you will dissolve your fat; you will maintain control of your appetite sufficiently to curb your urge to eat what you're not permitted; and you will eat healthy foods that you enjoy. Take the physical and emotional well-being promoted by ketosis/lipolysis and combine that with the gustatory pleasure of a rich, luxury diet. Result: One healthy, happy human being.

I think this result is much better than the sac recidivism of the bus rider I described just above.

In this chapter, you're going to learn how to do OWL. Let's start by determining your physical goals.

Take a Pause for Reflection

It's time to take a serious look at your body, and decide what you want to do with it and how you want it to look. Be realistic. Give some serious consideration to what you want to be physically. In all probability, you no longer expect to be an Olympic athlete or a fashion model. On the other hand, you may be looking to the other extreme, toward goals that are really too modest, like being *less* than fat and *relatively* healthy. I know that many of my patients come to me thinking that such goals would be quite all right—even more than they can hope for.

Frankly, I think you should set your sights higher than that. How about ideal weight, excellent health, and vigor that's surprising for your age and somewhat more than you ever expected to have again? Trust me, that's not overly ambitious. That's realistic. And when you achieve it, it's oh so satisfying.

The human body responds rather quickly to determined efforts to improve it. Pounds to drop off, blood pressure does drop down, cholesterol and triglyceride levels do begin to retreat from disturbing heights, blood glucose and insulin levels do stabilize speedily on a diet like this, and the whole human person does commence to feel better. This happens in response to a proper diet; it happens to people who stop abusing their bodies with caffeine, alcohol, and drugs; it happens to people who take large, intelligently chosen doses of vitamins and minerals; it happens with a proper, gradual program of exercise. *Your* body will respond just as other people's bodies respond. There's no mystery. Your body is a remarkably resilient, amazingly tough organism, and it will seize upon anything good that is done for it and make the most of it. If most of what you're done to your body is bad, then it has been hunkering down in a defensive position trying to survive the abuse. If you do all of the above things, then in the space of a few weeks, you will notice remarkable improvements in the way you feel. If you do even one or two or them, you're going to notice a positive change.

This book is primarily about diet, and quite frankly, my experience has been that diet matters more than any other single thing. As you know, I also lay out the basis for a sound program of nutritional supplementation in this book, and in Chapter 20, I describe the fundamentals of a good exercise program. So now, let us refocus on our first question.

When in your life did you look and feel your very best? How much did you weigh then? Can you comfortably weigh that again? Don't skip over the question. As I've always said, you're the greatest expert on your body.

Whatever your ideal weight was, you can almost certainly reach it again. 120? 140? 170? Why not go for it?

Reaching Your Ideal Weight!

It shouldn't sound like climbing Mt. Everest. I know that if you're metabolically similar to the 25,000 overweight patients I've treated during the last quarter century, you have an excellent chance of succeeding.

Once you reach your goal, you can look at yourself in the mirror and feel triumphant.

Do you have a clear conception of your ideal weight—the weight perfect for your frame and muscular development—when you were a young adult? Many people have a pretty good sense of that number. They held that weight for a good part of their lives and found that they gained weight only after specific events, such as getting married, having kids, stopping smoking, starting or stopping medication.

Many others have always been "stocky," and if you fall into this second category, you may have to resort to those not-very-accurate insurance tables. I reproduce a rather outdated but still serviceable insurance table below in Chart 17.1. Far from perfect, it at least gives you a ballpark figure to aim at.

Now, let's get back to sustaining that weight loss, which you've so happily begun.

Chart 17.1
DESIRABLE WEIGHTS FOR MEN AND
WOMEN AGED 25 AND OVER°
in pounds according to height and frame,
in indoor clothing, and shoes

HEIGHT		SMALL FRAME	MEDIUM FRAME	LARGE FRAME
		MEN		
Feet	*Inches*			
5	2	112-120	118-129	126-141
5	3	115-123	121-133	129-144
5	4	118-126	124-136	132-148

°*Adapted from Metropolitan Life Insurance Co., New York. New weight standards for men and women. Statistical Bulletin 40.3, Nov.–Dec., 1959.*

HEIGHT		SMALL FRAME	MEDIUM FRAME	LARGE FRAME
		DESIRABLE WEIGHTS (cont.)		
		MEN		
Feet	*Inches*			
5	5	121-129	127-139	135-152
5	6	124-133	130-143	138-156
5	7	128-137	134-147	142-161
5	8	132-141	138-152	147-166
5	9	136-145	142-156	151-170
5	10	140-150	146-160	155-174
5	11	144-154	150-165	159-179
6	0	148-158	154-170	164-184
6	1	152-162	158-175	168-189
6	2	156-167	162-180	173-194
6	3	160-171	167-185	178-199
6	4	164-175	172-190	182-204
		WOMEN		
4	10	92-98	96-107	104-119
4	11	94-101	98-110	106-122
5	0	96-104	101-113	109-125
5	1	99-107	104-116	112-128
5	2	102-110	107-119	115-131
5	3	105-113	110-122	118-134
5	4	108-116	113-126	121-138
5	5	111-119	116-130	125-142
5	6	114-123	120-135	129-146
5	7	118-127	124-139	133-150
5	8	122-131	128-143	137-154
5	9	126-135	132-147	141-158
5	10	130-140	136-151	145-163
5	11	134-144	140-155	149-168
6	0	138-148	144-159	153-173

Learn Your Levels

First, let's review your weight loss during the first 14 days of the diet and the degree of metabolic resistance it indicated. Chart 17.2 will give you a general sense of where you stand in the metabolic resistance framework.

Chart 17.2

Weight Loss During the First Two Weeks on Ketogenic Diet for Patients at Three Levels of Obesity

Degree of Metabolic Resistance for Males

Pounds Lost in First 14 Days When Metabolic Resistance is:

Pounds to Lose	High	Average	Low
Less than 20	4	6	8
20–50	6	9	12
Over 50	8	12	16

Degree of Metabolic Resistance for Females

Pounds Lost in First 14 Days When Metabolic Resistance is:

Pounds to Lose	High	Average	Low
Less than 20	2	4	6
20–50	3	6	9
Over 50	4	8	12

As I'm sure you've guessed, the degree of resistance to weight loss that your body shows corresponds to your degree of difficulty in getting well into ketosis/lipolysis. By definition, resistance to weight loss *is* resistance to ketosis.

Now, on the *Induction* diet, which you've just gone through, I asked you to go on virtually the strictest level of low-carbohydrate dieting. You were consuming 15 to 20 gms of carbohydrate. A smart strategy. If your body was capable of going into ketosis, it did. The diet was extremely low because I wanted to demonstrate lipolysis for everybody from the person who can really lose weight quite easily on almost any diet to the hardest case—the person who, until going on the Atkins diet, thought that losing weight was just about an impossibility.

And I am sure that better than 95% of you found that you were losing weight. The other 5% of you will have to look at the next chapter and work with the special diet I've devised for patients with extreme metabolic resistance.

But if you're a normal dieter, you're now going on to a somewhat more liberalized version of the Atkins diet, and you're entering a crucial stage for learning the parameters of your lifetime program. You'll find out what's *the most liberal level of carbohydrate consumption that corresponds to your own individual metabolic capacity to continue taking off excess pounds.* This is the carbohydrate maximum for the *Ongoing Weight-Loss* level of the diet—your Critical Carbohydrate Level for Losing (CCLL).

Naturally, you should wish to move into this phase of the diet with proper caution. I emphasize the importance of sticking to *low-carbohydrate* vegetables, nuts, and other meal accompaniments in these early days. The one thing we don't want to do is get you out of ketosis/lipolysis and put an end to the hormone-like elaboration of FMS. If that happened, we would have to resume the *Induction* diet again, or, as I must chide so many of my patients, "It's back to square one."

Remember, some very common foods have amounts of carbohydrate that aren't insignificant. A grapefruit has around 20 gms and an apple only slightly less. Measure that against the fact that approximately 40% of metabolically overweight women can't lose unless they're eating less than thirty grams of carbohydrate a day!

Therefore those foods that you may always have to eat with great moderation and restraint, so you must save them for a later date. There will be time enough to try them on your *Maintenance* diet.

Remember that most fruits are high in natural sugars and that your tendency to develop glucose and insulin disorders will always make fruit-eating somewhat risky for you.

A Private Personal Number Just for You

Remember two basic principles:

1. On this diet, your rate of weight loss is generally proportional to your exclusion of carbohydrates.
2. The level of carbohydrate you are consuming can be measured, and thus, *if you wish,* you can attach numerical quantities to the carbohydrate food you're eating and decide just how much of this or that you're consuming. See the Carbohydrate Counter in the back of the book, as well as Chart 17.2 in this chapter. For more food items, you'll find *Dr. Atkins' New Carbohydrate Gram Counter* available, quite inexpensively, at your favorite bookstore.

With that in mind, I'd like to refer to the level of carbohydrate consumption below which you can lose weight as your CCLL. Below this number, you will indeed have *ongoing* weight loss.

There are two ways to determine this CCLL. Which one you choose will depend on your personality. If you're a precise, methodical person who likes weighing, measuring, and numbering, then you'll find out the actual number. The way you'll do this is by increasing the quantity of carbohydrate you eat beyond that one salad you ate on the *Induction* level. And as you carry out this increase, you'll measure the grams of carbohydrate in each of your additions. Usually, I consider an increase in carbohydrates of five daily grams as representing a "level" of the diet.

You'll go up until eventually you'll reach a number at which you *stop* losing. That's your CCLL. Above it, you lose no more, or you begin to gain. Below it, you're definitely dieting in the popular sense of the word, i.e., you're losing weight. For those among you who are precise, numerically oriented people, the CCLL will be a fairly precise number.

You'll be able to say to another Atkins dieter, "My Critical Carbohydrate Level for Losing is 45 grams," or 32, or maybe only 19.

On the other hand, you may be a rule-of-thumb person—many of you will be. That's fine too. If you don't like to fuss about with numbers, then your mode of procedure will be even simpler. You'll increase your carbohydrate consumption steadily until your weight loss begins to become imperceptible and then you'll back down from that level. You'll be able to see roughly how much salad and vegetables you're eating and, as long as you have a good eye for constant quantities, you'll be all right.

If you go beyond your CCLL, your scale will herald the mistake, and you'll make adjustments accordingly. You may ask, where do the lipolysis testing strips (LTS) fit in? They generally fade out and do not change to purple at a point a little bit below your CCLL. When that happens, your CCLL will be only a few carbohydrate grams higher.

The only confusion is that everybody hits plateaus (periods where no weight comes off). The first few periods in which you fail to lose weight will most likely be plateaus and almost never represent the reaching of the CCLL. To identify your CCLL, you must ascertain that you are neither losing pounds nor inches for several weeks. If you feel chagrined about the length of time, then you may well begin to learn your first lesson: *Don't be in a hurry to get it over with; this is one weight loss program that doesn't have an ending.*

At a later stage of the diet, when you've lost almost all the weight you want to lose, you pass from the *Ongoing Weight Loss* diet, pass through (usually in the course of a few weeks, though for some people it might take a couple of months) the important *Pre-Maintenance* phase of dieting, and go on to the *Maintenance* diet. At that point, there will be another landmark level: Your Critical Carbohydrate Level for Maintenance (CCLM) will be the highest number of grams of carbohydrate that you can consume *without starting to gain the weight back*. For most of you now-slim Atkins dieters, that number will be somewhat in a wide range from 25 to 90 gms a day. Look at Chart 17.3.

Chart 17.3		
CARBOHYDRATE GRAM LEVELS AND METABOLIC RESISTANCE		
Metabolic Resistance	*Ongoing Weight-Loss Level* (CCLL)	*Maintenance Level* (CCLM)
High	15 or less	25–40
Average	15–40	40–60
Low	40–60	60–90

The degree of metabolic resistance is perhaps better estimated from the CCLLs than from data extrapolated from the response to a 14-day test diet. As you continue to do the diet, you will, by glancing at this table, have a more accurate idea of your degree of metabolic resistance.

The Wise OWL Mindset

Moving to the *Ongoing Weight Loss* diet presents you with an opportunity to progress toward your ultimate goal, which should be, in case I didn't tell you yet, to arrive at your ideal weight, at your all-time healthiest, and so happy with what you get to eat that you wouldn't change it for the world. If you're a diet veteran, ask yourself this: "Have you ever before reached your goal weight on a diet that was exactly what you wanted to eat?" You should see at a glance that the missing link between temporary and permanent weight loss is to be living on a diet that satisfies your body and soul so well that you have no desire to leave it. With low-carbohydrate eating, you can do just that, and this is your first opportunity to shift gears with that goal in mind.

As you, now full of new-found confidence that carbohydrate-restricting can bring you to your formerly elusive goal weight, savor the prospects of adding to your diet, you may begin to ask: "What would make my OWL experience most enjoyable?"

In addition to the obvious satisfaction you may derive from vegetables and nuts, there are very inviting recipes in this book and in companion books°(and there are unique products designed for the Atkins dieter. You may seek out products such as a bake mix to make low-carbohydrate pancakes, muffins, and bread, a shake mix for instant protein drinks, or meal replacements and those few protein bars low enough in carbohydrate to be usable on the OWL.

Choose the additions which best meet your individual needs for meal enjoyment, convenience, or hunger control, whichever the case may be.

Moving Up the Carbohydrate Ladder

If you do wish for a fairly easy and systematic way of increasing the quantity of the healthy carbohydrates that you can consume while still dropping poundage, my suggestion is that you do it by 5-gm increments. For instance, ½ avocado, 1 cup of cauliflower, 6 to 8 stalks of asparagus, and 1 ounce of sunflower seeds are all 5-gm carbohydrate increments. Thirteen average strawberries are a 5-gm increment, so are five ounces of hard cheese. Look at Chart 17.4 for other suggestions, or turn to the Carbohydrate Counter at the end of the book.

Chart 17.4
CARBOHYDRATE INCREMENTS

Food	Quantity	Grams of Carbohydrate
Almonds	15	4 gms
Brazil nuts	10	4 gms
Macadamia nuts	12	4 gms
Pecans	10 halves	4 gms
Pistachio nuts	50	5 gms
Sunflower seeds	1 oz.	6 gms
Walnuts	1 oz.	4 gms
Asparagus	6 spears	5 gms
Brussels sprouts	½ cup	5 gms
Cauliflower	1 cup	5 gms
Celery	3 five-inch stalks	4 gms
Endive	1 cup	2 gms
Mushrooms	10 small	4 gms
Radishes	20 medium	5 gms
Soybeans	½ cup	11 gms
Spinach	½ cup	5 gms
Cooked tomato	½ cup	5 gms
Turnip greens	1 cup	5 gms

---

*My favorite companion books are *Dr. Atkins' Quick and Easy New Diet Cookbook* (contains the bake mix recipes) and *Dr. Atkins' New Diet Cookbook.*

Chart 17.4 (Cont.) CARBOHYDRATE INCREMENTS		
Food	*Quantity*	*Grams of Carbohydrate*
Cottage cheese	1 cup	6 gms
Hard Cheese	1 oz.	1 gm
Lemon juice	½ cup	8 gms
Tomato juice	½ cup	5 gms
Blueberries	21 average size	5 gms
Raspberries	17 average size	5 gms
Strawberries	13 average size	5 gms
Bake mix	½ cup	5 gms
Shake mix	1 scoop	1 gm
Advantage bar	1 bar	2 gms

NOTE:
Read labels. All products have different carbohydrate counts. The figures listed refer to products available from Atkins Nutritionals.

Now that you've moved on from the one-salad simplicity of the *Induction* phase of the Atkins diet, why don't you get yourself a little notebook and keep track of the food you eat daily? Didn't I tell you you could replace your willpower with your brains? Well, now you can feed your brain this information. The more you know about the carbohydrate quantities of foods you eat, or want to, the better equipped you will be to plan an effective diet strategy.

Meanwhile, as you keep raising your level of carbohydrate intake (and even if you don't), you'll notice a slowdown in the rate at which you lose weight. How soon you notice those changes is another major tipoff as to how great your metabolic resistance to weight loss is.

On the fifteen grams of the *Induction* diet you may have been losing 5 pounds a week. In the first week to ten days, some of that loss may have been water weight, since the diet has a strongly diuretic effect. Perhaps your real level of weight loss on the strict level of the Atkins diet was 2½ pounds a week of actual fat, or approximately 10 pounds a month.

That isn't an unusual rate at which to lose. When Madge O'Hara came to see me, she weighed 156 on her 5'2" frame, and she planned to slim down to 115. She actually lost 21 pounds the first month, and my surmise is that six or seven pounds of that was water weight. The next month she lost seven pounds. By that time, she was at a considerably higher level of the diet, and she took off the last 13 pounds to her goal at a leisurely pace. Those pounds took ten full weeks to go, but, by the time they were gone, she knew exactly how she was going to eat for the rest of her life.

Now that you're liberalizing the diet, you too should expect to see a gradual diminishment of the rate of loss. An additional fact, observed on any diet, is that the rate of weight loss will also be slower as you get closer to your ideal weight. A very important rule is to plan to take two or more months to shed the last 10 pounds. This places you on the *Pre-Maintenance* level of the diet—an almost mandatory level if permanent weight loss is to be achieved. I cannot stress enough how advantageous it is to merge into your *Maintenance* diet, rather than have an abrupt transition. This is the point when formula diets fail their followers.

On the other hand, if you still have thirty or more pounds to lose when you complete the *Induction* diet, you certainly will not be happy with a major slowdown. To you, I would urge adding carbohydrate very slowly, staying for weeks at each 5-gm incremental level.

Let's say in your third week on the diet, you add that half cup of broccoli to the salad you were already consuming. You're up to about 20 gms a day. Perhaps your weight loss that week drops from 4 pounds to 2½. The difference may be water weight. In the fourth week, you add another 5-gm increment. You lose 2 pounds. The fifth week you add five more daily grams of carbohydrate. You lose 1½. And so on.

You may find that you can go up to 35 or 40 gms of carbohydrate a day and still lose a pound a week. This would put you at an average level of metabolic resistance. Your LTS should still be purple, even if only slightly so, and this, together with your continued weight loss, indicates that you're still in ketosis/lipolysis. But even if the sticks do not turn color at all, that does not mean the diet is not working. As long as there is a continued loss of inches (even weight loss need not happen) and continued appetite suppression, the diet is working.

Though the rate at which you want to lose is up to you, I think you might well be content with this state of affairs. As long as the pounds are disappearing, and you're heading steadily toward your goal, why worry? Let's suppose, though, that you are rapidly coming to the conclusion that the extra 10 gms of carbohydrate don't mean as much to you as the extra pound per week of weight loss does. You may opt to stay at a lower level of carbohydrate and be satisfied with the knowledge that you *could* have more if you chose to. Just remember to use a *Pre-Maintenance* phase as you near your ideal weight.

What If I'm Not Average?

If you can go up to 50 or 60 gms of carbohydrate a day and still be losing a little weight and showing ketosis, then you have a fairly low level of metabolic resistance. In all probability you weren't all that overweight, and staying permanently slim on the Atkins *Maintenance* diet is going to be a breeze for you. You're a person who's going to be able to eat two salads, two helpings of vegetables, and perhaps a fruit daily and still remain at a stable weight. If you're careful, and you find you don't go into a weight-gaining spiral, you may even be able to have an occasional potato and some wild rice. Considering you're already eating one of the world's most luxurious protein diets, I predict a great deal of pleasurable eating ahead. But I do ask this question: If so little of your problem is *metabolic*, how did you become overweight in the first place? You should be on the lookout for a pattern of self-destructive behavior. It could be that that is a component of your weight problem.

Some of you aren't so lucky when it comes to metabolic resistance. Those of you with a very high metabolic resistance to weight loss are most in need of this book. If you *stop* losing weight after you reach 20 or 25 gms of carbohydrate daily, you will have to adapt to eating not much more carbohydrate than is on the *Induction* diet. And you certainly will want to study the next chapter very carefully, even though it is primarily written for that 5% who can't lose at all on the Atkins diet.

If you're going to stay slim and healthy, then a significant increase in the amount of exercise—which I strongly recommend for everyone—is absolutely essential for those of you with high metabolic resistance. Without it, losing weight may actually be hard for you.

Moreover, with a high degree of insulin resistance, you're at serious risk of developing diabetes and heart disease, unless you ruthlessly control your consumption of carbohydrate. Obesity, because of these medical consequences, is your deadly enemy, and you must conquer or control it.

It's quite likely that I'm preaching to the converted, because those of you with a high metabolic resistance to weight loss are already well aware of how serious your problem is, and I've generally found that people with severe obesity problems can be among the most committed of dieters once they're shown a technique of weight loss that actually works and that doesn't force them to undergo the really horrific pain of semistarvation.

Here is where a low-carbohydrate diet's suppression of appetite reaps its most handsome dividends. As long as you remain at a keyogenic level of the diet, you'll be able to enjoy them.

Now I'd like to look at some possible solutions for those of you whose metabolic resistance is quite extreme.

18 | Treating Extreme Metabolic Resistance: The Unique Fat Fast

By the time you got to page 3 of this book, you noticed the emphasis I placed on obesity being metabolic far more commonly than it is the consequence of any gluttony. I hope that I provided some emotional comfort for those of you who had never been told that was true. It must be very unsettling to be told that the sole reason for your overweight is your enjoyment of and indulgence in food. It's no fun to think that one's overweight because one's gluttonous, and it's just darn seldom that that's the case.

Obesity *is* almost always a metabolic problem, and to be specific, the metabolic disturbance is hyperinsulinism. So far, so good. Now what happens when the metabolic obstacles are so great that it seems as though you *can't* lost weight?

The inability to lose weight, even on effective diets, does exist. I have seen scores of patients with this problem and thousands more who *tend* to have it. This very real condition doesn't have any official recognition, you can't find it in the diagnostic code index or in textbooks, and many doctors treating obesity have denied its existence, although an increasing number of them are just recently beginning to acknowledge the phenomenon.

So that leaves it up to me to give it a name. We'll call it "metabolic resistance to weight loss," or, for short, "metabolic resistance."

Let's define it. Somewhat arbitrarily, I'll say, "Inability to lose weight or to continue to lose until a reasonable goal weight is reached on either a diet containing 1000 calories or on a 25-gram carbohydrate diet." It is very rare to find someone who can't lose any weight on these dietary regimens, but it is not so rare to find individuals who get "stuck" short of their seemingly realistic weight goal. I would estimate that 4% of obese subjects have metabolic resistance, and this may be 1% of the total population. In the United States, that comes to two and a half million people, quite a crowd for a condition that could benefit from medical intervention and yet is not even an officially recognized condition.

I'll try to provide some consolation by offering you a chapter of your own.

How Can You Tell If You're Metabolically Resistant?

You can tell by doing. If you seem to be a slow loser and have had a prolonged "plateau" on some official carbohydrate-containing diet, ask for or find a 1000-calorie version of that diet and follow it for long enough (2–3 weeks) to ascertain that you are still not losing. If this happens, you would be judged "metabolically resistant" by most doctors (as long as they believed you) but not necessarily by me.

For I have found that 3 out of 4 people who do not lose on 1000 calories of balanced food intake *will* lose on the *Induction* diet. Your next step, therefore, is to do the *Induction* diet. There is the distinct possibility that you will lose on the 14-day *Induction* diet but will get stuck on it before you reach your weight goal. You then deserve the official diagnosis of metabolic resistance. The rest of you, who are getting there slowly and with difficulty, would carry my diagnosis of *relative metabolic resistance*.

What Should the Metabolically Resistant Do?

My first reaction would be to say find a doctor who treats metabolic resistance, for you certainly need some expert medical advice. But, alas, I doubt you could find such a person; *I* have never located one.

Yet there are medical questions that have to be answered at the outset, such as: Are you taking any medications? If you are, there's a very good chance they are the cause of your metabolic resistance.

The worst offenders are the psychotropic drugs; phenothiazines, antidepressants, including prozac, tranquilizers, lithium, and the like. Secondly, hormones such as estrogen, prednisone, and other steroids can cause weight gain and prevent weight loss. Many of the anti-arthritic medications, especially the NSAIDs, do it, too. Then there are the diuretics and, to a lesser extent, other cardiovascular medications. Insulin and oral antidiabetics surely have their effect. In fact, it has been said that when a person is metabolically resistant, *any* medications can aggravate the condition.

You Don't Expect Me to Just Stop My Medications, Do You?

I most certainly don't expect a reader to do that. The risk could be incredible. But for *my* patients that is exactly what we aim for. You cannot stop a medication deemed necessary unless you can provide an equally effective alternative treatment. It may surprise you to know that for each medication grouping I listed, there is an effective *nutritional* alternative. Since that subject is a little far afield of the subject of this book, I would like to refer you to *Dr. Atkins' Vita-Nutrient Solution*. (There you will learn about over 130 nutritionally-acting natural substances that have been shown in scientific papers to help overcome 60 of the most common illnesses and symptoms for which people are usually prescribed medications.)

The technique is the gradual replacement of the suspect drugs with the nutritional protocol (diet and supplements) that can adequately substitute for them. (*N.B.: This requires a nutrition-oriented professional with experience; not suitable for a do-it-yourselfer.*)

If you've attended to the medication problem, the next possibility is to look into your hormonal balance. Certainly a significant percentage of the metabolically resistant have underactive thyroid function.

I test for this with a standard battery of thyroid tests including one to test the TSH levels (an elevation of TSH is the most reliable blood test of all), and another to test the thyroid autoantibodies (there is a new technology for detecting these, much more sensitive than previously). But, if the metabolic resistance is associated with specific low thyroid symptoms such as sluggishness, brittle hair, coarse skin, irregular menses, depression, and difficulty keeping warm, I would do one more test—the basal body temperature.°

°This is accomplished by holding a glass thermometer under your arm for 10 minutes, before you get out of bed in the A.M. If the average of four or more different mornings' readings is 96.8 or less, that is *prima facie* evidence of sluggish thyroid. I actually find the average oral temperature more reliable. This is done by placing the glass thermometer under the tongue for 3 minutes, four times daily (before each of the meals and before bedtime) and averaging all four temperatures for 3 days. Here, a reading below 97.6 would be considered abnormal and evidence of sluggish thyroid function.

If you show any of these manifestations of underactive thyroid, then the administration of your corrective dose of thyroid hormone (by your doctor) is very likely to correct your metabolic resistance. If your doctor balks at this suggestion, please convey to him my experience—that I have never found a supervised therapeutic trial of thyroid in this situation to be risky.

There is a simple at-home test that you must do if the evidence seems inescapable that you are metabolically resistant. Use the lipolysis testing strips after you have done the strict *Induction* diet for several days—nothing but meat, fowl, seafood, eggs, cheese— this time without even the salad. Those who are truly metabolically resistant will be the only ones who do *not* turn the sticks purple.°

There are still those who do not get a measurable ketogenic/ lipolytic response and yet do not lose weight. In this instance, we are confirming that fat stores do break down, and we do anticipate a loss of inches. Those who can develop lipolysis but no weight loss usually turn up an explanation based on medication or a hormonal problem.

For the Hardest of Hard-Core Metabolic Resisters

But there will still be some of you who don't lose on the *Induction* diet or even on a low-fat diet of under 900 calories, and some who don't even get into a ketosis/lipolysis metabolism under any circumstances. The following discussion is for you.

When you are frustrated that things are not going your way, there are two common responses you might make, one destructive and one constructive. You might, and I've seen this response too many times, give in to your frustration and say to yourself, "Dieting is not worth it," and decide, "I'm going off this diet." The consequences are sad but predictable. If you are not losing on an extremely effective diet, you will surely gain—and rapidly— whenever you ease up on that diet. And since the diet was giving you control over your eating behavior (by suppressing your hyperinsulinism response), the loss of control can only accelerate that weight gain.

°At the Atkins Center, we can quantitate the degree of ketosis/lipolysis much more accurately, using the ketoanalyzer, which measures the amount of ketone excreted through the lungs, a quantity directly proportional to the blood level. In this manner, we can make hour-to-hour determinations of the ketone level in order to study our patient's metabolic responses.

The constructive response to "getting stuck" involves a dispassionate bit of self-analysis that leads to the conclusion that, "Whatever I must do, I will do." Going off the diet *is* the correct response, but it can only be for the purpose of going *on* to a more effective diet.

Remember there are two effective techniques for losing weight that we have been utilizing. One is the restriction of carbohydrate, the other, the restriction of the total amount of food, customarily measured (with some degree of metabolic inaccuracy) in calories.

You might study your response to eating less food; smaller portions, fewer calories, less calorically-dense foods (i.e., lower fat). Perhaps you were seduced by the concept of "eat all it takes," which you may have interpreted as "eat all you want," and the two means of determining your optimal quantities may be quite different. For you the most effective strategy might be to say to yourself, "I'll eat just enough that I'm physically free of intolerable hunger signals, and no more." No question, for the person who is stuck, that's the first thing to try.

So do that, and come back to this section after you've given your new quantity concept a fair try (several weeks, perhaps).

You now have to answer those questions. Is the newly modified diet working now? If so, am I as happy as I was on my *Induction* diet? Do I feel as well? Can I do this for a lifetime? If the answer is yes, then do it—you've found your answer. If the answer to any of these questions is no, read on.

The second principle of weight loss we work with (and the number one principle, overall) is carbohydrate restriction. I placed it second here merely because, if you are on the *Induction* diet, you are already quite restricted in carbohydrate. Of course, you're not at absolute zero in carbohydrate—there are the veggies, the salad, the lemon juice, and the other low-but-not-zero carbohydrate items that make this diet so livable. What would happen if you cut way down on them? (I shouldn't have to say this, but, if you're cheating occasionally, stop it instantly, and shame on you for entertaining the notion that your metabolism is at fault, when, more likely than not, it's your discipline).

Well, try retreating to zero carbohydrate, and then ask yourself the same question. Does the diet now work, and do you feel well, and are you happy, and could you spend your life on it?

If you're still not losing, you have hard-core metabolic resistance, and the worst part must be that nobody seems to understand what a prison you're living in. Stick with me, then. I'm probably one of the few people who understands you. What other professional has acknowledged the existence of your problem?

There was a time when I used to say to people, "Well, you can always cut down calories and carbohydrate, and go all the way down until you are on a fast." Not as bad an idea as it might sound to someone who has never tried it. The fasting state, once induced, is full of self-protective devices. A person on a fast liberates more FMS and other lipid mobilizers than on almost any other diet, and the FMS leads to ketosis/lipolysis, loss of hunger, and a variety of other benefits that make the average fasting person comfortable and often exhilarated.

The beautiful fact about fasting and the Atkins diet is that one can use the *Induction* diet to create a maximal outpouring of FMS and then, without an interruption, switch into fasting without going through the hunger/discomfort that characterizes the first two days of a fast. So by doing 2 to 3 days of a "nothing but meat, eggs, fish, and fowl" diet, you can being your fast already in an effective state of ketosis/lipolysis.

Now, as the Benoit study and other research has shown, fasting is accompanied by a loss of lean body tissue as well as fat, and some of the pounds you lose will not be the ones you want to lose. Plus, loss of essential minerals such as potassium make it dangerous for many people, and dozens of deaths (usually from heart rhythm disturbances secondary to potassium depletion) have been reported.

So I believe, as does most everyone in the field, that fasting should be modified. It should include lots of electrolytes such as potassium, so a dilute juice fast or a vegetable broth fast is preferable. (If I don't go into details, don't fret; I've got something better to tell you about presently.)

One of the current "rages" is the protein-sparing modified fast (PSMF) that you've heard of as "formula diets," the type that helped Oprah Winfrey achieve such a spectacular, albeit evanescent, weight loss. These diets maintain most of the efficacy of fasting and share with it many of the risks, but they do minimize these risks. However, because most of them contain carbohydrate, they still allow for a significant amount of weight loss as lean body tissue. That, plus the fact that they do nothing to prepare you for a lifetime *maintenance*, explains the notoriously rapid regain so often seen after such an experience.

So What's Your Answer, Dr. Atkins?

The best answer to metabolic resistance to date is not new. It has been known for 27 years. Remember the Benoit study that I described on page 62? Well, he studied a diet that outdid the total fast by 88% as far as loss of body fat is concerned. And Benoit, in turn, had simply used one of the experimental diets devised by Kekwick and Pawan.

That remarkable diet that provided results so spectacular that the closed-minded establishment spokesmen couldn't believe their data, contained 1000 calories, 90% of them as fat! The other 100 calories consisted of approximately 15 gms of protein and 10 gms of carbohydrate.*

I hope I'm not telling secrets out of school when I tell you that the subjects on Kekwick and Pawan's and Benoit's studies *didn't enjoy their experimental diets*, even though they did enjoy the way they felt. But you know how very interested in food I am. So as I read and reread their amazing results, I suddenly shouted "That I can do!" I knew I could make the Kekwick and Pawan diet enjoyable. I've tried it on my metabolically resistant patients, and they did very well. I have not used it on my usual patients, because I believe that the diet could be risky when applied to those who are not really metabolically resistant. Those of you who are simply dissatisfied that your rate of loss is too slow should be using the regular Atkins diet and keeping to it strictly. Don't use this one except for brief intervals of less than five days, or unless you are being followed by a physician experienced with this diet.

Now for the Fat Fast Diet

The first thing you will learn is that 900 calories of fat (90% of the 1000 calorie allotment) is provided by 100 gms of fat—not a lot of food. It's less than four ounces of butter, for example.

So let's see how that can be translated into foods you will actually enjoy.

Let's start with two foods which are in exactly the correct proportions and fill the 90%-fat criterion quite naturally—rich, luxurious cream cheese and sinfully delicious macadamia nuts. Ten ounces of cream cheese would be an entire day's food allotment, as would five ounces of macadamias.

---

*These numbers imply that the diet is deficient in protein and is therefore not suitable for long-term use, unless amino acid supplements are given periodically. Note that there is no essentiality of carbohydrate and, therefore, carbohydrate need not be supplemented.

Since a nibbler's diet works better than a gorger's diet—that is, frequent small feedings are preferable—it is better to divide the food allowance into four nibblings of 250 calories each, or five of 200 calories each. In effect, you will be on a fast modified by five handfuls of macadamia nuts (one ounce each), per day, or the equivalent. The fasting is modified by your intake of fatty foods, much as the protein-sparing fast is modified by a protein drink. And remember, this diet is only to be used by people whose body fat is as resistant to being lost as a color-fast fabric is resistant to losing its color.

That's why I call it the Fat Fast for the Fat Fast. It is not designed for those who want to lose fat fast. There. I said it, and I'm not sorry.

This is the way it could work. You might opt for two ounces of cream cheese at 7 A.M., 3 P.M., and bedtime, interspersed with one ounce of macadamias at 11 A.M. and 7 P.M. Or vice versa. It is worth trying that for two days, directly after the *Induction* diet, just to prove to yourself that you don't get hungry, that your blood sugar is remarkably stable, and that you feel quite well. What a wonderful feeling it will be to know how easily you can adapt to the most effective fat-losing diet ever described in a medical journal!

Is That All You Eat?

Well, there are a great many things you can eat—and here is where the food lover in me can help make your Fat Fast an enjoyable experience. I can show you modifications of the basic diet that are fun for all of you, and, for those of you who have been fat-deprived all these years because you thought it was the right thing to do, this can be an answer to wish-fulfillment dreams.

For each of your five 200-calorie fat feedings, you may have:

- 2 oz. of sour cream, containing 1 tablespoon of caviar, served on three or four crisp fried pork rinds.
- 2 deviled egg halves, served not in the whites, but on the pork rinds or on a thin slice of our soy bread recipe.
- Graham Newbould's Paté for Royalty (2 oz.) served on the soya bread.
- 2 oz. of chicken salad made with triple the usual amount of mayonnaise (or ham salad, egg salad, shrimp salad).
- 1 oz. of the above in a half avocado.
- 2 ½ oz. of whipped heavy cream, artificially sweetened, and

with ground vanilla beans.
• And then there are choices from the recipe section, including chocolate truffles.

The rest of your diet should consist of calorie-free beverages, taken liberally. See page 269 for list of permissible beverages.

So there we have taken a diet devised for an experiment to learn about why fat is less fattening calorie-for-calorie than protein or carbohydrate, and converted it into something enjoyable, extremely well-tolerated, and useful for overcoming metabolic resistance.

First, we must establish whether this program works for you. Those who go on the Fat Fast *must* study themselves with LTS before, during, and after. If you don't go into ketosis on this program, you should be seeing a doctor who specializes in metabolic disorders, for you surely have one. Since I don't expect more than a few hundred readers of this book to be in such a category, my staff can certainly take the time to talk to people in this elite group and answer your questions. But for most of you, I believe you will have found a tool that will finally allow you to be slim.

Now it remains for me to tell you how to use it.

I do not believe the Fat Fast should be used for more than one week at a time. This is simply a safety measure because the diet has not been tested for long-term use. It should, therefore, be interspersed with the *Induction* diet or some other strict level of the Atkins diet. The most important aspect of the switchdown is not to interpose any carbohydrate that would suppress the FMS production. Your strategy should be to lose on the Fat Fast and to use the regular Atkins diet to maintain that loss. An alternative to this when the Fat Fast works and the *Induction* diet does not is to modify the Fat Fast in such a way that you can stay on it longer. You may find that you can lower your fat percentage to 80% or so, as long as the other 20% contains mostly protein. You may find that you lose on 1200 calories and that you can change from 5 feedings to 3 meals of approximately 400 calories each. With a more liberal use of vita-nutrients, I would consider such a diet safe but *only for a person who has demonstrated total inability to lose on the Induction diet.*° (A person with metabolic resistance cannot expect to lose

---

°Powerfully effective diets, which the Fat Fast is, can be dangerous when they induce rapid weight loss. When they are just barely strong enough to overcome extreme metabolic resistance, they are rather safe.

rapidly and must develop the patience of Job. Figure it will take a year or two to reach your goal and be content if you proceed steadily on that schedule.

My Metabolically Resistant Patients

I have seen hundreds of metabolically resistant patients in my career, perhaps more of them than any other doctor. I wish I could tell you I discovered a cure for metabolic resistance, but I can only report that we are making progress.

I have discovered quite a few nutrients that have helped many of these people, but none that have helped all of them. Those of you with this problem should turn to Chapter 22, where I list them as well as discussing other advantages of an intelligent use of nutritional supplementation. The vita-nutrient most likely to help overcome metabolic resistance is L-carnitine. L-carnitine's biochemical role is especially suited for breaking the weight loss logjam. It catalyzes lipolysis, the reaction where fat can be used as fuel. The problem is that carnitine is expensive and some people are not benefited until 8,000 mg are given. Research is underway at the Atkins Center looking for ways to accomplish the carnitine effect with lower doses. Other nutrients we are studying are coenzyme Q_{10}, lipoic acid, chromium, vanadium and a variety of herbs.

If your metabolic resistance to weight loss is so severe that even this book isn't a complete solution to your problem, I hope you'll find a medical or nutritional professional who has some familiarity with supplementation and can help you with questions of dosages, durations, combinations, and risks involved in using them.

Your Problems Always Will Be More Severe

Just remember, if this chapter has been about you, then all the rest of the book is conditioned by that fact. For you, the occasional indulgences I offer to other dieters in the maintenance chapter are going to have to be very occasional indeed.

19 | Pre-Maintentance— *Your Preparation for Permanent Slimness*

If you've reached this stage of the diet, then you don't have a lot of weight still to take off. I tend to advise dieters to advance gradually toward their *Maintenance* diet when they just have five to ten pounds left to lose. Depending on how much your weight loss has slowed as you advance upon your goal weight, it could be two or three weeks, or one or two months before you'd naturally get there on the OWL diet.

Now, I'm telling you to slow down even further. The slower you lose that last five pounds the better. I think you should increase carbohydrates until you're losing less than a pound a week.

In effect, by the time you reach that "perfect" weight, you will be on the *Maintenance* diet, and your weight loss will be just cruising to a halt. The previous weeks will have:

1. Accustomed you to your lifetime eating plan.
2. Given you a good indication of what it will be like.

Constructive Deviations

One of the things you'll learn in *Pre-Maintenance* is what exceptions you can make to the diet you learned in the *Induction* and OWL diets and still go on losing weight, albeit slowly. Start with one or two deviations a week, such as a fruit and a starch dish—a plate of wild rice or a baked potato. Or you may simply want to eat more of the special recipes or dieters' specialty products you have been introduced to.

By the time you reach your goal weight and your *Maintenance* level, you might be enjoying three such deviations. A glass of wine, a couple of slices of whole wheat bread, a half a cantaloupe for lunch one day. Perhaps a chocolate mousse made with the shake mix and heavy cream or a stack of pancakes made with the bake mix. Or, if your metabolic resistance is at the low end, a few things more than that each week.

But be careful. There are a couple of reasons why people sometimes get into trouble on the *Maintenance* diet.

1. They don't recognize just how strict the *Maintenance* diet still must be.
2. They're startled to discover that without ketosis/lipolysis the wonderful advantage of appetite suppression has gone away.

That's why *Pre-Maintenance* is important. This is the stage in the diet at which you become acclimated to the rest of your life. As you do *Pre-Maintenance*, the protection of ketosis is beginning to vanish. You'll want to eat a bit more, so do. But try not to stuff yourself heedlessly. You have nothing to make up for. Unlike other diets, this one hasn't caused you any pain or hunger.

Nonetheless, suppression of appetite has made your life easy up to now. Now you'll have to think a little more about what you're adding on to your menu. Add the carbohydrates slowly and glide sweetly and safely into *Maintenance*. As you're about to learn, a proper lifetime *Maintenance* diet really involves using all four of your diets when appropriate. No ideal weight is constant, just as no person is constant.

There will be times in your life when you gain some weight back. Fortunately, you'll have developed the confidence to know that those small weight gains can be easily taken off. Most people find that on this diet, it's easy to control their weight. So let's see how it's done.

20 | Maintenance— *Slim Forever*

The bells should be ringing, the flags should be flying: You're there. You've arrived where millions of overweight people in this country have never been since they were children—at your ideal weight. The psychological uplift must be considerable. I really don't think there's anyone, man, woman, or child, who doesn't like to look good.

Glance in the mirror, try on some newly tailored clothes, or climb into duds you haven't been able to shoehorn yourself into for years, and then—O luxury—listen to the comments people make. I'll bet you've taken center stage. Losing weight sure attracts attention!

Have you won the battle of the bulge? Or have you only graduated from boot camp, where you got in shape for the battle ahead? As a part-time dieter and full-time gourmand, I can personally attest to the fact that you have only achieved the latter. And recidivism among dieters who have lost considerable weight is such a well-documented fact that many cynical doctors advise not even trying to lose. Which is why you *need* a maintenance diet and a determined approach.

I remember talking to Marjorie Burke, a 41-year-old nurse who first saw me when she weighed 254 pounds and who had never weighed less than 175 since she became an adult. She had tried all the diets, including a famous liquid-protein diet on which she started to go bald. She said that for more than twenty years she hadn't gotten up in the morning, gone in the bathroom, and looked at herself in the mirror without feeling disappointed and depressed. Now that is all gone, part of a somewhat grim past.

Was she ever going to fall off the diet? The answer was plainly *never, never, never*.

Protect Your Weight Losses

You, too, have invested a lot of effort and psychic energy in those lessons. Since you and I both know you have a tendency to gain, I want you to keep a sharp eye open for any resumption of weight gain.

If your metabolism can handle it, I'm about to allow you—in moderation—many of the foods you used to enjoy. (The outstanding exception is sugar.)

My experience treating overweight patients involves managing several thousand patients who have lost to their goal weight four or more times, only to gain it back every time. So I can assure you, you should not rush blindly back toward the way you used to eat, with the intention of getting as close to your former eating patterns as you can without absolutely violating the rules of the diet. That would show you really hadn't learned anything from this diet. (Which is to be expected, because diets are not teachers.) But this diet is an experience, and experience is supposed to be the best teacher. What I *hope* you've learned is how to make a lifetime commitment to a different way of eating.

The Nitty Gritty Of Maintenance

What you should be asking yourself is, "What level of carbohydrate consumption do I *feel* best on?" That's really a more rational goal than to find the most liberalized level of carbohydrate consumption you can manage without weight gain. Many people find they feel better on a quite low level of carbohydrates—perhaps only 25 or 30 gms a day—than they do on the most liberal version of the diet. That might be two salads and a large helping of vegetables. Together with the satisfying portion of protein and fat, that would provide for a very healthy diet.

Other people feel best on twice that carbohydrate consumption and have the metabolism to support it. This is your opportunity to individualize a perfect diet for you. *Remember, your best carbohydrate level is the one you can be happiest on without weight regain.*

A Delicious Lifetime

As you've seen, the Atkins diet is really four diets. The *Induction* diet, which is the most austere form of a low-carbohydrate ketogenic diet; the *Ongoing Weight Loss* diet (OWL), which is designed to continue weight loss over the long haul; the pivotal *Pre-Maintenance* diet, which thoroughly accustoms you to that all-important transition between losing and maintaining; and the *Maintenance* diet, which we are talking about right now, and which is intended to keep you slim and healthy for a long lifetime.

What most of my patients discover by the time they reach the maintenance phase of dieting is how endlessly varied, rich, and satisfying this way of eating is.

Donna Miller, who came to see me a couple of years ago drained of all energy, beset with allergies, and thirty pounds overweight, had always been a bread, bagels, and pizza freak. In four months, she went from being a size 12 (almost bursting out of it, as she admitted) to being a size 8. In addition, her energy had returned almost as soon as we had taken her off of wheat, sugar, and milk. But what was she going to eat?

She was a resourceful woman, and I hope her diet sounds as attractive to you as it does to me. For breakfast now, she often eats sliced raw tuna and a little salad. Or two scrambled eggs with tofu. For lunch, she'll stir fry or steam vegetables the way the Japanese do, and with it she'll have corned beef, or a lean hamburger patty, or some fish. For dinner, she likes zucchini, eggplant, or asparagus. She often mixes up minced garlic, herbs, and parsley in tomato sauce, and she frequently has chicken, rib steak, or salmon. She also finds she can have lentils, split peas, and kasha without gaining weight. She often has the kasha with cinnamon and a few apple slices.

Donna has been expanding her variety of salads since she went on the diet, and she told me recently that what she particularly appreciates about the diet is that it has a lot of alternatives, which she now finds she enjoys more than the rather repetitive high-starch menu she used to be on. What impresses me the most is that every item in her new eating plan is wholesome, fresh, and healthy.

Frankly, I defy anyone to propose a more luxurious diet on which you can stay trim and healthy than the Atkins program.

Of course, I've been promising you all along that this is a diet that boasts not so much of its instant weight loss—though it achieves that—but of its staying power. Instead of bouncing back into the land of the fat, the Atkins diet welcomes you permanently into the home of the slim.

But what if you get on the *Maintenance* diet, you're eating happily and feeling great, and suddenly you notice those awful pounds and inches have started staging a recovery?

Dealing with Weight Gain

Well, since you've started the *Maintenance* diet I know that, by definition, you've reached your ideal (or at least desired) weight. Therefore, you're probably no longer practicing a ketogenic diet, since ketosis/lipolysis by definition involves an element of fat loss. Newly slim people are no longer trying to shed pounds and so they don't burn fat. They're above their Critical Carbohydrate Level for Losing (CCLL).

But here's the catch that many dieters *don't* catch: There is very little leeway before you break through the *other* Critical Carbohydrate Level—the CCLM, the one at which you begin to gain. A typical person of average metabolic resistance may find he must stay between 40 and 60 gms of carbohydrate daily. Eating more than the 40 is preventing him from losing more pounds and becoming too thin; eating less than the 60 prevents weight regain.

At this ideal weight, you are, in fact, pretty finely balanced in the amount of your carbohydrate intake. Nothing is exact, of course. Since life is change, your weight will, in fact, be constantly shifting up and down by small increments. The most convenient way to maintain your best weight now is to not let that *up* get too far out of hand. If it does, then you may find yourself sliding down the uphill path, to coin a phrase.

I recommend that you know your weight—after all, it's one aspect of your general health that you can always easily keep track of. Getting on the scale daily (or at least twice a week) is a *must* for successful weight maintenance. *When you find that you've gone five pounds or more over your ideal weight, then you must promptly put things back on their proper course. And you must do it without delay.*

Doing so is as simple as going on the diet in the first place. But, when you discover you're five pounds overweight, don't put off dealing with it. Maybe Thanksgiving is coming up, or Christmas, or your birthday, or your spouse's birthday, or your vacation. By the time you celebrate any one of those with a bout of unrestrained indulgence, you may find that instead of being five pounds overweight you're fifteen pounds overweight and plummeting uphill fast. Instead of waiting, act.

Your action is as simple as BDK. *What you should do is go straight back to the Induction phase of the diet.* Do *not* go back to your *Maintenance* diet without first losing *all* you have regained. It's simple. A salad a day of carbohydrate and *voila!*, you've slashed your weight back to perfect in as little as six to eight days, or two or three weeks, if you have high metabolic resistance.

It is imperative that your baseline weight be something fixed indelibly in your mind as a goal you must always be at or near. It should not drift upward over the years of weight maintenance. If it does, then you're gradually compromising with the metabolic pull that leads most of us to reach equilibrium only when our lifetime high weight is reached.[°]

Your strategy here should be very much like the base runner who allows himself to take a lead off first base, but never so far that he cannot scurry back to the safety of touching the base, should the pitcher suddenly turn to pick him off. For you, your goal weight is the base you must touch between deviations. Getting to it provides you with the safety of never straying too far from your lifetime objective. Thus, after each five-pound bulge you notch, you must dust off and use the *Induction* diet again.

My experience has been that dieters who regain weight on the *Maintenance* diet are the ones who, when they put on some poundage, simply return to their maintenance level of carbohydrate consumption, instead of to the *Induction* level.

For consistent success, you simply must interpose the strict *Induction* diet between your weight gain and the eventual return to the *Maintenance* diet. If you don't do that, you're likely to gain the weight back by increments. You gain five pounds, you stop gaining for a time on *Maintenance*, then you gain five pounds more, and so on. If you let this happen, you gradually slip away from your goal weight until it begins to seem out of reach again. Simply put, you gain when you're eating too many carbohydrates—when you've

---

[°]Many obese people seem to have an appestat (or, more accurately, a ponderostat), which causes them to regain on balanced eating, up to a very specific point at which the weight stabilizes and no further gain takes place, even though the weight-regaining diet remains constant. For most people, the ponderostat is set at their previous lifetime peak weight. Medications can certainly elevate this equilibrium point, as can the cessation of cigarettes or diet pills.

exceeded your CCLM. And as the extra pounds slip on, the nagging metabolic misfortunes that you thought were behind you rise up again. Your energy level declines and the hyperinsulinism symptoms you experienced before start to come again. Those who got off medications may find they require them again. And those with yeast symptoms may find the bloating and brain fog returning. You're on the wrong road, friend.

Don't Reactivate Your Addictions

Naturally, in this situation, you may find yourself engaged in a real battle for self-control as your defenses crumble. Perhaps you've been indulging too much in the foods that got you into trouble to begin with. You may suddenly fall right back under their spell.

Hyperinsulinism and the resultant low blood-sugar levels plus specific food allergy/intolerances truly create an addictive situation. If you go back on sugar, or—for some of you—on bread, fruit, or fermented foods, you suddenly discover that you *must* have these foods, that no day or meal feels right without them. If this should happen, and you observe yourself carefully, you'll notice that the need that develops is genuinely physical. It isn't simply that a jelly donut tastes good to you, and you'd *like* to have it. No, your body absolutely roars with anxiety and passion for that jelly donut. And then you *know*. You've activated an addiction, just like an alcoholic with his bottle.

This isn't shameful; it's physical, it's chemical, it's metabolic, and that's precisely why you must avoid it. Most of you already know that for a significant portion of your life carbohydrates have been stronger than you. Don't trifle with them.

Nearly all of you will find that, if those carbohydrate cravings return, you can cure them with several days of *Induction* dieting. But this simple maneuver is, for many hard-core recidivists, more easily said than done. A professional recidivist, for reasons known only to him or herself, will not return to the *Induction* diet, until he or she has regained *all* the weight or is experiencing intolerable symptoms. But I think recidivists are made, not born, and if you catch yourself procrastinating, or worse yet, not even thinking about nipping your regain while it is still a bud, you can avoid this behavior by recognizing that your decision to lose any regained weight *immediately* is the best way to manage this lifetime plague.

Back to Maintenance

Meanwhile, how's it going to go while you're cruising along at your desired weight?

On the *Maintenance* diet, you can add in most vegetables, nuts, and berries. You can cautiously reintroduce the vegetables containing more than 10% carbohydrate, as well as whole grains such as oats, barley, millet, wild rice, couscous, or buckwheat. You may even be able to handle an occasional potato and a fruit a day. You can begin to use recipes that contain some carbohydrate ingredients (breaded veal chops, etc.). But the last choice for you, the truly hazardous indulgence, is sweets. Frankly, my suggestion to you is that you restrict your consumption of sweets made with real sugars to the occasional slice of birthday or wedding cake. Those of you who have had a sizable chunk of your life made miserable by sugar may even decide, after graciously accepting them, to quietly deposit those pieces on somebody else's plate.°

Your Metabolic Tendencies Are Never Cured

You never are, you know. Your fat is one symptom of a lifetime chronic illness. You do have and always will have a metabolic tendency to overweight. The problem of hyperinsulinism that I identified for you will not go away because you have taken a nutritional path that circumvents it. If you go back to eating the way you once did, or even partly so, you will arouse the sleeping demon. In very short order, your body will secrete large quantities of insulin, you'll suffer the symptoms of low blood sugar, and your insulin resistance will lead to the production of more insulin and that, in turn, to weight gain.

If you want to be healthy and free of surplus body fat, then you cannot return to a perfectly random and careless pattern of eating. Thus one of the chief purposes of this book has been to build good habits into your lifestyle.

°My other suggestion is to create your own personal world of sweets made with artificial sweeteners or stevia or tagatose. The recipe section at the end of the book will introduce you to the concept and give some of our most successful ideas. By using sugar substitutes, you really have the ability to create sugarless versions of your favorite sweets.

But What About My Bad Habits?

Of course, we all have them. Food is so confusing, so delicious, so psychologically essential even at times when it's not physiologically necessary. We all eat for pleasure and for reassurance, as well as nutrition.

It may have been a hard week at work, and when you get to the weekend one of the things you definitely intend to get into is a little modest pigging out (or perhaps not so modest).

I, too, enjoy binges. The question really is what type of binge. *Parade* magazine did a food survey in November 1991, and, when they asked people what foods they usually binged on, the first five answers were chocolates, desserts, cookies, ice cream, and candy.

I would prefer that you binge on protein/fat foods. I say that not because you can't gain a pound or two if you put away too many two-inch-thick steaks, but because protein foods are fundamentally self-limiting. Everyone has eaten thirty cookies at one sitting at some time in their life, and many carbohydrate addicts have done it hundreds of times, but how many people have eaten ten hard-boiled eggs at one sitting? People just don't do it. Protein and fat foods satiate appetite quite quickly. It really isn't possible to go on munching them endlessly, and hardly anyone desires to. That doesn't mean that a chicken breast doesn't make a delicious snack, and that, combined with a few other things, it doesn't make a delicious minor binge.

The crucial fact about protein foods is that they don't unleash a metabolic tidal wave in your body. Very few people get a protein addiction. Your blood glucose level doesn't sharply rise and fall when you sit down to eat a western salad. But it does just that when you sit down to eat a slice of pie. That leads to the need for another slice and then another.

I don't want to scare you with the prospect of never eating another piece of Grandma's pumpkin pie. If you weren't an uncontrolled carbohydrate addict with severe obesity that only this diet has been able to cure, then you could probably indulge occasionally.

Only you know how *addicted* you are to the sweet stuff—and that's the real test. If you aren't addicted, then you have room to maneuver. The occasional slice of pizza or the ice cream everyone seems to enjoy just might be permissible. But be careful: When those first five pounds go back on—and they will—take yourself firmly in hand and get back to your ideal weight.

And remember, the way you're eating now is healthful. Junk food isn't, and it isn't going to make you feel good. After you've been off them for a while, the ice cream or the pizza go down nice, but once you've eaten them, you may notice a temporary return of some familiar old symptoms. I don't recommend such compromises, I simply recognize that human nature demands them now and then. And in case you're worried about the fact that *your* personalized, metabolically corrective, heart-healthy diet is quite different from the high-carbohydrate, 30%-fat diet that the government agencies and their food-industry-supported advisers are recommending, just look back at Part 3 of this book. The facts should provide some comfort.

Some Parting Recommendations

For those of you who have been successful, your diet voyage seems to be almost over. In fact, it continues, but you're going to be at the helm, and the boat will be responding to your guidance. So, I want to leave you with a few basic principles for your lifetime on the Atkins diet:

1. Be food aware—remember that fresh meat, fish, fowl, vegetables, nuts, seeds, and occasional fruits and starches are the foods nature designed you to eat. That packaged stuff in the supermarket puts money in somebody's pocket. But try not to put it in your stomach. This is the only body you've got. Notice how good it feels now. Notice how much better it looks. Keep it that way.

2. Be wary—endlessly wary—of sugar and corn syrup, and white flour and corn starch. Look at the labels of whatever packaged foods you find yourself obliged to buy and avoid like the plague the packages that contain sugar, corn syrup, honey, maltose, dextrose, fructose, lactose, sorbitol, and all the other variations and inventions of the modern sugar-refining industry.

3. Individualize your diet. Try new foods. Increase the variety of foods that you like and enjoy. Use the recipes provided in Part 5 of this book, or in one of the companion cookbooks. This will help to prevent you from going back to eating foods that you have enjoyed in the past, but which simply aren't good for you. I most strongly recommend that you develop a menu that's appealing, tasty, and satisfying to you. You need to be happy

with the food you eat. Once you're happy with eating healthy foods, your dietary future is almost assuredly going to be a healthy one.

4. Continue your already established and effective program of vita-nutrient supplementation. I've told you some of what you need to know. Chapter 22 provides further details.

5. Use caffeine and alcohol in moderation.

6. Remember that addictions can only be managed through abstinence.

7. Take care of weight regain promptly and effectively by returning to the *Induction* phase of the diet for as long as it takes to get all the way back to the weight you have designated as your goal weight. Swear that you will *never* allow yourself to be more than a two-week diet away from that goal weight.

8. Exercise.

One final word. You may have noticed that a National Institutes of Health consensus panel recently reported that the record of the best low-calorie diet programs suggests that "90 to 95% of dieters regain all or most of their hard-lost pounds within five years."

But when a program changes the *composition* of the diet, not the quantity, and when pre-maintenance teaching and the five-pound rule are consistently applied, recidivism is a rare phenomenon, indeed. Our patient files resoundingly confirm this fact.

21 | *Exercise— A Pleasant Path to Slimness*

Since I thrive on controversy, I haven't mentioned exercise. My stand on exercise (I applaud it and encourage it) is the least controversial part of the book. Which doesn't mean exercise isn't important for you. Not only is it an essential part of the program, but in cases of severe metabolic resistance, it's likely to be the difference between success and spinning your wheels.

Of course, exercise really ought to be a part of any diet program. I've helped many people become slim who didn't want to exercise and therefore never did, but all of them would have been much better off if they had been willing to incorporate a reasonable amount of healthy exercise into their lives.

When you go on a diet, you're trying to change the shape of your body. It's pretty clear that exercise is complementary to this, for exercise is the only other normal activity that actually alters the size, thickness, contours, etc., of the physical you. In our society, the number of people who want to lose weight so they'll feel better is probably exceeded by the number who want to lose so they'll look better. Exercise is important for both purposes. It's just plain good for you.

Take Out Some Heart Insurance

I suspect that the modest decline in the rate of heart disease that we say in the 1970s and '80s is directly attributable to the fitness boom. Dr. Kenneth Cooper's *Aerobics* and the many running, jogging, stretching, and jumping books that came after it really touched a nerve in America. People saw that this was something good, something entirely positive in a time of great negativity—the era of Vietnam and Watergate—and they went right after it.

Exercise's time had come, and a good thing too. What a bunch of couch potatoes we were becoming! I was as guilty as the next person. It's so easy to sit down in front of the TV and let gravity have its way with you. But I've discovered like millions of other people that there's a great deal of exhilaration to be gotten out of moving one's limbs. I didn't need to be convinced about the health benefits.

Population studies—what the medical world calls epidemiological studies—can clarify your thinking quite a bit on this point. Coronary artery disease has been shown to be almost three times as likely among Washington, D.C.'s sedentary postal clerks as among its physically active mail carriers. In another study, North Dakota's non-farmers were found to be twice as much at risk as its farmers.

Nor is heart disease the only area in which exercise functions protectively. Obesity, hypertension, adult-onset diabetes, osteoporosis, and even cancer are all significantly less common among the physically active.

And What If You're Having a Hard Time Losing

Meanwhile, you want to lose weight. If you fell into that category of metabolic resistance that I've just been discussing, then exercise can be tremendously important. You're going to need every edge you can get—not just the dietary edge I've been teaching you but the physical movement edge I'm discussing now.

It has been calculated that you could lose 15 pounds a year just by doing thirty minutes of aerobic exercise three times a week. After all, each mile you walk burns a hundred calories. It doesn't sound like much, but those miles add up.

Moreover, even modest quantities of exercise build muscle mass, especially if you've been sedentary, and the cellular structure of muscle is so constituted that it burns more energy than do your fat cells. That's true even while you're being inactive. Therefore, a person who exercises is slowly but steadily shifting his body toward greater energy consumption and therefore greater slimness. This, too, is a form of metabolic advantage, and I hope you'll seize it.

What Are the Advantages to Exercise?

1. Exercise can be fun.
2. Exercise can make your body look better and help you lose weight.
3. Exercise can (indeed, almost certainly will) make you healthier.
4. Exercise can make you feel good. After the first few days of fatigue, it will give you more energy, and it will make you fitter for any and all of life's challenges.
5. Exercise reduces the output of insulin, "the fattening hormone."[1]

What Are the Drawbacks to Exercise?

1. There are none.

What Are the Reasons Given for Not Exercising?

1. Laziness. This is usually the real reason, and I can hardly criticize you with a straight face since, for much of my life, I've been guilty myself. The solution for you may be what it was for me: Find an exercise you really like (in my case, tennis) and build your fitness program around that. I still don't like many forms of exercise, but I do some of them, because I tell myself they'll help me to play tennis better.
2. Lack of time. Oh, how often I've heard this one. Please, tell it to the Marines. Listen, folks, if you sleep 8 hours a night, that still leaves you with 16 hours a day. Subtract 8 hours for working and 2 for eating and personal hygiene, and there are still 6 hours left. You can find *some* time in those 6 hours for exercise. Your body is one of your most serious responsibilities, since you're going to have an extraordinarily difficult time fulfilling your other responsibilities without it. If you can't squeeze out half an hour a day, you know whose throat you're cutting.
3. Age and/or poor physical conditioning. If you're over a hundred, call me for a special consultation to discuss the possibility of your not exercising; the rest of you won't get away with this lame excuse. As for poor conditioning, that's exactly what we're trying to remedy.

4. Ill health. That's a reason to start slowly and proceed cautiously, not a remission of sentence. An exercise program can be tailored to any condition, and the sickest person can start at a level appropriate to his condition. If you still have the use of your limbs, then you can exercise.

What Are the Types of Exercise?

> Remember, if you're over 35, before you undertake any exercise program more strenuous than brisk walking, have a doctor examine you and conduct a stress test to check for cardiovascular problems.

Aerobic Exercise

Aerobic exercise is exercise that challenges your heart rate and causes increased oxygen consumption. Walking is only very mildly aerobic because the level of exertion is so low. Aerobic dancing, cross-country skiing, simulated skiing, running, swimming, speed walking, rowing, and bicycling are all highly aerobic. The benefits of such exercise are immense, quite apart from weight loss. Every cell in your body requires a constant supply of oxygen, and if you've been a couch potato for years, then many of them are being starved of their proper supply. *This means that once you accustom yourself to a regular routine of aerobic exercise, you will positively begin to feel physically better than you did before.* Except for death and taxes, nothing is more certain than this fact.

If you take up some form of vigorous aerobic exercise, then I'd urge you to get some form of professional advice or at least buy a self-help book on the type of exercise you want to do. It's important to learn how to do limbering and stretching exercises, so you can loosen up your muscles, prevent tightness, and reduce the chance of injuring yourself. Running, because of its impact on your knees and ankles, requires care *and* a good pair of running shoes.

Those of you who haven't exercised in a long time, or who want to prevent osteoporosis, might want to try an exercise trampoline. The purpose here is to increase the vertical stress on the weight-bearing skeleton such that the vertebrae respond to a signal that more calcium must be laid down along the stress-bearing planes. The springs in the trampoline allow you to absorb a cushioned major impact. The more calcium you accumulate premenopausally, the better you will withstand the involutional calcium loss.

Anaerobic Exercise

This term refers to any type of exercise that isn't significantly aerobic. This includes many types of exercise that build muscle mass, like weight lifting and indeed many forms of physical work. Such exercise is not nearly as healthy and heart protective as aerobic exercise, but it can have two benefits: It will help to shape your body and make you more attractive, and because it builds muscle, it will make it easier for you to maintain an ideal weight. If you increase your musculature by a considerable degree, then you will find that the ideal weight is somewhat higher than an insurance table would lead you to expect, since muscle weighs more than fat.

Mildly Aerobic Exercise

Exercise such as walking, golf, tennis, horseback riding, ping-pong, and dancing may only mildly increase the pumping action of your heart and the activity of your lungs, but they are still tremendous improvements on the lifestyle of a non-exerciser. If you want to feel good and live a long life, then I think the least you should do is accustom yourself to taking a half-hour walk each day, preferably at a brisk pace.

For the life-long non-exerciser, walking is just simply the best way to begin. I know that many of my readers will be people who for years haven't traveled further than two blocks except in an automobile. Great! Tremendous improvements in your well-being lie just ahead of you. Walk five blocks. Then try six. If a ten-minute walk is hard on you today, stiffness will ease, breathing will improve, and relaxing endorphins will be released into your body. Before you know it, you'll be walking a mile. All you need do is break through the initial crust of bad habits. Feeling good when you move is natural. Not feeling good is a highly artificial state. Remember that Mother Nature would certainly consider today's "modern" lifestyle an aberration.

What Do You Do to Get Started?

1. Work with your own schedule and figure out what part of the day you're going to reserve for exercise. Many people who

have busy lives find that the only way they can consistently get in their exercise is to do it first thing in the morning. If that's the case with you, then why don't you lay out your clothes and your walking or running shoes before you go to bed at night, and when you get up in the morning simply step into them and get going. You can always wash and eat after you've put in your half-hour.

2. Start your exercise plan slowly for the first few weeks. Begin by doing less than you think you can do. If a ten-block walk seems hard, then do eight. You'll find that progress is rapid. Each successive day, you can do a little more. Lots of people start too aggressively. The purpose of an exercise plan is not to exhaust yourself. If you do vigorous aerobic exercise, then you should not do it seven days a week; five should be the maximum. If you start a weight-lifting program, *never* do it two days in a row.

3. If you're very overweight, you should start with walking. That will be challenge enough. After all, until you get that weight off, your chance of injuring your joints with some form of highly active exertion is *much* greater.

A Few Final Comments

When you exercise, there should be a normal elevation of your pulse rate. If you feel dizzy or have chest pain, *STOP*. It is obviously time for you to check things out with your personal physician.

If everything goes normally, you will probably find that you can increase your exercise by 10 to 20% each week.

Many people will discover after just a couple of weeks of exercise that they're pleasantly addicted. This is one of the few addictions in this life of ours that you need never fear.

Even the most confirmed non-exercisers among you will find that after two or three months, you've formed a habit that can remain pleasantly and easily part of your life forever.

Go to it. The only things you have to lose are the chains of inactivity.

22 | *Nutritional Supplements— The Secrets of the Atkins Center*

The essential fact you must know for this chapter is that the best doctors I know actually *treat* their patients with vita-nutrients. By that I mean they use what I call a "nutritional pharmacology" and they prescribe what Dr. Stephen de Felice calls "nutraceuticals."

These terms may lead you to ask, "Is there a system of treating illness with nutrients and natural substances, instead of the drugs and pharmaceuticals that nearly every doctor prescribes?"

Well, I'm glad you asked; I was afraid you never would. There indeed is such a system. It is rapidly growing in popularity and has been embraced by over a thousand physicians and a hundred times that many non-physician health practitioners. I call it Complementary Medicine, because the basic tenet is that all healing arts can and should be made to complement one another. Another basic tenet is that the practitioner of Complementary Medicine should select the safest therapies first. That's why the Complementarist is so likely to use nutritional therapies; their safety, when compared to the drugs they replace, approaches infinity.

Now, I certainly am a Complementary physician. In fact, there are a few plaques on my wall suggesting that there are those who think I'm one of the leaders of this movement. And so I have a confession to make. Mary Anne Evans, Harry Kronberg, and all the other patients of mine whose case histories help personalize this book were all given something more than the Atkins diet.

All my patients—and my case examples were no exceptions—receive a fairly significant amount of vitamins, minerals, essential fatty acids, nutritional agents called intermediary metabolites, and herbs that work nutritionally—the entire group referred to as vita-nutrients. I prescribe them because I have learned from my clinical experience, my reading, and my attendance at medical meetings, to say nothing of interviewing around one hundred of the world's greatest health science leaders every year for my daily radio broadcasts, that nutrients can impact anyone's health.

I have found so many vita-nutrients to be valuable, conferring health advantages *even for healthy people*, that I no longer consider that a person following a theoretically optimal, even "perfect," diet could live as long or as healthfully as he could were he also to take nutritional supplements.

I'll cite just one example to prove my point. The antioxidant group of nutrients, when tested scientifically, are consistently shown to confer significant protection against damage caused by free radicals, violently active, environmentally-engendered electrons implicated in the causation of cancer, heart disease, and aging. Even a person with a perfect diet is not living in a perfect environment, and so he can maintain his good health longer if he takes the effective doses of vitamins A, C, E, plus selenium, glutathione, cysteine, CoQ_{10}, and bioflavonoids.

Studies have been done seeking to find the maximal effective doses of nutrients. Two-time Nobelist Linus Pauling concluded that most of us should be taking 10 gms of vitamin C daily. In fact, when all the useful nutrients are considered and we ask the question *What is the optimal dose for each,* the best scientific answer might lead us to take over 100 vitamin pills per day.

Since that clearly isn't practical, I was led, of necessity, to devise a system of nutritional prescribing I called Targeted Nutrition. This allows me to prescribe (and individuals to select for themselves) a variety of formulations targeted to the nutritional needs appropriate to certain clinical problems. For instance, if a person is subject to frequent colds and viruses, and wants to make sure that he has the nutritional support to help prevent one, he might opt for an acute infection formula such as the one we at the Atkins Center call "Colds & Flu." Such a formula contains the vitamins C and A, plus zinc, bioflavonoids and the B-complex constituents that published studies have shown to make a nutritional difference in our ability to fight off such invaders.

Unlike drugs, the nutritional agents are not directed against the disease. Rather, they are in support of the host's ability to mount a defense against the disease, which he can do so much better when his nutrition is provided for. The world has been programmed to believe that one fights illness by attacking it with a combination of killer drugs, but, since I have been using nutrition, my patients get well much faster and much more thoroughly when their own resistance is supported nutritionally.

The application of Targeted Nutrition certainly extends to those whose chief concern is the loss of weight, and, for this purpose, I have devised a dieter's basic formula, a sort of companion piece to the Atkins diet. I'll tell you about it, so you won't necessarily have to get it from Atkins Nutritionals (in the sale of whose vitamins, I, of course, have a personal financial involvement) but can simply provide yourself with a collection of vitamins providing the equivalent nutritional support.

Our Atkins Diet Basic #3 Formula contains all the ingredients in our basic multiple vitamin, although in somewhat different dosages. It was designed to be taken in a dose of three to six a day (the larger dose for 200-plus pounders), but even double that would present virtually no risk of overdosing. It differs from the usual basic formula in that it contains greater amounts of chromium, pantethine, selenium, vanadium, and biotin. This group of nutrients is emphasized because of scientific reports suggesting that they all play nutritional roles in glucose, insulin, and lipid metabolism. Our Dieter's Formula (Basic #3) follows.

Dieter's Formula
Basic #3

Vitamin A	200 IU
Beta-Carotene	500 IU
Vitamin D-3	15 IU
Thiamine (HC1) (B_1)	5 mg
Riboflavin (B_2)	4 mg
Vitamin C (buffered)	120 mg (150 mg)
Niacin (B_3)	2 mg
Niacinamide	5 mg
Pantethine (80%)	25 mg (30 mg)
Pantothenic Acid (B_5)	25 mg
Pyridoxal-5-Phosphate	2 mg
Pyridoxine (HC1) (B_6)	20 mg
Folic Acid	200 mcg
Biotin	75 mcg
Cyanocobalamin (B_{12})	30 mcg
Vitamin E (D alpha tocopherol)	20 IU
Copper (Sulfate)	200 mcg
Magnesium (Oxide)	8 mg
Choline (Bitartrate)	100 mg
Inositol	80 mg
PABA	100 mg

Manganese (Chelate)	4 mg
Zinc (Chelate)	10 mg
Citrus Bioflavonoids	150 mg
Chromium Polynicotinate	50 mcg
Molybdenum (Sodium)	10 mcg
Vanadyl Sulfate	15 mcg
Selenium	40 mcg
Octacosanol	150 mcg
N-Acetyl-L-Cysteine	20 mg
L-Glutathione (reduced)	5 mg

In a base of intestinal flora and growth factors to facilitate uptake in the lower intestine.

Suggested Dosage: 3 to 6 tablets daily with meals.

Chromium deserves the most attention. First discovered as the unique mineral constituent of the Glucose Tolerance Factor (GTF), a molecule which serves as a sort of catalyst for the action of insulin at its receptor sites, chromium was beginning to be thought of as an essential nutrient, and GTF was being considered for recognition as a true vitamin. In many ways this was a frustrating state of affairs, because finding a food source for chromium is actually quite difficult. Only brewer's yeast seemed to qualify, and, as you learned in Chapter 13, the 30% of the population deemed to be overstocked with *Candida albicans* would not do well on such a food. However, it has recently been discovered that the picolinate of chromium is well assimilated, and a spate of studies have shown that chromium will build muscle (an anabolic effect) and decrease body fat, plus lower the cholesterol levels.[1]

You are probably best served by taking in chromium in dosages of 300–600 mcg per day.

Pantethine is the intermediary between the B vitamin pantothenic acid and the important coenzyme A. It plays a pivotal role in many metabolic pathways and is a remarkable cholesterol-control nutrient. It is valuable in allergy, colitis, and stress, and in yeast infections. I use 100 to 400 mg daily.[*2]

Selenium is valuable as an antioxidant and its deficiency seems to provide an increased cancer risk. In addition, a recent animal study by McNeill suggested that it plays a beneficial nutritional role in diabetes prevention. I think 200 mcg is a proper adult daily dose.[3]

---

[*]Pantethine poses problems for the vitamin manufacturer since it exists as a liquid form. We have seen products where pantethine was listed on the label but, on assay, contained none. Make certain that the product you use contains adequate pantethine.

Biotin is one of those unsung B vitamins whose nutritional role was recently emphasized when J.C. Coggeshall and his associates noted a significant drop in diabetics' blood-sugar levels when biotin was given.[4]

And just another good word about vitamin C supplementation. G.J. Naylor and his associates did a double blind placebo-controlled study on 41 extremely overweight women who had failed at previous weight-loss efforts. After six weeks, the control group had lost an average of 2.1 pounds, but the group receiving 3 gms of C daily lost 5.7 pounds.[5] Not earth-shattering to be sure, but when combined with vitamin C's advantages in shoring up our resistance to infections, I want to make sure you are all adequately provided with ascorbic acid.

After you decide on an appropriate multiple vitamin and mineral preparation, the next most important nutritional group for long-range supplementation is the essential fatty acids. You won't find these in a multiple vitamin because they exist physically as oils. Oils and dry powders mix very poorly, and so they must be taken separately. There are two types of essential fatty acids that most of us really do need. One type is the omega-3 series, which occurs in animal sources (fish and marine mammals primarily) and vegetable sources (linseed or flax oil), providing the essential oil, alpha-linolenic acid. Another type if a special omega-6 subdivision called gamma linolenic acid, found useful in atopic eczema, PMS, cholesterol elevation, and many other deficiency situations and contained in EPA, borage oil, and black-currant oil.

Essential-oil administration is best done individually by a nutrition counselor, but, for general purposes, I might suggest 2 capsules of borage oil, 2 of fish oil, and 2 of flaxseed oil. Convenience lovers may opt for 6 of the Essential Oils Formula, which contains all of the above and which I prescribe to my patients.

Then there are nutrients whose deficient supply sometimes causes a nutritional logjam. Occasionally metabolic resistance can be explained in part as a nutritional shortcoming. I would like to mention three such nutrients. You may want to study the effect of these upon your dietary responsiveness.

The first of these is L-carnitine. Carnitine is involved in fat transport, and, when it is deficient, overweight people have difficulty getting into ketosis/lipolysis. Carnitine's primary use is in heart disease, where it corrects a common type of cardiomyopathy, helps stabilize heart rhythm, lower triglyceride levels, and increase

HDL cholesterol. For these conditions, the dosage ranges between 1000 and 2000 mg daily.[6]

Coenzyme Q_{10} is another nutrient essential to heart function. It is also essential to proper working of the immune system and is a specific nutritional correction for periodontal (gum) disease. But overweight readers might be interested in a Belgian study, headed by Dr. Luc Van Gall, which showed that over half of a group of obese patients had *deficiency* levels of CoQ_{10} and compared them with a similar group without deficiency.[7] After nine weeks, the formerly deficient group lost 29.7 pounds on a standard diet, compared to the nondeficient ones who lost 12.7 pounds on the same diet. If this work mirrors the incidence of CoQ_{10} deficiency in all overweight subjects, then one out of two of you will benefit considerably from this single nutrient. Van Gall used 100 mg daily in his research.

Pyridoxine alpha-ketoglutarate (PAK) is less well studied, but it does seem to have a favorable effect on diabetes. Any nutrient capable of facilitating the action of insulin should quite logically be helpful for those who are struggling to lose weight. I use between 500 and 1500 mg daily.

So the basic supplementation consists of:

Basic formula for dieters—6 times a day.
Chromium—300 mcg daily or slightly more, unless it is in your basic formula.
Essential oils—3 to 6 a day, or individual GLA, EPA, and flax.
L-carnitine, CoQ_{10} and PAK—if you determine that they help.

Additional Advantages

Now that I've laid out the basic framework of supplementation for all of you, here are specific nutritional answers to common dieters' problems:

- For constipation: You may use magnesium oxide, extra vitamin C, or a variety of vegetable laxatives and bulking agents. My favorite choice is psyllium husks. Start with 1 tablespoon in one full glass of water and increase or decrease the dose until the optimal bowel movement is obtained.
- For sugar cravings: L-glutamine, 500–1000 mg before meals and perhaps right at the point in time when craving is

greatest.[8] Extra chromium is valuable here, too.

- For hunger not assuaged by being in ketosis: L-phenylalanine or acetyl L-tyrosine, 500 mg of the former, or 300 mg of the latter, before meals.[9]
- For fluid retention: Pyridoxal 5 phosphate, 50–100 mg, plus taurine 1500–3000 mg daily.[10] Asparagus tablets work very well here, too.
- For fatigue: Octacosanol, 5–10 mg, PABA, 600–2000 mg, dimethylglycine, 3 to 6 sublingual tablets per day, sublingual B_{12} tablets, 1–3 daily, or 1–3 B complex tablets daily (50 mg strength).[11]
- For nervousness: Inositol, 500 to 2000 mg daily, and herbal teas such as camomile, valerian, and passion flower.[12]
- For insomnia: The above taken at night, plus melatonin, 3 to 6 mg before bed (ties your sleep cycle into day/night cycle; counterproductive for night workers). Calcium, magnesium, niacinamide, pantothenic acid, and 5-hydroxy tryptophan may all be useful here as well.[13]

Nutrition and Health Problems

Now let's talk about a supplement program for common medical problems that affect a significant portion of my dieting patients.

Let me simply list what I prescribe. I make no claims that the nutrients below have a direct therapeutic effect on the conditions for which they are used. The effects they have are accomplished through nutritional pathways. Since I have been prescribing in this manner, my patients show clinical improvements four or five times more frequently than they did when I practiced a very competent brand of orthodox internal medicine. This fact can only be attributed to the high percentage of my patients who have specific nutritional deficiencies.

- For hypoglycemics, I use the basic formula, Blood Sugar Formula, plus chromium, L-glutamine, zinc, selenium, magnesium, all of the B complex, PAK, extra biotin, L-alanine; or else I use Atkins Formula HF-12.[14]
- For diabetes, I use the basic formula, Blood Sugar Formula, plus extra chromium, zinc, selenium, inositol, CoQ_{10}, PAK, biotin, vanadyl sulfate, magnesium; or else I use Atkins formula DM-17.[15]

- For the lowering or prevention of cholesterol elevations, I use lecithin granules, chromium, pantethine, niacin and other B complex factors, garlic, vitamin C, GLA (borage, primrose, or black-currant oils), EPA (fish oil), beta-sitosterol, glucomannan, guar gum, pectin, psyllium husks, dimethyl glycine, CoQ_{10}, phosphatidyl choline, or I use the Vita-Nutrient "Cholesterol" formula plus the Essential Oils Formula.[16]

- For elevated triglycerides, the slate is similar to the list for cholesterol, except that L-carnitine and EPA are emphasized. Also, because of the correlation of triglycerides and hyperinsulinism, the nutrients helpful in diabetes will prove to be helpful here.[17]

- For hypertension, I use magnesium (preferably as orotate, taurate, arginate, or aspartate), taurine, pyridoxal 5 phosphate or pyridoxine, garlic, essential fatty acids (GLA and EPA), CoQ_{10}, potassium, or I use the Atkins Essential Oils Formula and the Blood Pressure Formula.[18]

- For coronary heart disease, I use one of the above-mentioned magnesium compounds, L-carnitine, vitamin E, CoQ_{10}, serrapeptase and/or bromelain, garlic, chromium picolinate, or I use formula CV-4.[19]

- For arthritis, I use shark cartilage, superoxide dismutase, calcium EAP, pantethine, niacinamide, pyridoxine, PABA, vitamin C, bioflavonoids, vitamin E, SOD/catalase, copper sebacate, or I use the Atkins formula AA-5, plus the Essential Oils Formula.[20]

The roster of nutrients which have been studied favorably in these conditions should provide a glimmer of insight into how much published work there is on nutraceuticals. Consider at the same time the almost obscene profit margins consistently reported by the pharmaceutical industry and you may get a flash of recognition as to why all these bona fide medical studies supporting a competing therapy are not widely disseminated. When your doctor doesn't tell you about them, it's only because nobody told him about them.

The restriction of carbohydrate gives you an edge and, similarly, the targeted use of nutritional supplements gives you another kind of edge. Learn about them, learn how to use them, and use them properly. When you do, the Edge will surely be with you.

23 | *Eating Your Way to Permanent Slimness in the Real World*

I have thoroughly explained the glorious experience of discovering the Metabolic Advantage, inducing a hunger-free state by the unrestricted eating of protein food, advancing level by level into more and more interesting meal plans, merging happily, yet imperceptibly, into a lifetime of eating luxuriously and healthfully while keeping at your goal weight. But does it really happen this way?

You can be sure it does, but ask me how often the scenario unfolds in precisely this sequence, and I would have to estimate about once in ten times. On the other hand, how often is that goal of slimness reached and kept through a more circuitous course involving starts and stops, and recoveries and snafus and thrills and disappointments and surprises and frustrations and the need to resort to willpower and discipline, *and* the cleverness and wisdom to use the metabolic edge to your own advantage? Put another way: How often is the trip to slimness more like something planned by a very inept travel agent? My patient records indicate this happens more like six times out of ten.

We don't all get there the way it was worked out on the drawing board because we are confronted with a gigantic obstacle called the Real World. In the Real World, there can be sad events that can upset us so that we turn for solace to our old reliable friends, the foods that have always comforted us. There can be happy events—vacations, holiday times, let's-bring-out-the-Champagne celebrations, family weddings, and unrestrained dinner parties. There can be business traveling, unexpected illnesses or surgery, or financial squeezes. In all of these situations, that chain of events I outlined will be broken and we determined dieters will have to find ways to right ourselves and get back on course. And, with the tools I'll give you, you will.

Please note that the Real World problems I just mentioned are not intrinsic built-in obstacles to our program, as they are when you use diet centers that provide you with food or formulas. At such establishments, trying to maintain weight loss *without* the pre-packaged food or protein drinks requires an entirely new technique of adapting to rearranged hunger signals. That transition must be thoroughly provided for in the program; when it is not, it is truly appropriate to call such a program a scam.

Our program starts in the Real World, continued in the Real World, and endures in the Real World. Once you learn to apply the basic principle of staying at or below your CCLs, you never have to change. You make your adjustment at the beginning, and that's that. If the connotation of the word "diet" is "something with a beginning and an end," then this is not a diet, it's simply a new and better way to adept your eating to your metabolism for the rest of your life.

I, for example, have perfected dieting down to the point where there is only one thing I cannot resist. That one thing is temptation.

I hope that last line got a chuckle, because it contains so much of the truth. The real obstacle in the real world is, for most of us, temptation.

Dealing with Temptation

So, let's overcome temptation, not with our willpower, which is so often in short supply, but with our brains, a potentially unlimited resource.

Imagine that you're doing great, losing weight, feeling better than ever, thrilled with yourself, hearing compliments from friends and semi-strangers alike, and *you want something you're not supposed to have*. What to do?

There are three long-range strategies you can employ:

1. You can talk yourself out of your momentary passion and stay the course.
2. You can bend the diet, but not break it.
3. You can fall into the non-strategy strategy and break the diet, in which case you'll have to act quickly to get yourself out of trouble. Or alternatively, you can break the diet *as a strategy*, which occasionally can be quite a useful technique.

The First Strategy

Staying on the diet is your first line of defense. But what if you want something to eat, and it isn't just any food you want and certainly not more of the same, but quite specifically something *you're not allowed to have*? Worse yet, it may even be something you were allowed to have on all those other diets. You remember, the ones you gained on or couldn't stay on. What now?

My advice is: Never ignore a craving; it may pass, but it is likely to reappear momentarily when your resolve is weak. And then you break the diet. Since craving is part and parcel of addiction, that could trigger a cycle of addictive eating behavior. If this has ever happened to you, then you yourself may actually be an addict.

The correct response, I've learned from experience, is to *change your physiology*. Let me elaborate, because this point might save your diet—and your life. Your craving appeared, most likely, in a relatively fasting state; it was triggered by a fall in blood glucose and your body perceived a need to brake the falling glucose level and gave a signal that sweets were needed. (This theory only applies when you crave some form of quick-fix carbohydrate.)

Your strategy will be to change your physiology from a fasting to a fed state. In layman's language that means *eat something*. In Atkins diet language, food, rich food, and plenty of it, but, of course, fat and protein food with very little or no carbohydrate. This will stabilize your blood glucose and all the other constituents that give rise to the craving signal. Presto! No more craving.

The best foods to do this with are macadamia nuts, the dieter's best friend. Other nut choices are walnuts, pecans, or brazils. Other foods for stopping cravings are cream cheese or rich dessert cheeses like mascarpone, St. Andre, or Explorateur. You can also do this with something sweet—either artificially so or with stevia, I must emphasize—and with heavy cream. Put three or four tablespoons of heavy cream into a glass and make an instant farmer's soda by topping it with your favorite diet soda, or you could learn to make my personal favorite by whipping up 3 ounces of heavy cream and adding in ⅔ of a scoop of my Shake Mix and create a chocolate, vanilla, or cappuccino mousse. Or you may opt for diet gelatin dessert slathered generously with whipped heavy cream (not the pre-made, sugar-added type, of course).

I'm sure you already understand the basic principle of this kind of eating. Macadamia nuts, for instance, may be on every conventional diet's no-no list because they are so calorically dense, but what counts is the effect they have upon your body chemistry. Macadamia nuts, by having such a high ketogenic ratio (fat divided by carbohydrate) suppress the appetite and tend to result in your eating fewer calories per day. Moreover, let's not forget convenience—all nuts are extremely portable; they can easily be kept in your purse or shirt or coat pocket. If your business or travel schedule forces you to miss meals or be frequently exposed to unacceptable meals, you've got a meal substitute at hand, a perfect tide-me-over.

Another favorite of mine now that we're beyond the level of *Induction* dieting is the avocado. As the only fat-containing fruit in common usage, most of it in the beneficial monounsaturated category, this unique vegetable product provides a welcome taste departure for those who crave something fresh, natural, and filling. A half avocado, with the big hollow where its giant seed resided, can serve as an edible cup in which to place shrimp or crabmeat or tun salad and thus provide that elegant lunch that makes the time between your filling breakfast and your satisfying dinner pass so happily. A California avocado contains about 12 gms of carbohydrate, about the same as ½ an apple. And then there's guacamole; you'll find my favorite recipe on page 316.

At the other end of the spectrum is a convenience food that sounds terribly fatty but, in fact, contains nearly none. Those are the maximizers of crispness, fried pork rinds—the zero carbohydrate consolation price for corn or potato chip addicts. Virtually all the fat has been rendered off, leaving you with the protein matrix that held the pork fat together. Your paté, sour-cream-based dips, and guacamole find an exceedingly crisp and comfortable home atop a fried pork rind.

But what if we're not talking about an addictive craving or a simple impulse that can be satisfied by a change in body chemistry? What if we're talking about long-term desire? Something you always knew was one of your favorite foods and now is on your no-no list. You know, things like French fries, pizza, bagels, tacos, egg rolls, pancakes, linguini, and . . . well, why torture you any more.

Finding Food Passion Substitutes

One of the best don't-fall-off-the-diet techniques is to eat foods that substitute for a desired food. If your not-so-secret desire is for any of the above, or for blintzes, lasagna, Yorkshire pudding, or even sweets, from chocolate truffles to ice cream, cheesecake, or strawberry shortcake, then the answer is in using the ingeniously developed substitutes for these foods I've provided in the recipe section or through Atkins Nutritionals.° Learn to use them. They are just as much a part of your diet as is a grilled chicken and tossed salad.

Spend as many months as you can integrating these recipes into your new diet and lifestyle and keep absolutely clear in your mind that *our* cheesecake is not *their* cheesecake, and *our* pizza is not *their* pizza, because their foods can be ten times more dense in carbohydrate content. Calorie-restricted foods may be legally called low calorie if the calorie level is reduced by 33%, but our carbohydrate alternatives are down a whopping 90% in carbohydrate. Great, isn't it? It is unless you deviate. There is enough carbohydrate in the real thing that it will change your body's chemistry around completely. One full portion of real pizza or ice cream will send your fat mobilizers, ketones, and lipolysis to a screeching halt.

But there are also carbohydrate-containing foods that are among my favorites. They break the steak-and-salad prototype quite dramatically and yet don't contain enough carbohydrate to do more damage than raise your carbohydrate count a 5-gm level or two.

First and foremost among these discoveries are the crisp breads. My dieting life improved considerably when I found something crunchy and toasted to pile my cream cheese or cold cuts upon or to serve as finger-size appetizers at parties. These toasted rye or wheat-bran delicacies, based on a popular Scandinavian concept, are mostly carbohydrate, so unlimited use of them would be a dieter's disaster. But, because they are baked so thin, they provide so much crisp surface area per carbohydrate gram, they are quite an ingenious way to spend your carbohydrate allowance. There are many brands and each has a different carbohydrate content per crisp, ranging from 3 to 6 grams, some of which is fiber. (Fiber is good for your digestive system and a legitimate deduction from your carbohydrate totals.)

I won't repeat this again, but every food idea I mention could be off limits for those of you who demonstrate food intolerance to one

---

°Formed in response to this very need voiced by thousands of low-carbohydrate dieters, Atkins Nutritionals product line, at this writing, includes cheesecake, protein energy bars, a bake mix, shake mixes, and crunchy cheese chips, all in a variety of flavors with negligible amounts of carbohydrate. Numerous other products are currently in development and each may provide a low-carbohydrate alternative for many dieters' taste preferences.

of its ingredients, and what and rye are two of those foods that turn up rather frequently as food intolerance items.

The Second Strategy

Bending the diet? How can one bend a diet a clearly defined as this one, Dr. Atkins? Well, you can.

By now, you're into the *Ongoing Weight Loss* diet or perhaps the *Maintenance* diet, and you're personalizing your food strategy. You should be using the Carbohydrate Gram Counter at the end of the book to help you decide what foods you can add. Or you may find considerably more usable information in the mini-book titled *Dr. Atkins' New Carbohydrate Gram Counter*.

Study the lists with regard to a) how much you would enjoy the food item, and b) how many grams of carbohydrate it would contain in the portion size you would be content with. You might even want to make a mathematical ratio—enjoyment value/carbohydrate grams—to help you select candidates for your next diet level. Although I would hope that your response would be a little more spontaneous, such as, "Hey, that sounds good to me, and only *x* grams of carbohydrate!"

At any rate, select those candidates for addition to your diet that to you have a high enjoyment-per-gram ratio—and don't forget our recipes! White the selected items down on some note paper and list the gram counts beside them. If you are doing well, and you have found some five or six gram items, you will immediately recognize that adding one of those items per day simply means that you will have moved up one full level on your OWL diet. You're still on track.

But suppose your favorite diet fantasy has ten grams—or twenty. An alternative system for advancing a level is to add forty grams a week. So you might opt for a ten-gram "extra" on Tuesday and Thursday and a twenty-gram diet bender on the weekend. If your CCLL is fairly high, you may even, a few weeks or a month later, add another forty grams per week, or even another after that.

What you are doing is creating your own personal diet plan, based on your demonstrated degree of metabolic resistance and your favorite foods, perhaps the very items you thought would never get on a diet. You are not on the Atkins diet; there never was an Atkins diet; you're on the "Atkins and I" diet. I contributed the principles; you contribute the personalization and execution.

But Sometimes Bending Becomes Breaking

Sometimes, of course, one does more than just bend the diet's carbohydrate quantities—one eats something one is supposed to be avoiding. Every time a dieter does that I am concerned that the food in question may turn out to be the trigger mechanism for an addiction. Then, look out! A full-blown binge usually begins right then and there.

Binges come in all shapes and sizes, and can prove so disastrous they can turn a seemingly sure fire diet success story into an instant failure. The weight regain is usually so profound it can be measured in pounds-per-day, and sometimes in pounds-per-hour. And the time that you're on the binge is certainly an essential question. Don't let it run its course, because all too often that course is not run until you are at your lifetime high point.

To stop a binge, your first responsibility is to know you're in trouble and immediately apply an effective technique. The best way I have found to stop a binge is to take certain nutrients: chromium (picolinate or nicotinate) 400 mcg, 3 times daily for 2 days; plus L-glutamine 500–1000 mg, 3 times daily; plus B complex, 50-mg strength. At the same time, overwhelm the cravings by instituting a high-fat, zero-carbohydrate diet. Fatty red meats, cream cheese, the shake mix or diet soda with heavy cream—and nothing with carbohydrate. Two days after you induce ketosis/lipolysis, the cravings should be done, you should be once again in control, and the weight gained so rapidly during the binge should already be falling to its previous level. And congratulations, you just dodged a bullet.

Back in control again, you had better be figuring out what food or food combination was the binge trigger. You certainly won't want to play with that again.

But there is a hard-core problem that arises when you discover there's something about dieting you don't like. Or more specifically, that there's something you like too much, and you're not getting it. Naturally, you're thinking, "Why did I promise that I would never have that food again? I'm no longer willing to keep that promise." Must always be *always* and never be *never*?

This important question has several answers. In one answer, I ask you to consider the plight of a recovering alcoholic. Most of us realize that when an addiction such as alcoholism is the problem, it is far, far better that never really be *never*. So if your proposed carbohydrate deviation involves something you're addicted to, I sadly must give you that never-never advice. But most of us feel deep down that when we enjoy a lifetime favorite food we're doing it for the sake of pleasure and not out of addiction. So I guess I must allow you to try it and find out.

Breaking with Intent: You Might Try a Reversal Diet

And there is yet another answer—a strategy that will allow you to break away from the constriction of your own successful diet. This strategy is simple, and, I'm sure, to the careful readers of this book, startling. Suppose your favorite missing foods are on *another* diet, but not on this one. You merely have to announce to yourself, "I'm ready to go on the XYZ diet right now." Then do it.

Suppose you develop a longing for a specific food category such as fruit or pasta? You may want to go on an all-fruit diet for three or four days, or an all-pasta diet. This radical departure from what you've been doing so successfully for quite a stretch may seem counterproductive, but it serves a few purposes. It allows you not to have to say to yourself, "I can never eat my favorite food again," and it acts as a metabolic reversal technique, which can sometimes jump-start the low-carbohydrate diet, if it has shown any signs of slowing down. Let me explain.

After many months on a diet which works by virtue of forcing the body to take inefficient metabolic pathways, and thus dissipating hundreds of calories as heat (which presumably is what happens on a strict low-carbohydrate diet), the body may begin to adapt by becoming more efficient, thereby slowing the rate of weight loss. Don't panic as you read this—this adaptation to the lipolytic pathway has never been scientifically demonstrated. Most of you will be able to reach your goal weight and stay there without ever noticing the adaptation phenomenon. But some of you will get the sense that the rate of weight loss has slowed inordinately. You should consider a period of time on a reversal diet.

On the other hand, those of you who cleared up a variety of symptoms on the Atkins diet may have to think twice before embarking on diet reversal, because it's highly probable all (or most of) your symptoms will return on the reintroduction of high-carbohydrate items.

But I think all of you should know the principle of a reversal diet, and many of you should try it somewhere along the line. In reversal dieting, you should go on a regimen very low in fat and protein and high in complex carbohydrates. The aforementioned all-pasta diet, if not mixed with an oily/creamy sauce, qualifies; the all-fruit diet, because its carbohydrates are not complex, does not. (But for three days, why not?) And there are more serious diets that make for ideal reversal techniques. The extreme low-fat version of Dr. Julian Whitaker's diet, or Dr. Dean Ornish's diet, are examples.

The main purpose of reversal dieting is to reestablish the dramatic effect that you must have noticed when you first went on the *Induction* diet, namely, rapid, sustained weight loss. You do it to break up a logjam. Please note that the reversal diet itself is an austere program; it is not a balanced diet, and it most certainly is not taking a break from dieting for a while. When you try to interpose a period of balanced dieting, the result is all too often a rapid regain of weight. The lesson you must learn is that if you "go off the diet," you don't go off into a vacuum, you go *onto* another diet. Make sure that other diet is also one in which *you are in control*.

The Mini-Binge

There is another technique for breaking the diet deliberately, yet remaining in control. It is the 60-minute mini-binge popularized by Drs. Rachel and Richard Heller, and designed for carbohydrate addicts. The Hellers called this carbohydrate binge a reward meal and allowed it every single day. In their program, an austere low-carbohydrate diet could be interrupted by an hour of unrestricted eating, as long as the food was nourishing and well-balanced. The operative principle behind that technique is that insulin is released in two phases when carbohydrates are consumed, and the second and greater amount begins about 75 minutes after your first contact with carbohydrate. You must be sated before that and must have stopped eating within the hour.

If the Hellers' system can be made to work for you, its advantages would be obvious. The disadvantages are major; they are: no emptying of glycogen reserves, therefore no fat mobilization, therefore no ketosis/lipolysis, therefore no metabolic advantage. Those whose overweight is metabolic, in contrast to addiction-based, would not do well. I would suggest, then, that you not do any Hellering until you are close to your goal weight and then to do it little by little, so that you will have familiarized yourself with the effect it has upon your subsequent diet control, your appetite level, and your weight. But you should be aware of the principle because, in case carbohydrate happens to jump into your mouth uninvited, you can do considerable damage control by finishing it before an hour is up. And whatever you do, don't do it in a dining establishment with slow service.

You, Your Diet, and Your Environment

You will note that I have given you a series of strategies for bending the diet or reestablishing it, but that one common denominator can be found in all of them: You are the master strategist. You are in control. Believe me, I've seen a lot of potentially successful dieting experiences fall apart, and almost all of them do so for the same reason—the dieter's loss of control of himself or his environment.

We've just run through some strategies teaching you how to control yourself, so now what's needed is an awareness of what you must do to control your environment.

There can be no doubt that your immediate external environment is much less hospitable to low-carbohydrate dieting than it was at the time the first Diet Revolution was proclaimed 20 years ago. The combined counterrevolution of fat phobia and pharmacophilia has made it difficult for the person who recognizes his own individual differences from the masses and who demands his freedom of choice in matters involving his own health. Instead of being swept up in the hysteria, you now have to fight for the privilege of being different, enlightened and effective at self-preservation.

Training Those Special People

Your first obstacle is people. People whom you normally rely upon for advice—spouses, family members, well-meaning friends, even health professionals with expertise in other areas—are all likely to share the all-too-human trait of being "knee-jerk reactors"—people influenced by buzzwords they've heard so often that they cease to question how the conclusions came about. "Oh, that's a high-fat diet; that can't be good for you" is their reflex response, but you can bet they've never heard of Yudkin or Kekwick or Reaven or Benoit, nor have they ever made an in-depth study of my life's work.

So how do you take charge and teach them? Because, valuable as these persons' advice has been to you in the past, you must remind them that you don't *know* something until you look into it. If your naysayer is someone you live with or must deal with every day, then you know you need their total cooperation as much as you need your own singleness of purpose. If I were you, I would start by insisting that they read this book. "I'm impressed that Dr. Atkins has used his program on so many thousands of people and that he still stands by it," you might suggest, "and I want to know if I can make it work for me. Since I need your support, why don't you study his arguments and his backup carefully and see if you can poke holes in his argument."

You must gain the cooperation of everyone in your immediate environment; resisting temptation is a lot easier if you don't see and smell your favorite carbohydrates. I've mentioned the problem with nonbelievers, but what about those who feel "Dieting is *your* problem; eating is *my* privilege?" Here you must use the pragmatic take-charge person's motto: "If you can't lick 'em, get 'em to join you."

My recommendation is to get your significant others to join you in dieting. If that person in your life is also overweight, you will have a very good selling point—the prospect of *painless* weight loss. But, if he's locked into the low-fat-will-do-it fairy tale, you may suggest: "Why don't we try both diets and see what is best suited to our metabolisms?"

Now suppose you're in the situation where you're the only one who has to lose weight. You should suggest our "meat and millet" diet for normal weight people whose objective is to become healthier. You can get the instructions in *Dr. Atkins' Health Revolution*. It's a diet allowing unlimited complex carbohydrates, but because meat is allowed and sugar is not, it makes for dieting compatibility with the "Atkins and I" diet.

One more very important message. Suppose the temptation takes the form of the sugar-laden junk food that's in the house "for the kids": "Kids like that stuff, you know." If you think that the most dangerous food additive on the planet is proper nourishment for growing members of the human race who happen also to be your loved ones, then perhaps you should rethink your position. Who more than someone with virtually their whole lives ahead of them stands to be damaged the most by a substance that helps create diabetes, hypertension, and heart disease? Allowing kids to eat according to the pleasure principle and not according to the principle of health maintenance is probably not the kind of parenting you wish to do. So, make the resolution now: *Sugar is not going to enter my home.*

Dieting in the Big World Outside Your Home

But how do you control your work environment? With common sense. The coffee and danish cart at 11 and 3 smells so good! Not if you've had scrambled eggs and bacon for breakfast and a satiating lunch as well. Your sales-resistance is at its greatest when you're sated. Does the cafeteria or luncheonette nearby serve suitable food? Check it out, because if they don't, you start packing your lunch.

Low-carbohydrate dieters will find restaurants to be much more friend than foe. They stay in business because of their ability to make food taste better than most of you manage to achieve in your kitchens. So most of their main courses qualify. The trick is not to be seduced by all the extras. If it's at all possible, know what you're going to order before you walk in. And don't go for the carbohydrate extras just because you're "entitled."

The fun comes when you discover restaurants that do great things with the diet automatically. It shouldn't be too difficult to find a good cut of meat, fish, or fowl with the right seasonings, pre-pared well, and still having no carbohydrate. I've had well over 5000 wonderful restaurant meals—100% on the diet. I know where to get the best steaks, roast beef, rack of lamb, crispy duck, and poached salmon in my hometown. But I also know the best trout with a macadamia nut crust, the best veal a la Triestina, saltimbocca a la Romana, Chinese shrimp and lobster, Mexican fajitas, guacamole, and chiles rellenos. Ladies and gentlemen, this is the true gourmet's diet. I always say, "If you're going to lose a hundred pounds anyway, you might as well do it with generous quantities of luxurious food."

The trick in restaurants is not to start eating until the appetizer or main course that *you ordered correctly* arrives. If you can get a celery and olive tray instead of bread and butter, you do have an alternative. Remember, too, never same room for dessert.

Dinner parties can be real obstacle courses. The present gener-ation is the first in history wherein hostesses are not embarrassed to have an all-pasta dinner party, and so there is a possibility that you may find nothing desirable to eat. Let me warn you about going off the diet for just one meal. That figures to set back your dieting for nearly a week in regard to weight loss. The better policy is to let the host(ess) know you're on a doctor's diet, so that you may ask what is being served. If the meal simply does not qualify, either ask for a raincheck or for permission to bring your own food. If you fear that there won't be enough protein food to last you the duration of your stay at the party, make sure you bring something portable along—those macadamia nuts, for example.

Airline travel can be another diet-breaker. Whenever possible, call in advance and ask for a special diet meal. Tell them you're on a diet that is all protein and no carbohydrate. Their response will probably be, until more of you demand it, that they don't have such a diet meal. Often it is the kosher meal that is the lowest in carbohydrates of those they offer, so, O'Shaughnessy, order the kosher meal. (But first, ask what they intend to serve.)

Master Your Strategies and Be Slim for Life

Remember, you have more tools at your disposal than you think. Besides the four diets, there are a variety of levels of each diet, there are combinations of intense dieting on weekdays, with liberal eating on weekends, diets for holding the line and for getting a job done, high-fat and low-fat variations, high- and low-calorie variations. There is even the Fat Fast for short bursts of accomplishment. (See Chapter 18.)

With these tools, you become a master strategist. You are like a star quarterback, grinding it out for a while, going for a big gain (or loss in this case) when the time is right but always keeping your eye on the goal line—and ultimately the victory.

24 | *The First Seven Years of the New Revolution*

In addition to treating patients with all kinds of medical problems and writing books about our experience with them, I write a monthly health newsletter, *Dr. Atkins' Health Revelations*. This has allowed me (actually forced me) to keep absolutely current on the many health-related subjects I must write about.

In the seven years since this book was first written, there have been many changes in the knowledge and experience that relates to understanding overweight and how to control it. I would like to take this opportunity to share them with you.

The major discoveries during this time span are focused on powerful evidence that the mainstream endorsement of low-fat diets, combined with appetite suppressants and/or fat blockers are seriously in error. And the most significant popular reaction is the beginning of an *en masse* rejection of this deeply entrenched belief system. More and more people are willing to cast aside their fear of time-honored food standbys such as meat, eggs, and butter in order to achieve the good health results that had, until then, eluded them.

Lessons from Fen-Phen

Untold millions were "burned" by the "fen-phen" fiasco and quite a few paid with their lives. The use of the drugs fenfluramine and phentermine, and the resulting heart damage and death, was the direct result of two fallacies pushed upon us by corporate interests. The harm wrought by the first fallacy, "Drugs are good for you," is self-evident. The second fallacy, "We must all follow a low-fat diet," the real fen-phen killer, needs some explanation.

A low-fat diet is virtually devoid of satiety value; to lose weight on it, you must exercise like a demon, and either experience intolerable hunger or have your appetite suppressed. And the latter is what the victimized millions chose to do. The crime was the ruthless suppression of true information about low-carbohydrate diets, which provide their own appetite suppression. How can there be a better appetite suppressant than a ribeye steak? Why would anyone need appetite suppressants when they can lose up to a pound a day eating real food in satisfying quantities? Could these fallacies have been promulgated because there is a lot of profit in selling diet pills? Well, there may be even more profit in switching people from steak and eggs to white flour and cornstarch.

Statistics That Don't Lie

The failure of the low-fat experiment is heralded by the statistics compiled by the U.S. Department of Agriculture. As we cut fat from 40% of our calories to 33%, we found that our total caloric intake jumped up 10%, even though the food we ate was far less dense in calories. It turns out that more than 100% of the increase took the form of refined carbohydrates—sugar, corn syrup, and white flour, the essence of junk foods.

I doubt that you are an authority on food policy, but would you not deduce from this that perhaps fats curb the appetite and that without them, our cravings for junk food might get out of control? Well, no Federal food policy advisor has ever admitted culpability; they persist in blaming us. They attribute the 32% increase in obesity, in a ten-year span, not to their failed experiment, but to our losing interest in dieting. They may be partially right. Many of us have given up trying after learning the hard way, that it may be easier to be fat than hungry.

The New Diet Revolution's Impact

But the word is getting out, and people by the millions are making the changeover from low-fat to low-carbohydrate. Even more millions are experiencing doubt over whether everything they've been taught about nutrition could be wrong and whether all their successfully dieting friends may be onto something worth trying.

I'm sure this very book had a great deal to do with the change in people's approach to dieting, not only by helping its readers, but by the successful imitators it has spawned. Moreover, the scientific community has made some significant contributions, which I'd like to fill you in on.

What Triglycerides Mean To You

The first of these, in my view, centers around the newfound respect that researchers give to the role of triglycerides as a cause of heart disease. And matched with that is the role of the beneficial HDL cholesterol.

Late in 1997, Michael J. Gaziano, M.D., and his Harvard associates looked at a group of men to determine their risk for heart disease. They found that the ratio of triglyceride to HDL was so highly correlated with coronary events that those whose ratio was in the upper 25% of the entire group were 16 times more likely to have a heart attack than those in the lowest 25%. There never has been a combination of risk factors anywhere this highly correlated with heart disease. And it is not a fluke; many previous studies, including major ones in Muenster, Germany, and Helsinki, Finland, showed pretty much the same thing.

Now this is why this information is so important to a group of dieters. High triglycerides, especially when combined with low HDL cholesterol, are a surrogate marker for a high insulin response to carbohydrate intake. That's the very thing that also causes you to be overweight, and the very thing that the Atkins diet corrects.

True, there are many behind-the-times, pharmaceutically oriented cardiologists who will still insist that a low-fat diet and a panoply of drugs is the answer for this treacherous combination. If they do, they will be wrong. That is unequivocal. The connection between triglycerides and insulin and its response to cutting carbohydrates has been demonstrated in so many scientific studies published over the last 30 years that it deserves to be an accepted fact. We would not be consistently seeing 80% drops in triglyceride among people who needed them if the Atkins diet were not precisely corrective of the problem. Here is an example of the success of a treatment proving the cause of the condition.

Even if the general cause of the disorder cannot be agreed upon, there will be little doubt of what works for an individual. If you have either high triglycerides or low HDL (and every overweight person must know his/her levels) and your triglycerides are three times higher than your HDL (must be drawn after a 12-hour fast) then do the *Induction* diet for 3 to 4 weeks and recheck your levels. You will almost certainly see a major improvement. Even though there is no proof that you will extend your life that way, you will never meet a doctor who does not feel that making major improvements in major risk factors will very likely do so.

Diet Comparisons—The Battle That's Never Waged

With all the millions of dieters and diabetics who have turned to low-carbohydrate eating, you would think that some researcher would do a study to compare the effects of such a diet against a standard offering. Apparently, the powers-that-be are not ready to chance their diet in competition with one that has a powerful winning record. What will they say when it fails miserably to measure up to the contender?

Therefore, all studies of comparison diets were done with diets very similar to one another—often a 60% carbohydrate diet was compared against a 40% diet. As expected, there was little to choose between them. Finally, in 1998, we are beginning to see a few studies moving toward looking at lower carbohydrate diets. One such study began with a diet quite similar to this one, but halfway through the three months, the carbohydrate restriction was moderated to a 36% level. Even so, a 19% drop in triglycerides with a 15% increase in HDL was reported, the subjects lost weight, and nothing worsened. One day, when researchers have the courage to study diets low enough in carbohydrates to produce lipolysis, they will prove how dramatically beneficial such diets are.

The Mediterranean Diet—Sort Of

However, about a dozen studies were published comparing what they called the Mediterranean diet with a diet espoused by the American Heart Association. The difference was that some of the carbohydrate was eliminated and replaced with olive oil. The olive oil variation won each and every comparison study concerning lipids, blood sugar, and other risk factors. The lower fat diet was repeatedly proven to be inferior to its comparison partner, yet there still has been no movement from the concerned organizations to change their recommendations.

Instead, we hear faint praise for the olive oil, but no one deigned to point out that the diet victorious in this head-to-head struggle was simply higher in fat and lower in carbohydrate.

But enough evidence about the failure of the low-fat diet has been amassed to get the attention of important voices in mainstream medicine. The most important epidemiologist of our generation, Harvard's Walter C. Willett, wrote that "a substantial decline in the percentage of energy from fat consumed during the past two decades has corresponded with a massive increase in obesity."[1] It's nice to see a leader of mainstream medicine echoing what I have long said is the most important cause (the low fat diet)–and–effect (the upsurge in obesity) relationship in all of bariatrics (the study of obesity).

25 | *Questions Most Frequently Asked*

In the seven years since this book was first written, I have stayed in touch with tens of thousands of my readers. During my daily radio call-in broadcasts, my public lectures or in-patient care, I have heard thousands of questions, and now that my website is interactive, I have been receiving even more questions through e-mail. From all of this, I have a pretty good idea what it is that you may need to know of me.

Here are the questions I see (hear) most frequently:

Q. I started the diet off really well, but now I seem to have stopped losing and I still have a lot to lose. What's wrong and what do I do?
A. There are many possibilities. The first is that you may be on medications that prevent weight loss. (See page 176 for that discussion) Virtually every medication is replaceable with vita-nutrients, and a doctor familiar with the information in *Vita-Nutrient Solution* should be able to lower your dosages or wean you off those medicines.

Secondly, in going beyond the *Induction* diet and creating the *OWL*, you were permitted to add some carbohydrate items. The new level of the diet may have been adequate to achieve some weight loss, but not enough to break through the plateau you are at now. The solution is to return to the *Induction Diet*, and if that works, don't add so many extras the next time.

Then there is the possibility that you are doing a low-fat version of the diet, meaning that much of your diet is protein. Protein, more often than not, follows the same metabolic pathway as carbohydrate, which may thus inhibit fat mobilization. A brief trial using foods with a high fat-to-protein ratio will, if weight loss resumes, tell you if this is your problem. Sometimes, low-fat foods are the culprit; they tend to have much more carbohydrate than the original they replace. Also, remember that "sugar-free" is not synonymous with "carbohydrate-free." *Any* carbohydrate can hold back weight loss. Read labels.

Fourthly, remember that prolonged dieting (this one, low-fat, low-calorie, or a combination) tends to shut down thyroid function. This is usually not a problem with the thyroid gland (therefore blood tests are likely to be normal) but with the liver, which fails to convert T4 into the more active thyroid principle, T3. The diagnosis is made on clinical grounds with the presence of fatigue, sluggishness, dry skin, coarse or falling hair, an elevation in cholesterol, or a low body temperature. I ask my patients to take four temperature readings daily before the three meals and near bedtime. If the average of all these temperatures, taken for at least three days, is below 97.8 F (36.5 C), that is usually low enough to point to this form of thyroid problem; lower readings than that are even more convincing. It may be appropriate for those of you who fit these criteria to be prescribed thyroid by your doctor, and if so, a natural form of the hormone, which contains T3, is far superior to the most popular form of prescription thyroid, synthetic T4.

Other possibilities include the use of aspartame, which in large quantities may inhibit weight loss. If you take in three or more servings of aspartame-containing foods or beverages daily, it may be worthwhile to switch to another sweetener to see if weight loss resumes. If none of the above apply to you, reread Chapter 18, because you seem to have extreme metabolic resistance. But there may be a way to break up metabolic resistance by certain vita-nutrients. (See page 177)

Q. No matter what I do, I can't seem to get into ketosis; my testing strips never turn purple. What should I do?
A. A low grade of ketosis/lipolysis can take place without the LTS ever turning color. (The ketone analyzers we use on our Atkins Center patients often demonstrate this phenomenon.) If weight loss (or inch loss) is taking place, there is no need to do anything different. But make sure you are not taking in hidden carbohydrates (the sugar in coleslaw or salad dressings are two examples) and read my answer to the previous question to see if any of it applies to you. If you are not showing ketones *and* not losing, and are following the strictest version of the diet, you should reread Chapter 18.

Q. I am taking medications and not losing—and I cannot find a doctor interested in helping me get off medications. What do I do?

A. There is no easy answer to this question, because you certainly do need such a doctor. There is good reason why it requires a medical license both to prescribe and to *de*prescribe medications— pharmaceuticals pose risks, both coming and going. Yet, as my latest book, *Dr. Atkins' Vita-Nutrient Solution,* points out, the switching from medications to safer, more appropriate nutritional therapies can be accomplished in most instances.

Even though the number of doctors able and willing to help in this way is growing month-by-month, they still represent a decided minority of physicians. Mainstream medicine seems to have unwittingly painted itself into a pharmaceuticals-only corner.

The only answer is to "ask around." Perhaps other Atkins dieters know of such a doctor. This is why I am solidly behind the concept of creating community or neighborhood chapters of my followers, so that each community can "train" one or more doctors to be responsive to our needs and to utilize our collective wisdom.

I can help with those of you who take drugs to control symptoms or have easy-to-follow abnormalities such as blood pressure or sugar elevations. Take the appropriate vita-nutrients and call or visit your doctor and state: "I have made major lifestyle improvements and they are working—my symptoms (or elevated sugar or pressure) are gone. Would you please supervise a small reduction in medication dosage so that we can both see if my improved lifestyle will allow me one day to get off medications?"

Hopefully, those of you who have good rapport with your doctors can help them help you and their other patients by showing them a copy of *Vita-Nutrient Solution,* emphasizing the parts that provide them nutritional options for drugs with undesirable side effects.

Q. Could the medications I'm taking interfere with the diet's success?

A. You bet! Most medications, it seems, have an adverse effect on weight loss if you tend to gain weight in the first place. For a list of major offenders, refer to page 176.

Q. What medical conditions should be monitored by a doctor during the diet?

A. Every condition requiring medication should be monitored, because the improved nutrition frequently renders the medication unnecessary. A partial list of these are diabetes, hypertension, heart conditions, rhythm disorders, heart failure, edema, gastritis, heartburn, colitis, Crohn's disease, Meniere's disease, depression, panic attacks and headache.

On the other hand, the program is capable of aggravating certain conditions, notably: Gout and uric acid kidney stones, gall bladder colic, constipation, digestive deficiencies involving ability to digest fat or protein, and a small percentage of lipid disorders. (See Chapter 15, "Testing for Fat Sensitivity.")

Those taking multiple medications need particularly careful monitoring because the balance among these drugs may be upset by improvements in underlying conditions caused by the diet, which can potentially lead to dangerous drug-drug interactions.

Q. I can't just stop the medications, can I?
A. Not without considerable risk. Stopping medication requires a doctor's knowledge just as prescribing it does. But if your health care practitioner is willing to monitor you during the tapering process, you will find that the information in *Vita-Nutrient Solution* will point you to natural alternatives to every category of drug I singled out as leading to weight gain.

Q. I've found a doctor willing to get me off medications, but he is not experienced at finding alternatives. What can I tell him?
A. A vita-nutrient solution requires a whole new course in medical therapy, but here are some important concepts.

Depression: Most psychotropic medications, including Prozac, Zoloft, and lithium, are extremely weight-inducing. Alternative therapies include St. John's wort, kava-kava, 5-HTP (hydroxytryptophan), acetyl tyrosine, GABA, S-adenosyl methionine and others.

Arthritis: The NSAID drugs and prednisone-type drugs all tend to put weight on. Dozens of alternatives work; outstanding are cetyl myristoleate, MSM, glucosamine sulfate, chondroitin sulfate, pantethine, niacinamide, copper, and the essential fatty acids— GLA, EPA and DHA.

Water Retention, Heart Failure: Diuretics, the drugs usually used here, cause problems for dieters by causing loss of vital minerals, such as potassium and magnesium. The natural therapy that is preferred over kidney-suppressing diuretics is taurine. Vitamin B$_6$ helps, too.

Asthma: Most asthma medications do not inhibit weight loss, but when it is severe enough to require prednisone, it then involves using a weight-gaining drug. Your vita-nutrient checklist includes pantethine, vitamin C, quercetin, grape seed extract, magnesium, essential fatty acids, and DHEA plus pregnenolone to help reduce the prednisone requirements.

Space doesn't provide the opportunity to list more problems and solutions, but all the information your doctor may need can be found in my *Vita-Nutrient Solution.*

Q. I seem to have gained and am unable to lose since my gynecologist put me on hormone replacement therapy. Is that possible and what can I do about it?

A. Yes, hormones, especially estrogens, are one of the best examples of medicines that make losing weight difficult. Fortunately, high doses of the B vitamin folic acid (30–60 mg), along with boron (6–12mg) and natural progesterone, can allow for a significant dosage reduction of the Premarin or other hormone without allowing for the side effects usually seen with estrogen withdrawal.

Q. The Atkins diet makes me light-headed and faint but I am taking blood pressure medicine. Which is causing it and what should I do?

A. The diet has a profound blood pressure lowering effect and a profound diuretic effect. It routinely turns the blood pressure medications into an overdose. If the drug is a diuretic, it should be stopped and replaced by taurine (1500–3000 mg) even before the diet is started or you will be at risk of low potassium and other minerals lost by the diet-diuretic combination. In any case, it is better to continue the diet (it is beneficial) and reduce the dosage of the blood pressure medications (they are dangerous) than to do the opposite.

Q. Can a person with kidney problems be put on the diet? If so, how is the diet adjusted?

A. It takes a lot of kidney disease to be unable to handle the protein in the diet. People with creatinine levels below 4 generally have no problem. To be safe, anyone with creatinine levels above 3 should have a repeat level checked after 2 to 4 weeks on the diet. If the creatinine is not increased, it appears safe to stay on the diet. I have had to treat several high-creatinine patients with carbohydrate restriction because of its many benefits. In these cases, I used a high-fat, low-protein variant of the diet.

Q. Can a patient with gout be put on the diet? If so, what adjustments are made?
A. Gout *can* be aggravated by this diet. The problem is neither the protein nor the fat, but the rapid weight loss. (A total or partial fast often causes a threefold elevation of uric acid.) Two alternatives are to advance to a higher carbohydrate, slower weight loss level of the diet or to take a prescription drug, allopurinol.

Q. Can Type I and Type II diabetics both follow the diet?
A. For a type II diabetic, the diet is a godsend. In fact, it is usually "curative," allowing for normal blood sugar without medication. For type I, it usually helps to at least cut down on the insulin requirements, but this can only be done if managed by a doctor extremely familiar with treating type I diabetics with this diet.

Q. Should overweight cancer patients be on this diet? Won't it overburden the body and cause toxicity?
A. My overweight cancer patients have done extremely well on this diet, but the decision rests on whether the severity of the obesity problem may handicap the patient's cancer-fighting reserve. The diet's main advantage is that it provides very little fuel to cancer cells, which require glucose for growth. Toxicity is not a problem, but vegetables with high phytochemical content can be very valuable, so most of my cancer patients are given a diet combining the healthiest of protein foods with an extremely liberal use of those vegetables known to be high in cancer-fighting phytonutrients.

Q. How long can a person be on 20 gms or less carbohydrates per day?
A. As long as that person remains overweight and feels well.

Q. Why do I have bad breath on the diet and how can I improve this problem?
A. This "bad breath" is from the production of ketones as you burn body fat and is a good sign that the diet is working. Ketone production is necessary for continuing weight loss. To counteract the odor, you

may increase to a slightly higher carbohydrate level; however, this will slow down weight loss. You may also use chlorophyll (must be sugarless), eat more parsley and dark green, leafy vegetables, and be sure that your water intake is at least 8 or more glasses daily.

Q. I can't start my day without coffee. Why can't I have it on this diet?

A. Simply this: Caffeine stimulates the insulin mechanism, and that's your vulnerable spot. It raises blood sugar at first and then allows it to crash. This could mean fatigue, irritability, cravings, increased appetite, or the like. If you try the diet for two weeks without caffeine, and would then like to re-introduce it to see if you notice any of these effects, and you do not, you may find it acceptable to have a small amount of coffee from time to time.

Q. Will the diet work if I continue my wine? My favorite wine has almost no carbohydrate.

A. Here's the problem with all alcoholic beverages, and the reason I recommend refraining from alcohol consumption on the diet. Alcohol, whenever taken in, is the first fuel to burn. While that's going on, your body will not burn fat. This does not stop weight loss, it simply postpones it: since the alcohol does not store as glycogen, you immediately get back into ketosis/lipolysis after the alcohol is used up.

If you must drink alcohol, wine is an acceptable addition to levels beyond the *Induction* diet. If wine does not suit your taste, straight liquor such as scotch, rye, vodka, and gin would be appropriate, as long as the mixer is sugarless; this means no juice, tonic water, or non-diet soda. Seltzer and diet soda are appropriate.

Please note: if you have added alcohol to your diet and suddenly stop losing weight, it would be wise to discontinue your alcohol intake.

Q. What's the difference between your diet and the other popular ones—*The Zone, Sugar Busters,* and *Protein Power,* and may I choose the one I like best?

A. Two of the diets you mentioned are quite different and do not share the advantages of the Atkins diet. The third, *Protein Power,* is eerily similar to mine.

The Zone is simply an untested version of a low-fat diet. Its recommendation for 30% fat calories is identical to the government-issue diet and is less than the average American now eats. The only difference between the government diet and *The Zone* is that *The Zone* shifts 20% of the calories from carbohydrate to protein.

But there are very few palatable choices among protein main courses whose protein calories equal their fat calories. Steaks, roasts, chops, whole chicken, cheese, scrambled eggs, scampi, and sauteed fish—all fall outside *The Zone*. Worst of all, *The Zone* never allows you to switch over to your stored fat as your primary energy source; there is a constant influx of carbohydrate. Therefore, there is no ketosis, no appetite suppression, and no automatic weight loss. If you want to lose weight with *The Zone,* you'll have to experience the hunger.

Sugar Busters is somewhat more permissive of main courses despite many admonitions to readers to keep the fat intake low. However, it contains considerable carbohydrate. Six breakfasts a week are made of cereal, not eggs, and bread and starches are liberally presented each day. It, too, would not allow for ketosis/lipolysis or automatic weight loss.

Protein Power claims to be the first low-carbohydrate diet book to present a scientific explanation of why it works. Yet the book you are now reading was published three years before *Protein Power.* I'll ask you to be the judge of whether I have explained the scientific basis of this rather miraculous diet plan.

As to which diet you should choose, it should be *yours*. It should be based on *your* critical carbohydrate level, first to allow for automatic weight loss and then for automatic maintenance of *your* goal weight. And it should be based on the food choices *you* find most satisfying.

Q. Is your diet suitable for serious athletes?
A. It *should* be used by every athlete who needs to lose weight. It is *not* suitable for an athlete who cannot afford to lose. Carbohydrate loading has been recommended for stamina in endurance competition, but a recent study casts doubt on that dogma. Trained cyclists were able to pedal for nearly 80 minutes on a 7% carbohydrate diet, but only 42 minutes on a 74% carbohydrate diet.[1] The trick is to wait two weeks after the adaptation to the high-fat diet to occur, so don't expect instant extra energy.

26 | Debunking the Fallacies About The New Diet Revolution

It is almost certain that you are reading this book because you know or know of someone or of many people who have lost weight and overcome other health problems by following the individualized diet program you've read about here. And you may be wondering why everyone does not acknowledge the fact (and it is a fact) that cutting carbohydrates is far and away the ideal eating pattern for correcting overweight.

In largest part, the reason why this diet plan is not part of mainstream teaching (as it certainly should be) has been the constant barrage of misinformation repeatedly disseminated through the media hell-bent on convincing everyone within view or earshot that the Atkins diet is downright dangerous, as well as ineffective.

If you've encountered these critical reviews, I'm sure you have mixed feelings about the advisability of going on or staying on the diet plan that seems otherwise so perfectly suited to you. So I will take this chapter to address every criticism I've seen in print, answering them with the wisdom gleaned from 35 years of clinical experience with the program.

I do not know of a single example in all of modern medicine where the discrepancy between what is said in print and what actually takes place is so vast. At the end of this chapter, I'll tell you why I think this is so.

ONE—Ketosis is harmful, dangerous, an abnormal state that leads to acidosis. Ketones are toxic waste products, they come from muscle breakdown, they damage the brain, yada, yada, yada.

Of this, I am certain: anyone who makes such a statement has not researched the subject. The role of ketones in our bodies is a well-researched bit of scientific data, and it has never been questioned—it is not controversial. These are the scientific facts:

Ketones are one of the two fuel-delivery substances in our bodies—the other is glucose. Whenever your body sees fit to utilize your alternative metabolic fuel, your stored fat, the biochemical agents it uses are ketones.

To illustrate this point, let me describe the seminal study done by Dr. George Cahill and his Harvard associates, a group considered so authoritative that their conclusions have never been challenged. They incubated slices of living brain with the two brain fuels, glucose and ketones. The brain cells, in their instinct to stay alive, actually utilized more of the ketones than the glucose, which had been erroneously considered to be the only fuel the brain could use. Similar studies were done with heart muscle and other tissues; thus, ketones were convincingly established as a preferred fuel for vital organs, and soon all the textbooks described them as such.[1]

Other research made an even more convincing point. Obese individuals were shown to be unusually "ketoresistant." This term means they find it unusually difficult to develop ketones, as those who lose weight easily do. (That's why I talk about ketosis/lipolysis as the dieters' principal objective.) It has been repeatedly demonstrated that overweight subjects produce just enough ketones to meet their immediate needs for fuel—and no more. Therefore, the very people who need a ketogenic diet are the people in whom ketones will never accumulate. A dieter will have no more ketones after three months of cutting carbohydrates than after 3 days. So people, except insulin-dependent diabetics, simply do not build up ketones.

The confusion comes from the unhealthy ketosis (actually ketoacidosis) seen in a type I diabetic, a person who cannot produce insulin. Since people are overweight because of too much insulin, it is essentially impossible for ketoacidosis to happen to them.

So the next time you read that the ketosis produced by the Atkins diet is dangerous, challenge the writer (in a letter to the editor, if necessary) and ask "What is so dangerous about using up your stored fat in the very way Nature intended us to do it?"

TWO—*The Atkins diet only works because it is a low-calorie diet.*

If the first criticism is an indicator of ignorance, than this criticism is an indicator of subnormal intellect. If a cheese omelet has 600 calories, two scoops of tuna salad 600 calories, a 12-oz ribeye steak 1100, and the olive oil on the salad another 300, how can such an effective weight loss diet be called low in calories?

To be sure, it is true that the vast majority of Atkins dieters note a big drop-off in hunger, which does lead to eating less, but the caloric density of the food that accomplishes this dieters' godsend hardly qualifies the end result as low in calories.

Furthermore, would you not wonder whether that statement is, in reality, a criticism? To be able to eat until you are no longer hungry, avoid diet pills, and still be low in calories—just how bad is that?

THREE—On the Atkins diet, all you lose is water weight.

Read that one and you'll know why so many political leaders adopt a strategy of lying to the public. They believe the public is gullible enough to believe anything; so do the perpetrators of this whopper.

A good portion of any initial weight loss on *any* diet is water weight. However, by now, there are probably millions of American citizens who have lost two sizes or more and many who have lost over 100 pounds on the Atkins diet and kept it off indefinitely. There is no way to accomplish that except by losing unwanted body fat, period.

I've seen the water-weight argument in print scores of times but never have I heard it uttered in an open forum where someone could easily rebut the critic by showing off their belt with six new notches.

This is not to deny that the Atkins diet has a diuretic effect. It does for those who need it, making it an invaluable natural therapy for all forms of water retention, high blood pressure, and congestive heart failure.

FOUR—The Atkins diet is unbalanced and lacks basic nutrition. That's why supplements must be provided.

The Atkins diet is certainly unbalanced; that is done deliberately to make it a corrective diet. (Please reread the beginning of chapter 8.) The evidence that insulin over-release is responsible for most overweight is quite impressive, and the best way to correct an insulin disorder is to bypass the problem. Don't eat foods that will stimulate insulin activity—they are the carbohydrates.

The second part of the criticism is more thought-provoking. I for one, am deeply committed to finding a vita-nutrient solution for most health problems. This means that I believe that no eating pattern contains optimal nutrition, and that all of us can improve our health by taking vita-nutrients targeted for problems to which we, as individuals, are vulnerable.

That said, let's look at the contribution of the food components of various diets to essential nutrients. Those on a low-fat diet need supplementation desperately. They are low in the fat-soluble vitamins A, D, E and K and the essential fatty acids, our number one deficiency. They may be low in nutrients we get from meat, such as vitamin B_{12} and carnitine. And if people fall for the Food Pyramid fallacy and overdo white flour, they will be low in half the B complex (the part that's not in the mandatory enrichment) and most of the essential minerals.

On the other hand, all animal foods eaten without processing contain a balanced variety of vitamins and minerals. Add to that all the vegetables which constitute the majority of the carbohydrate on the *OWL* and *Maintenance* diets, which are, after all, followed 99% of an Atkins dieter's time, and you have a diet providing better underlying nutritional values than any other diet used for weight loss purposes.

In point of fact, a proper Atkins dieter follows the entire program, including the supplements I outlined in Chapter 22. With that, you have the most vita-nutrient rich intake of any weight-loss program—bar none.

FIVE—The Atkins diet leaves you tired, weak, low in energy, unable to function, blah, blah, blah.

This is another example of people not doing their reality-checking. Well over 95% of Atkins dieters report more energy than when they were on their usual diet, be it for gaining or losing weight. The reason is that the diet stabilizes the blood sugar and provides consistent energy throughout the day. Perhaps the basis of the criticism was the AMA's widely publicized observation that an all-pemmican diet made Arctic-based soldiers tired on bivouac in 1943. You heard me! That's how far the opposition had to fetch to come up with ammunition to use against the World's Greatest Weight Loss Diet.

SIX—There is too much protein on the Atkins Diet, which makes it bad for the kidneys.

There are probably millions of people who believe this untruth simply because it has been so often repeated that even intelligent health professionals assume it must have been reported somewhere.

But the fact is it has not. There never has been a single case report, not even in a foreign language, describing even an isolated example of a protein-containing diet causing any form of kidney disorder.

If you have ever heard this one, think of it! Someone just repeated to you a total fabrication with less chance of being true than the present veracity gold standard: "But I didn't inhale."

The only remotely related phenomenon is the fact that with far-advanced kidney disease already established, it is difficult to handle protein. But protein has nothing to do with the *cause* of the kidney problem.

SEVEN—The Atkins diet is high in fat, and we all know that fats cause gallbladder disease.

There is now overwhelming scientific evidence that gallstones (responsible for over 90% of gallbladder disease) are formed when the fat intake is low. Two separate studies showed 25% of subjects on an ultra low-fat diet developed gallstones, and a third study on a 27-gm fat diet, produced gallstones in 13%.[2]

The reason is that the gallbladder will not contract unless fat is taken in and if it does not do so, the bile salts will crystallize into stones. Our gallbladders need to be kept active to prevent stone formation. The scientific name for the reason stones form is "biliary stasis."

It is true, however, that people with existing stones may have trouble with high-fat meals. Such individuals may have to follow a low-fat variation of the Atkins diet.

EIGHT—The Atkins diet causes calcium excretion, and thus osteoporosis.

At least this one is not totally out of left field. There were several studies showing that people who took in protein powder did excrete more urinary calcium than those who did not.

However, Herta Spencer, M.D., repeated the study with meat. Her research concluded that calcium loss lasts only two weeks; the body then readjusts itself, returning to a regular state of homeostasis, and the calcium loss stops.[3]

There is neither clinical nor epidemiological evidence that people who consume a high protein diet develop more osteoporosis; so we should place this complaint into the "Needs More Evidence" category.

NINE—High fat diets cause cancer.

The evidence says otherwise. All of it is epidemiological so it could never prove anything, but this is what the studies show: As I pointed out in Chapter 16, it certainly does not cause breast cancer. The low-fat diet seems like the worst one of the lot. And it is logical that it should be. Breast cancer is associated with being overweight and the low-fat, high-carbohydrate diet has been shown to cause overweight. Why should it not increase the risk of breast cancer?

But the colon cancer is more interesting and may even provide a clue as to how to order your food. Dr. Willett's group, who provided the most usable epidemiology to date, conducted a study on nearly 48,000 male health professionals to parallel their Nurses Study. Neither total fat nor animal fat related to the incidence of colon cancer but the frequency of red meat did (hamburgers did, but hot dogs didn't).[4]

The Harvard researchers must have regretted that their questionnaires didn't ask the doctors *how* their meat was prepared, because it is almost certain from two other studies that the culprit is over-frying the meat. In one, only those who like their meat "well-browned" had the increase in colon cancer, the rest did not.[5] There is research showing that carcinogens (cancer-causing chemicals) are formed when red meat is charred. Tentative conclusion, pending further research, is broil your meat, do not pan-fry, and have it medium rare.

Other researchers take a different slant. For example, Dr. Silvia Franceschi, writing in *The International Journal of Cancer*, concludes: "As a dozen studies report, there is solid evidence that it is sugar or refined starch that may be a main cause of colon and rectal cancer."[6] Perhaps that is why I have seen so few of my patients come down with this very common form of cancer.

TEN—It is a known fact, acknowledged by every major health organization, that fats are the major cause of cardiovascular disease.

I certainly do not deny that every major health organization, as well as the United States government, endorses a low-fat diet in the unquestioned belief that fat causes heart disease. But are they right? There is compelling evidence pointing in the opposite direction.

Let's start with the work out of Framingham, Massachusetts, the community studied for fifty years by Harvard researchers to glean meaningful information about the cause of heart disease. They did show that the risk of heart disease correlated both with cholesterol levels and overweight, but, and too few health organization leaders will tell you this, their data showed that weight gain and cholesterol levels *moved in the opposite direction* to the dietary fat and cholesterol intake!

More recently, the Framingham group reported on a study in which the young healthy male population of the community was followed for several decades to see which dietary patterns would lead to having a stroke. They found to their amazement that those with the highest intake of saturated fats (no less) had the fewest ischemic strokes (the most common kinds), actually 76% less than those with the lowest intake of saturated fat.[7]

Or look at it this way: in 1910, a coronary event was a rare find, so rare that it had never been described. (The first description of a coronary occlusion was published in 1912.) By 1970, it was the cause of death of a majority of Americans. What were the dietary changes in the U.S. between 1910 and 1970?

Our intake of cholesterol was unchanged, our intake of animal fat fell by 25% and of butter by 77%. This is what went up: Our consumption of trans-fats such as margarine (the fat we don't allow) went up by 400%, and more important, because of its high percentage in the American diet, our intake of sugars and refined carbohydrates went up by 60%. Why don't the organizations finger refined carbohydrates and trans-fats as the culprits?

Plus, look at the logic I presented in Chapter 15. If a diet lowers your bad cholesterol and your triglycerides while raising your good cholesterol, then why would it be expected to increase your heart risk? All you have to do is make sure you, like the vast majority of my patients, get those satisfactory results. I've never known a critic of my diet that could find a coherent reason for telling someone whose heart risk factors had improved dramatically to get off the diet.

ELEVEN—The Atkins diet is considered the "most severe" of the carbohydrate-restricted diets, and most likely to have immediate adverse effects.

"Severe" may be a synonym for "effective," but from the standpoint of ease and comfort of following and of unbridled enjoyment of eating, it is the most permissive. The idea of severity must come from the extremely low level of carbohydrate provided by the *Induction* diet. But it would be quite apparent merely from reading this book that the *Induction* diet was never meant for any purpose except to jump-start the body chemistry into fat mobilization. Throughout the dieting experience, each individual seeks the most permissive level of carbohydrate intake that gets the job of weight loss or maintenance done.

The diet is individualized; it is only "severe" when anything less severe would not work. I know from treating patients that the diet is capable of succeeding over 99% of the time, and I wanted to make sure that no one missed the opportunity to succeed.

The question arises: Could the diet work too well for certain people and cause symptoms? The answer is that such a result could take place, although it is rare. That is why I instruct my readers to advance to the next stage of the diet should that happen.

TWELVE—The bad thing about the Atkins diet is that it makes you crave sweets!

The fact is that whoever the "you" in the above statement is, that person is probably a sugar addict. The diet merely allows "you" to realize that an addiction exists. It is very much like an everyday drinker realizing, when no liquor is available, that he is an alcoholic.

Craving is a symptom of addiction, and the most effective sure-fire cure for addiction is abstinence. The Atkins diet, with the help of chromium and glutamine, allows you to get on with the project of dealing with your addiction.

For almost everyone with sugar cravings, the Atkins diet is the most effective treatment for this addiction. I have treated thousands of patients whose cravings come back only after a few unfortunate derivations from the diet, to be brought under control only when the diet is adhered to. Incidentally, research (and my experience) shows the low-carbohydrate diet to be an extremely effective adjunct to breaking other addictions, including alcohol, cigarettes, opiates, and other illicit drugs.

THIRTEEN—The Atkins diet causes bad breath.

It can. It actually will, when it is working at full efficiency, cause ketone breath. Without our bodies manufacturing ketones, there would not be any rapid weight loss.

Here's the issue. Ketones, which impart a sweetish smell, do not cause what I would call "bad breath." A different breath smell to be sure, but not an offensive one. I have not noticed it among my patients for years; perhaps I simply consider it normal.

FOURTEEN—The Atkins diet is not suitable for vegetarians.

It is only unsuitable for people who wish to—or must *remain* vegetarians. Yet I have prescribed this diet for hundreds of vegetarians who felt so much better on the special vegetarian version of the *Induction* diet that they abandoned their vegetarian conviction simply in order to continue feeling so much better.

For a conforming vegan, the diet is not worth trying. For a ovo-lacto-vegetarian, it can be done, with difficulty. The problem lies not in the impossibility of making meal plans with tofu, olives, avocados, and the like, but in *creating a diet enjoyable enough to stay on for life,* a point I consider to be essential to dietary success.

Vegetarians with extreme obesity and/or type II diabetes or hypoglycemia will simply have to choose between remaining vegetarian or overcoming their condition.

FIFTEEN—People on the Atkins diet learn to eat fatty foods like bacon and eggs, so when they go off the diet, they are worse off than before.

Look at the prejudice that must lie behind such a criticism. The Atkins diet provides an overweight person the single best opportunity he has ever had to find a lifetime diet he can live with, without a desire to abandon it. There is no intent to make it a diet that someone goes off of; that's why it asks you to follow only the rules that count the most.

If someone opts to go off this diet, they are no worse off than if they abandon any diet. At least this one could win the competition entitled "Most Likely to Acquire Lifetime Adherence."

Now that you've had a chance to review the 15 most commonly voiced criticisms of my diet, along with my answers, perhaps you are struck as I am by the closed-mindedness, or even the intent to mislead the public, by these many voices hell-bent on dissuading you from even trying this diet. I trust you are equally impressed with the nearly complete lack of substance behind their allegations.

Do you know of another example in all the health sciences where such a vast discrepancy exists between what actually takes place and what is said to take place? I sure don't.

I hope some of you are outraged enough to do something about this effort to suppress information about your health choices. (Actually, I hope all of you are.) If so, perhaps the next chapter will point you in the right direction.

27 | *The Self You Serve Will Be Yourself*

The low-carbohydrate diet has not been one of the standard diets for a number of years, and, in many ways, that's a bit of a mystery.

If a doctor has to decide whether or not to use a drug—let's say prednisone—to treat his patient's rheumatoid arthritis, he legitimately has a conflict in his mind. He knows the drug will have a positive effect on the arthritic symptoms; he also knows it might have damaging side effects. There's no mystery there. The choice is difficult, the evidence divided.

A low-carbohydrate diet is a very different matter. The scientific evidence is *not* evenly divided. It is quite one-sidedly in support of the effectiveness and the health enhancement potentialities of such dieting. So what could possibly explain the reluctance to give this diet its place in the sun? I'm afraid I don't have an answer, but I tend to agree with cynics who point to the influence of the giant food companies, for not only are they deeply committed to selling junk carbohydrates, they are also among the chief funders of nutritional research. The Germans, on the other hand, might call it the *Zeitgeist*, or, as we would say, the spirit of the age.

Certainly high-carbohydrate diets have had it all their own way for the past two decades. I can't say that I've noticed people becoming any slimmer—or healthier, either. Frankly, I think it's high time the dissenting point of view roars to a crescendo, and I hope you'll become a part of a very necessary crusade.

What the Success of This Book Will Mean to You

I can't think of anything more gauche than an author encouraging his readers to talk up his book and mention its merits to others.

How utterly self-serving it sounds, but, in point of fact, the self you will be serving is yourself.

That statement should prove to be readily apparent to those of you who are like thousands of successful dieters who e-mailed or wrote to thank me for providing the diet that changed their lives. Along with their expressions of heartfelt gratitude, most of their letters expressed another, less pleasant theme, which usually read: "Why has virtually everyone told me I had to do things quite the opposite to what works?" or "Why was I allowed to suffer so much frustration when the easy answer I was looking for was never offered to me?"

These millions of individual dieters succeeded against all odds, not because the answer was difficult, but because it was kept from them by a quarter-century of negative statements about carbohydrate restriction that had no basis in fact, but a major basis in economics.

I tell you this because the suppression of low-carbohydrate dieting is, in reality, the tip of the iceberg of health misinformation that has not merely been robbing overweight people of an easy way to be slim and healthy, but robbing your family members and neighbors of a chance to overcome heart disease, or cancer, or arthritis, or a chance to grow old without the usual manifestations of aging. My patient care experience reemphasizes that, beside junk food being foisted upon us as better than meat, eggs, and butter, so too, are pharmaceuticals and surgery presented as better than safe natural, nutritional treatment options.*

Sooner or later, most every one of us is threatened by the conspiracy of silence regarding better health choices that fail to support corporate economic interests. Historically, the media and the government have sided with these interests and there is no one to get the message to our fellow citizens except you and I. The truth must be disseminated person-to-person, through word of mouth or e-mail or letter or merely by you standing up to be counted and announcing: "I am a *bona fide* member of the revolution."

Do you benefit from this? In myriad ways: For the dieter, the recognition that there are millions of us promises to lead to the availability of more and more low-carbohydrate options in restaurants and supermarkets as well as on airlines or in ballparks.

---

*For more information, please see the following article: Goodwin, James, et al., "Battling Quackery: Attitudes About Micro-Nutrient Supplements in American Academic Medicine." *Archives of Internal Medicine* 1998: 158 (9): 2187-2191.

For the family member concerned with the health of our loved ones, it may mean the availability of alternative therapies for cancer or heart disease or multiple sclerosis that work better than the invasive therapies consensus medicine would limit us to. And it may mean that health insurers and HMOs will no longer discriminate against those of us who are seeking a healthier way.

Over 25 years ago, I dedicated my first book to the "Diet Revolutionaries" who would make a difference in the world. Then, that was just a vague concept, but now it has real meaning. The world does indeed need Diet Revolutionaries, people who will organize into groups with meetings and membership rosters. Our purpose would be not only to help one another to be successful dieters, but to find others who promise to benefit from our experience and to enjoy the economic advantages that accrue to members of groups with large numbers of people. And there can be another altruistic attribute that makes us revolutionaries, not merely dieters. We can strive for a political presence that will lead to all citizens having a fuller range of health choices than the limited menu we are now being forced to accept.

If these words strike a responsive chord in you, then you may wish to make yourself available for membership into such a yet-to-be-formed group. I will leave others to work out the details; I simply am certain that it is an idea whose time has come.

All I ask of you now is to let me know who and where you are. You can keep myself and my staff abreast of your situation via phone or e-mail (listed at the end of this chapter). For those of you who are content merely to make your personal dietary experience as fulfilling and long-lasting as it can be, the message is not very different. Keep in touch with us through the aforementioned channels, let us know of your progress, send us pictures if you like, tell us your story. I and my staff love to hear about experiences of Atkins dieters throughout the country and the world.

On a consistent basis, there is no better way to stay in touch with all of our current activities and key nutritional and medical information updates than through our website (www.atkinscenter.com). We began the site less than two years ago with the simple goal of providing some basic information on The Atkins Diet, The Atkins Center, and some key products and services. As the monthly number of hits to our site has soared well into the millions, we have correspondingly raised our expectations for what this site can offer the obviously growing contingent of Internet-savvy Atkins dieters.

At present, visitors to our site will find a wealth of information on The Atkins Diet (including a long list of research excerpts), The Atkins Center, a frequently asked questions (FAQ) database, an opportunity to e-mail The Atkins Center with your questions/comments/testimonials (while we can't respond to all e-mails, we continually update our FAQ with responses to the most popular questions), an events calendar of my upcoming media/personal appearances, information on my nationally syndicated radio show, my monthly newsletter, and our increasingly popular "New Diet Revolution" cruises and resort weeks, as well as an online product catalog of Atkins food items and nutritional supplements.

By March of 1999, we will be adding even more great features to the site, including an Atkins Diet recipe database, a retail locator for Atkins products, postings from website visitors, a database of key questions to ask your doctor about chronic health conditions, and even a small, but hopefully growing, doctor referral list.

I have always believed that fully understanding your nutritional and medical options is an incredibly empowering experience, one that I have tried to facilitate through my books, lectures, medical practice, and now through our website. I hope you share my passion for this information, and that it helps you and others with whom you interact.

If enough of you talk about the Atkins diet and the effect it has had on your life, then all that you need to make your diet a breeze will begin to appear. Airlines will begin to serve low-carbohydrate meals, restaurants will instantly understand what you're asking for, hostesses will no longer offer you a choice between various forms of pasta, and hand-held ketone analyzers giving you an instant digital readout will be on the market—I've seen the prototype. Most important of all, low-carbohydrate foods will appear in the supermarket. Instead of low-fat ice cream filled with sugar, you'll find, in the same freezers, low-carbohydrate ice cream filled with cream.

Twenty years ago, when the original *Diet Revolution* was in full stride, this was exactly what did occur. The temporary triumph of the low-fat dogma in the 1980s did away with many of these conveniences, but it only takes a push to see them all return.

I wish I had had time to talk at greater length in this book about all the other aspects of the health-promoting regimen my patients are taught. I have given you a hint of what can be accomplished with vitamin supplementation, but the herbs, homeopathy, bioelectric techniques, and the rest of complementary medicine can all contribute to better health.

What I hope you'll go away with is the notion that only through the free play of ideas and therapies can people attain the greatest level of good health. I don't expect that the whole world will change over to low-carbohydrate dieting, but I do demand that the world permit those treatments to flourish that may not be mainstream but which nevertheless promise to get the health-promotion job done better than can consensus medicine.

To that end, let me introduce you to a foundation that I helped establish, and of which I served as its first president. Its name is FAIM (Foundation for the Advancement of Innovative Medicine), and its main purpose is to secure more health freedom for you and for the doctors who treat you. If you'd like to get more information about FAIM, please write:

FAIM
100 Airport Executive Park, Suite 105
Nanuet, NY 10954

The fact is, I'd just appreciate hearing from you. In the past, these communications from my readers have let me know that I wasn't tilting at windmills, but fulfilling a real need.

So here are the may ways to reach me:

1. *Website:* Check out our interactive website with the latest news and information, including appearances, book signings, cruises and resort weeks, etc. When you visit us, you may drop an e-mail, which is reviewed every working day.
   www.atkinscenter.com
2. *Call our office:* Make an appointment for a telephone nutritional consultation or schedule to see us in person as a new patient (which includes a follow-up in person or via telephone) at 888-ATKINS-8.
3. *Products:* For information on purchasing Dr. Atkins' vitanutrients, especially low-carbohydrate food products, call 800-6-ATKINS.
4. *Dr. Atkins' Health Revelations:* To subscribe to our monthly newsletter, please call 800-981-7162.

But don't just enjoy your sucess in silence—let us know who you are and how you are doing.

PART FIVE

Menus and
Recipes

The "Dr. Atkins and I" Menu

I've looked at many diets, and I've seldom seen one so dedicated to involving the dieter in his own eating as this one. That's because no diet works better than the one that you've helped create.

I thought of presenting you with a meal plan to help you in making your daily selections, but instead I decided to do something different. I've often been struck by the fact that some of my diet failures were people who, when confronted with a meal plan, were excessively literal-minded about it and felt that if the plan said pork chops on Tuesday, they had to have pork chops on Tuesday—even if they *hated* pork chops.

The truth is you don't have to eat any one thing, but you can and should eat everything that's on the menu below and that you love—and everything that's not on the menu but that's permissible (i.e., that doesn't contain inappropriate levels of carbohydrate).

I've divided these menus according to whether they apply to your time on the *Induction*, *OWL*, or *Maintenance* diets. Once you start doing your lifetime eating on this diet, some of you will find that you do best on the *Maintenance* diet, some of you will get best results on the *OWL*, and, of course, there are a few of you whose metabolic resistance requires a lifetime on a diet almost as strict as the *Induction*. Nonetheless, I'm willing to bet that the menus following will light a warm culinary fire in the pit of your stomach, no matter what diet you plan to be on.

Let me remind you that any foods on the *Induction* menus are included on the *OWL* and *Maintenance* menus, and any foods on the *OWL* are included on the *Maintenance*.

My general advice about doing the "Atkins and I" diet for a

lifetime is that you stick with basics most of the time and go to the recipes when you want a special treat. As you'll instantly see, many of the recipes are loaded with butter, cream, and egg yolks. This might give the misleading impression that that's what I want you to eat all the time, which is not the case. Unless you're on the special Fat Fast, eating lean foods is quite appropriate. The recipes are high in fat so that they'll be especially delicious on special occasions. As a general rule, however, only a small percentage of dieters should be on a high-fat diet, and that's limited to people who don't do well when the diet is lean.

There's also one general principle I'd like to recommend to you because it may save you a fair amount of physical discomfort, and that's the principle of meal rotation. There's a tendency for dieters to stick with a pattern of eating that they feel comfortable with and to repeat the foods that consistently please. But I think that the habit of eating certain foods every day is one you should take pains to avoid. In fact, I would recommend that you never have the same food on successive days. This is a technique of avoiding the ill consequences of food allergies and food intolerances, and it's well worth the effort. Therefore, I suggest you rotate your food choices. Among other things, have meat, fish, fowl, and shellfish on successive days but always according to your taste, seeking out the foods most convenient and enjoyable for you.

After all, the principal lesson of the book is that good food can be both enjoyable and healthy. Make it your goal.

The "Atkins and I" Meal Prototypes

The nine meals below give you the prototypical combinations of foods on each of the three main diets—*Induction, OWL,* and *Maintenance.* These foods are not fancy; they're intentionally typical and basic. If you don't like some of these meals, that's fine; after all, what you'll be doing in your actual daily eating is choosing meals that you do like from the extensive meal lists or adding appropriate meals that are your own choice or your own creation. You don't have to eat anything that's listed here.

I hope, however, that the prototypes will give you a quick illustrative sense of what the scope of your eating can be at each stage of the diet.

Typical Induction Menu

Breakfast:
Eggs, scrambled or fried, with bacon, ham, sugarless sausage, or
   Canadian bacon
Decaffeinated coffee or tea

Lunch:
Bacon cheeseburger, no bun
Small tossed salad
Seltzer water

Dinner:
Shrimp cocktail with mustard and mayo
Clear consommé
Steak, roast, chops, fish or fowl
Tossed salad (choice of dressings)
Diet Jell-O with a spoonful of whipped, artificially sweetened heavy
   cream

Typical Ongoing Weight Loss (OWL) *Menu*

Breakfast:
Western omelet
3 oz. of tomato juice or V-8 juice
2 carbo grams of bran crispbread
Decaffeinated coffee or tea

Lunch:
Chef's salad with ham, cheese, chicken, and egg—zero carbohydrate or oil-and-vinegar type salad dressing
Iced herbal tea

Dinner:
Seafood salad
Poached salmon
⅔ cup of vegetables from permitted vegetable list
½ cup of strawberries in cream

Typical Maintenance *Menu*

Breakfast:
Gruyère and spinach omelet
½ cantaloupe
4 carbo grams of bran crispbread with butter
Decaffeinated coffee or tea

Lunch:
Roast chicken
⅔ cup of vegetables
Green salad, creamy garlic dressing
Club soda

Dinner:
French onion soup
Salad with tomatoes, onions, and carrots, any sugarless dressing
1 cup permitted vegetables
½ small baked potato with sour cream and chives
Lightly breaded veal chops
Generous cup of fresh fruit compote
Glass of dry wine or two wine spritzers

Typical Breakfast, Lunch, and Dinner Selections

Snacks and Breads

Induction

All snacks that are made exclusively from meat, fish, fowl, and eggs.

From the Recipe Section of *New Diet Revolution*:

Basic protein bread
Sweet cheese snack
Chipped beef balls
Basic pancakes—This deserves special mention. The recipe will work as crepes as well as pancakes and can be used as the basis for blintzes, tacos, dessert crepes, or pork or chicken mu shu. It is an enormously adaptable snack ingredient.

Ongoing Weight Loss (OWL)

All foods on the Induction *diet are also included on the* OWL *diet*

From the Recipe Section of *New Diet Revolution*:

Bran-Soy muffins
Swiss snack

Maintenance

All foods on the Induction *and the* OWL *diet are also included on the* Maintenance *diet*

From the Recipe Section of *New Diet Revolution*:

Pizza
Walnut butter cookies

Breakfast

Induction

Main Dishes:

Eggs, scrambled or fried in butter, with bacon, ham, sugarless
    sausage, or Canadian bacon
Smoked Nova Scotia or sturgeon or whitefish or mixed smoked
    fishes and 2 oz. of cream cheese
Pancakes (see recipe section) and 2 oz. sour cream
Leftovers from properly prepared dinner
Snacks from snack list
Basic omelet:
    a) Gruyère and spinach
    b) Goat cheese and chives
    c) Western omelet
    d) Spanish omelet
    e) Corned beef or pastrami omelet (pancake style)
    f) Or any other low-carbohydrate omelet of your invention

From the Recipe Section in *New Diet Revolution*:

Cheese omelet
Scrambled eggs in cheese sauce with sausages

Ongoing Weight Loss (OWL)

All foods on the Induction diet are also included on the OWL diet

Main Dishes:

Eggs benedict, using diet bread instead of an English muffin
Welsh rarebit on diet bread

Breakfast on the *OWL* diet may also include:
3 oz. of V-8 juice or tomato juice, freshly prepared, when possible
½ cup onion rings, pan fried to a crisp (onions only, no breading)
2 slices GG bran crispbread or other similar product (2 gms of carbohydrate) or 1 slice of a 4-gm crispbread
1 slice of fresh orange (sliced to ¼-inch thickness) as a garnish
2 slices of diet bread recipe, toasted and buttered
Decaf cappuccino

From the Recipe Section in *New Diet Revolution:*

Cheese pancakes

Maintenance

All foods on the Induction *diet and the* OWL *diet are also included on the* Maintenance *diet*

½ grapefruit, may be baked with artificial sweetener
1½ cups of honeydew, cantaloupe, Spanish, Persian, casaba melon
1 cup of berries, any or all kinds, with a dollop of sour cream or whipped heavy cream (not pre-sweetened); may add cinnamon, chocolate, almondine, amaretto flavors, as presented by Wagner's Natural line
½ cup unflavored yogurt
Corned beef hash, using diet bread in the recipe, instead of the standard recipe
Creamed chipped beef on diet toast
Blintzes, using crepe recipe

From the Recipe Section in *New Diet Revolution:*

Eggs Florentine
Mushrooms, onions, and eggs
Broccoli frittata

A Maintenance Breakfast Special

For cereal lovers, 2 to 4 slices of GG bran crispbread or other similar product, crumbled by hand to smaller than bite-size consistency. Place in skillet, cover with water, boil off the water until the consistency of moist gruel is reached, add 2 different kinds of sweeteners, extracts like banana or coconut flavors if desired, and add 2 to 3 oz. heavy or light cream or half and half.

Lunch

Induction

Cheeseburger or bacon cheeseburger, no bun
Sour pickle
Clear chicken consommé (read label)
1 to 2 cups of tossed salad with a selection of the salad greens and with oil and vinegar, ranch dressing, blue cheese dressing, or creamy garlic dressing—make sure all salad dressings are sugar-free; better yet, ascertain that carbohydrate counts are below one gram per serving
Assorted cold cuts—ham, cheese, tongue, salami, roast beef, chicken, turkey, and salad as above
Chef's salad
Cucumbers in sour cream (see recipe section)
Chicken parts, broiled, no breading
Tuna salad, chicken salad, egg salad, ham salad, crabmeat or lobster salad (made with the named ingredient plus pure mayonnaise, not imitation mayonnaise or "salad dressing," plus chopped celery, onions, scallions, capers, etc., and hard-boiled egg, if desired)

Ongoing Weight Loss (OWL)

All foods on the Induction *diet are also included on the* OWL *diet*

Shrimp or crabmeat or tuna salad stuffed into a fresh tomato or into ½ avocado

Pizza (see recipe section)
Guacamole
Chicken salad (see recipes, also in dinner section)
Leftover meatloaf
Baked spinach

Maintenance

All foods on the Induction *and* OWL *diets are also included on the* Maintenance *diet*

Spinach egg pie

Dinner

Induction

Appetizers and soups:

Seafood salad (Frutta di mare)
Prosciutto
Shrimp scampi
Cold shrimp in mayonnaise and mustard or mayonnaise and
    horseradish
Beef tartare
Caviar and sour cream
Paté (see recipe section)
Steamers
Mussels provençale
Smoked trout
Smoked salmon
Quick bouillon soup

Salads (and dressings):

Tricolore
Arugula and deep-fried goat cheese
Country salad—mixed greens with bacon chunks and crumpled
blue cheese
Caesar salad (no croutons)

From the Recipe Section of *New Diet Revolution:*

Salmon salad
Bacon and egg salad
Mushroom salad
Avocado dressing
Russian dressing
Basic French dressing

Main Courses:

Steaks, roasts, chops—all kinds
Roast chicken, turkey, duck—in natural gravy
Spareribs—no glazing
Rack of lamb
Grilled, poached, broiled, panfried, baked fish—all varieties
Scampi
Lobster in drawn butter

From the Recipe Section of *New Diet Revolution:*

Roast leg of lamb
Chicken salad
Meatloaf
Warm beef, mushroom, and watercress salad flavored with
horseradish

Side Dishes:

1 cup of steamed vegetables, assorted or individual, from permissible vegetable list
Giant mushrooms (porcini, morels, portobello, etc.) sautéed in olive
oil

Desserts:

Diet Jell-O (plus a dollop of whipped, artificially sweetened heavy
   cream)

Ongoing Weight Loss (OWL)

All foods on the Induction *diet are also included on the* OWL *diet*

Appetizers and soups:

Avocado cream soup
Lobster soup

Salads:

Guacamole
Celery root salad (see recipe section)

Main Courses:

From the Recipe Section of *New Diet Revolution:*

Poached salmon
Blackened beef with a basil and parsley cream
Fried fillet of sea bass with leeks and tomatoes
Sauerkraut with variety of cooked meats
Beef stroganoff
Coq au oui

Side Dishes:

From the Recipe Section of *New Diet Revolution*:

Broccoli frittata
Eggplant balls
Brussels sprouts crisps

Desserts:

From the Recipe Section in *New Diet Revolution*:

Fruit mold
Italian sponge cake
Blueberry ice cream
Vanilla ice cream
Lemon mousse

Maintenance

All foods on the Induction *and* OWL *diets are also included on the*
Maintenance *diet*

Appetizers and soups:

Chilled marinated oysters
Stuffed fried mushrooms
Cream of onion soup

Salads:

From the Recipe Section of *New Diet Revolution*:

Cold salad of scrambled egg and cottage cheese with asparagus
Baked spinach flavored with basil and ricotta cheese
Stuffed fried mushrooms with goat cheese

Main courses:

From the recipe section of *New Diet Revolution*:

Chicken cacciatore
Chicken paprika
Cassolette of shrimp flavored with vegetables and bay leaves
Chicken curry
Chicken with okra and peanuts
Veal stew
Warm avocado pears and lobster glazed with béarnaise sauce

Stuffed veal chops with wild mushrooms
Warmed lobster salad with tarragon butter dressing
Escalopes of veal stuffed with a puree of mushrooms
Mousseline of queen scallops with saffron sauce
Medallions of lamb with green lentils and bacon

Side dishes:

From the Recipe Section of *New Diet Revolution:*

String beans with walnut sauce
Stuffed peppers

The Atkins Psychological Advantage Meal

Take advantage of your new-found liberty to eat all you want by going to somewhere where you can do just that. How about going to a smorgasbord restaurant and filling up on the protein and salad food? Fill your plate and then go back for seconds. Maybe even thirds. Make sure there's no sweet taste in any of the food you eat. Experienced dieters will recognize that taste instantly.

Desserts:

From the Recipe Section of *New Diet Revolution:*

Chocolate truffles
Rum truffles
Strawberry torte
Zabaglione
Italian sponge cake

Beverages

For all diets

Water (especially spring water, mineral water)
Club soda and seltzer
Essence-flavored seltzers (black cherry, raspberry, etc.; must specify no calories)
Hot or iced herbal tea (no barley, figs, dates, honey, etc.)
Decaffeinated coffee or tea

On *Induction* or *Maintenance* diets:
Artificially sweetened orange soda containing some natural juice

Recipes

Ah, you must all have noticed the number of times I said the Atkins diet is fit for a king. I am convinced that this is one slimming regimen on which you'll think you're royalty.

One of the reasons low-carbohydrate dieting did not sweep through the planet like a brushfire is that its early proponents, although agog with excitement over its capacity to melt down body fat stores, were very disparaging about the palatability of the diet. They described their experimental subjects as being unhappy with the monotony of the diet, and they suggested it would never be suitable for long-term use.

That's where the then-young Dr. Atkins entered the picture some 30 years ago. All my life I have been a cross between a gourmet and a gourmand. I loved and still do love to eat. I have read magazine articles titled, "How the Diet Doctors Eat," and I came to the conclusion that the world has never known a diet doctor who loves food as much as I do. This is bad news for me, but wonderful news for you. It caused me to create an Eater's Diet, a Hungry Man's Diet. If *Dr. Atkins' Diet Revolution* was an international success, it must have been in part because I succeeded in communicating my own excitement over food.

Well I couldn't allow this book to achieve any less in the food line, so I had to find a chef to match the royal pleasures I was planning for you. Vacationing in Barbados, fortune smiled upon me. I sampled the cuisine of Graham Newbould, master of the kitchen at the famous Treasure Beach Hotel. For six years, Newbould had been one of the chefs for Prince Charles and Princess Diana, and I soon understood why. Once you sample his recipes, so will you. Chef Newbould's recipes are distinguished, appropriately enough, by a crown, 👑. Compared to our standard recipes, they are admittedly more elegant—and more spectacular when served—and they are basically not meant to be daily fare. As you can see by the gram count, most are appropriate on the *Maintenance* diet—at those dinner parties where you simply want to show off how luxurious dieting can be. The other recipes were devised by my wife, by the dietitians at the Atkins Center, or come from *Dr. Atkins' Diet Cookbook.*

If Newbould is the jewel in this section's culinary crown, I can't pretend I'm anything but proud of our other recipes, loosely grouped according to meal and purpose. I haven't attempted to include everything. After all, most of you have been preparing protein main courses all your life, and it would be superfluous to tell you how to broil a steak or cook up bacon and eggs for breakfast.

I have, however, included the sort of rich recipes that dietary committees have been leading you away from but that will certainly produce a direct and immediate effect on your salivary glands. Since the Atkins diet is mainly a main course and salad diet, make those dishes as scrumptious as possible. If that extra touch of richness is what makes the dish a success, then don't feel constrained against using these rich things—the rule is: If dieting is inevitable, you might as well enjoy it.

Meanwhile, we all know there are certain things you aren't going to get on this diet. The most frequently dreamt of include sweet desserts, pasta, French fries, and bread.

And yet, over the years, we have learned substitutes for those much desired starches and sweets. I am able, because of my wife Veronica's imagination and the contributions of many of the culinarily-inclined patients I've known, to have desserts that are better than the real thing. I've eaten chocolate nut bars of an excellence that could not be equaled by all the cooks in the entire city of Hershey, Pennsylvania, even if they had the assistance of a special panel sent over from Switzerland. I've been able, in moments of need, to enjoy coconut custard pie or piña coladas—and all without indulging in an ounce of sugar.

I simply don't feel deprived. These are the things I want to share with you.

Let me now deal with a few specific ideas, so that you will know how to use this section. Turn your attention to the basic pancake recipe. This can make it possible for you to enjoy your own variations of pizza, blintzes, and tortillas, or you can roll them up with pork packed inside, as the Chinese do.

And then there's our bread, an exceptionally tasty, low-carbohydrate creation that can be used for sandwiches, croutons, toast, finger foods, garlic bread, or even pseudo–matzoh balls in chicken soup. Or how about, with the proper additives, creating ginger bread, banana bread, or Boston brown bread; not to mention the bread's most elegant use of all—as something that can mop up the exquisite juices of your sunny-side-up eggs.

As you taste these recipes and taste Graham Newbould's gourmet delights, I believe you'll become convinced you're not going to go on any other diet. Where would you find a diet that allows you to be a gourmet while you still go on dieting?

Soups

Avocado Cream Soup Barbara

8 servings (½ cup each)

1 medium avocado
2 cups heavy cream
1 cup water
½ teaspoon celery salt
¼ teaspoon seasoned salt
½ small clove garlic, minced
8 slices bacon, cooked crisp

Peel avocado and remove pit. Place it in blender with heavy cream, water, celery salt, salt, and garlic. Blend at medium speed for 15 seconds.

Pour into saucepan. Cook over medium heat for 5 minutes, stirring constantly. Do not boil.

Serve warm or cold garnished with crumbled bacon.

TOTAL GRAMS 31.5
GRAMS PER SERVING 3.9

Lobster Soup

6 servings

2 cups fresh or canned lobster meat
3 tablespoons butter
3 cups heavy cream
¼ teaspoon onion powder
1 cup water
½ teaspoon seasoned salt
¼ cup sherry

Cut lobster meat into bite-sized pieces. Melt butter in skillet and add lobster. Cook for 5 minutes over low heat.

Separately mix heavy cream with water. Add to skillet, stirring constantly. Do not boil. Add salt and onion powder. Refrigerate overnight.

Reheat. Add sherry. Serve in soup bowls.

TOTAL GRAMS 29.7
GRAMS PER SERVING 5.0

Quick Bouillon Pickup

1 serving

1 cup hot bouillon
1 egg
dash of Tabasco sauce
dash of salt

Blend egg in electric blender until light and foamy. Add bouillon slowly. Blend in Tabasco sauce and salt.

Serve hot in mug.

TOTAL GRAMS 0.8

Cream of Onion Soup Lightly Perfumed with Curry

4 servings

3 cups sliced onions
1 tablespoon butter
2 cloves garlic, peeled
2 bay leaves
2 cups heavy cream
1 cup chicken stock
1 tablespoon curry powder
1 tablespoon chives, chopped
salt and pepper (optional)

Melt the butter in a warm saucepan. Add the onions, garlic, and bay leaves. Sauté until golden brown.

Add the curry powder and cook for 1 minute, stirring so that the curry powder cannot burn.

Add the chicken stock and boil until the liquid has reduced by ½, then add the cream and simmer for approximately 15 minutes. Remove bay leaves.

Allow the mixture to cool, then place in a blender or food processor. Pass the soup through a fine strainer and season with salt and pepper according to taste.

When serving, reheat the soup (do not boil) and sprinkle the snipped chives and a little heavy cream on top.

TOTAL GRAMS 67.8
GRAMS PER SERVING 17.0

Egg Dishes

Basic Omelet

1 serving

2 eggs
1 tablespoon chives
1 tablespoon fresh parsley, chopped
⅛ teaspoon salt
1 tablespoon heavy cream
1 tablespoon butter
1 pinch freshly ground pepper

Combine all ingredients and beat lightly.

Melt butter in non-stick omelet pan.

After foam subsides, pour egg mixture into pan. Cook without stirring for about 1 to 2 minutes until sides and bottom are set but center is still wet. Carefully flip one side of omelet on top of other side to form a half moon.

Slide onto plate and serve.

TOTAL GRAMS 1.9

Cheese Omelet

2 servings

4 eggs
½ cup grated Cheddar cheese
1 tablespoon chopped parsley

Follow recipe for Basic Fluffy Omelet (see above). Before folding omelet over, add grated Cheddar cheese and chopped parsley.

After folding omelet over, continue cooking for 2 minutes to be sure cheese is melted.

Serve hot.

TOTAL GRAMS 3.5
GRAMS PER SERVING 1.8

Scrambled Eggs in Cheese Sauce with Sausages

6 servings

12 link sausages (be sure they contain no sugar)
1 3-ounce package cream cheese (full-fat)
1 tablespoon butter
¾ cup cream
¼ cup water
1 teaspoon seasoned salt
2 teaspoons parsley
8 eggs, beaten

Sauté sausages in skillet until brown. Drain.

In double boiler over simmering (not boiling) water, heat cream cheese and butter. Add cream, water, salt, and parsley.

Stir in beaten eggs with fork. Cook until eggs have thickened.

TOTAL GRAMS 19.2
GRAMS PER SERVING 3.2

Cheese Pancakes

6 servings

1 cup cottage cheese
6 eggs
3 tablespoons soy protein isolate (or soy flour)
3 tablespoons butter, melted
1 teaspoon seasoned salt
oil

Put all ingredients except oil in blender. Blend until smooth. Heat oiled griddle until very hot. Drop batter by tablespoonfuls onto griddle. Brown on both sides.

TOTAL GRAMS 11.0 (16.0 WITH SOY FLOUR)
GRAMS PER SERVING 1.8 (2.7 WITH SOY FLOUR)

Mushrooms, Onions, and Eggs

3 servings

1½ cups mushrooms, sliced
1½ cups chopped onion
4 tablespoons butter
seasoned salt to taste
6 eggs
2 tablespoons heavy cream

Sauté mushrooms and onion in butter until well browned. Add salt.

Beat eggs with heavy cream. Pour over mushroom mixture and stir until eggs are cooked (about 4 stirs). Serve immediately.

TOTAL GRAMS 16.1
GRAMS PER SERVING 5.4

Eggs Florentine

6 servings

2 cups cooked fresh spinach or 1 package frozen spinach
6 eggs
salt to taste
1 recipe Cheese Sauce (see below)

Preheat oven to 350 degrees.

Cook spinach. Drain well. Chop fine.

Place hot spinach in shallow baking dish.

Make hole for each egg in spinach. Break egg into each hole. Sprinkle with salt.

Prepare cheese sauce. Pour over eggs and spinach.

Bake in moderate 350-degree oven for 25 minutes.

TOTAL GRAMS 26.5
GRAMS PER SERVING 4.4

Cheese Sauce

18 tablespoons

¾ cup cream
⅓ cup water
¾ pound (1½ cups) Cheddar cheese diced
1 teaspoon mustard
1 teaspoon salt
½ teaspoon paprika

In double boiler combine ingredients for cheese sauce. Simmer slowly. Stir constantly until smooth.

TOTAL GRAMS 10.5
GRAMS PER SERVING 1.8

Bacon and Egg Salad

6 servings

9 hard-cooked eggs
9 slices bacon, cooked crisp
½ teaspoon seasoned salt
¼ teaspoon dry mustard
¼ cup mayonnaise (sugar free)

Chop eggs and bacon together in wooden chopping bowl. Add salt and mustard.

Fold in mayonnaise and mix well.

TOTAL GRAMS 9.0
GRAMS PER SERVING 1.5

Broccoli* Frittata

6 servings

4 eggs
1 cup cooked broccoli florets
1 cup thinly sliced onion
1½ cups mushroom caps, thinly sliced
½ teaspoon salt
½ teaspoon freshly ground pepper
4 tablespoons butter
3 tablespoons grated Parmesan cheese
1 teaspoon baking soda
¼ cup minced fresh parsley for garnish

Put 2 tablespoons butter in skillet. Sauté onion and mushrooms until golden. Remove from stove.

Put eggs, baking soda, salt, and pepper in a bowl and thoroughly beat. Add onions and mushrooms and broccoli. Mix well.

Add remaining butter to skillet and pour in egg mixture. Tilt pan to cover bottom with mixture. Fry on top of stove until eggs start setting. Sprinkle Parmesan cheese on top and broil until golden. Remove from heat.

Cut into wedges and serve. Garnish with minced parsley.

TOTAL GRAMS 31.8
GRAMS PER SERVING 5.3

*You can use any non-starchy leftover vegetable instead of broccoli.

Poultry, Beef, Seafood

Coq Au Oui

6 servings

4 pounds chicken parts
¼ pound bacon, diced
½ stick butter
1 cup red wine
1 cup chicken stock
3 cloves garlic
1 bay leaf
2 cups minced onion
3 cups mushroom caps, sliced
salt to taste

Sauté diced bacon in butter until golden. Remove from skillet and save.

Thoroughly wash and dry chicken. Brown in bacon fat. Remove and set aside.

Sauté onions and mushrooms. Return chicken and bacon to pan. Add chicken stock, garlic, wine, and bay leaf. Simmer gently 40 minutes to 1 hour in uncovered skillet. Add salt to taste.

TOTAL GRAMS 46.1
GRAMS PER SERVING 7.7

Chicken Curry

4 servings

1 chicken, cut into 8 to 10 pieces
1⅓ cups minced onions
3 cloves garlic, minced
1 tablespoon turmeric
1 tablespoon cumin
1 tablespoon ground ginger
1 tablespoon chili powder
4 tablespoons butter
1 cup heavy cream
1 cup hot water
salt to taste

Sauté chicken pieces in butter until golden. Remove.

Gently sauté onions, garlic, and all remaining condiments 2 to 3 minutes, stirring constantly.

Place chicken parts into sauce. Add 1 cup hot water and 1 cup heavy cream. Simmer until chicken is tender and reduce to about half original amount.

For variety, you can substitute lamb for the chicken.

TOTAL GRAMS 45.4
GRAMS PER SERVING 11.4

Chicken with Okra and Peanuts

4 servings

1 large chicken
3 carrots
2 leeks
1 whole onion
salt to taste°

½ pound small okra
½ pound shelled peanuts
1 tablespoon unsweetened tomato paste
1 stick butter
1 tablespoon fresh parsley, chopped

Combine first 5 ingredients. Cover with water and simmer 45 minutes. Remove chicken from stock and let cool. When cool, debone chicken completely and shred.

In Dutch oven, heat butter until foam subsides. Lower flame. Put in the shredded chicken, okra, tomato paste, and peanuts and sauté gently until golden. Stir often.

Sprinkle with parsley and serve.

TOTAL GRAMS 62.0
GRAMS PER SERVING 15.5

°The first five infredients constitute the stock, and are not consumed. Approximately 25% of the carbohydrate may be present on the chicken.

Chicken Paprika

8 servings

3 pounds chicken parts
½ stick butter
¼ cup vegetable oil
2¾ cups chopped onions
4 cloves garlic, chopped
4 tablespoons good Hungarian paprika
½ cup chicken broth
1 cup white wine
2 cups sour cream

Preheat oven to 375 to 400 degrees.

In a Dutch oven sauté chicken parts in oil-butter mixture on all sides until golden. Remove to plate.

Add onions and garlic to Dutch oven and sauté until golden. Add paprika, chicken stock, wine, and sour cream and simmer gently about 10 minutes.

Replace chicken parts into Dutch oven and coat with sauce. Bake covered in oven at 375 to 400 degrees about 45 minutes or until chicken is well done.

TOTAL GRAMS 68.0
GRAMS PER SERVING 8.5

Chicken Cacciatore

8 servings

5 pounds mixed chicken parts
½ cup olive oil
½ stick butter
1⅓ cups chopped onion
3 cups mushroom caps, thinly sliced
4 cloves garlic
1 cup white wine
2 bay leaves
2 teaspoons oregano
1 teaspoon freshly ground pepper
3 tablespoons brandy
1 cup sun-dried tomatoes
salt to taste

Soak tomatoes in hot water and set aside.

Sauté chicken in half olive oil, half butter, on all sides until golden. Set aside.

Heat remaining oil and butter in skillet and sauté onions until light golden. Add mushrooms and garlic. Continue sautéing until soft.

Place chicken parts in Dutch oven and pour onion-mushroom mixture on top of chicken. Pour in wine and add drained tomatoes and remaining ingredients. Cover lightly and simmer 30 minutes or until chicken is thoroughly cooked through.

TOTAL GRAMS 65.0
GRAMS PER SERVING 8.1

Meat Loaf

6 servings

3 pounds chopped mixed meats (lamb, veal, beef, pork)
2 tablespoons chili powder
3 eggs
3 cloves garlic, mashed
3 tablespoons cilantro or Italian parsley
6 ounces sharp cheddar cheese, shredded
2 tablespoons Worcestershire sauce
salt to taste

Preheat oven to 375 degrees.

In large bowl, thoroughly mix all ingredients. Place meat into oiled loaf pan and bake 45 minutes to 1 hour.

TOTAL GRAMS 19.1
GRAMS PER SERVING 3.2

Parfait of Chicken Livers with Braised Sultanas*

♛

4 servings

Chicken Livers:
1 tablespoon butter
8 ounces warm clarified butter
8 ounces chicken livers
1 whole bulb peeled garlic (or 8 large cloves)
1 cup sliced onion
1 cup ruby port
1 cup brandy or cognac
10 thin slices bacon
1 pinch grated nutmeg
1 pinch ground cinnamon
1 bay leaf
1 sprig thyme

Braised Sultanas:
4 ounces sultanas
2 tea bags
1 tablespoon Grand Marnier
½ teaspoon orange peel

To Prepare Chicken Livers:

Place the raw chicken livers and peeled garlic into a bowl and cover with plastic wrap. Warm gently on the side of the stove.

Meanwhile, take a terrine or a 1-pint casserole and line it with thin slices of bacon.

Place the tablespoons of butter into a warm saucepan. Add the sliced onions and steam them until cooked. Add the port, brandy, bay leaf, and thyme, and simmer uncovered to reduce the liquid by two-thirds. Strain the liquid onto the warm chicken livers and garlic.

Place the mixture into a food processor and puree it.

While the mixture is being processed, add the warm clarified butter slowly. It is important to add it slowly, otherwise the mixture will curdle. Add the nutmeg and cinnamon. Pass the mixture through a fine sieve.

Then place the mixture into the lined terrine/casserole. Cover the top with bacon and then cover the whole dish with aluminum foil. Place the terrine into a basin/bain marie and cook in a slow oven for 1 hour.

When cooked, remove from oven and allow the parfait to cool for 24 hours. When cool, slice the parfait and serve with a mixture of lettuce leaves and braised sultanas.

To Prepare Braised Sultanas:

Simmer the sultanas in 1 pint of water with the tea bags and orange peel. Allow to cool in the tea mixture, then add a tablespoon of Grand Marnier. The sultanas can be served warm or cold as an accompaniment to the parfait.

TOTAL GRAMS 80.9
GRAMS PER SERVING 20.2

°Braised sultanas can be replaced with 1 ounce of finely shredded leeks sautéed in butter seasoned with black pepper.

Stuffed Peppers

8 servings

8 medium green peppers
1 cup finely chopped onion
2 pounds meat loaf mixture (lamb, veal, beef, pork)
1 teaspoon dried dill
3 tablespoons vegetable oil
1 teaspoon salt
1 teaspoon white pepper
½ cup chicken broth
3 tablespoons unsweetened tomato paste
1 cup sour cream

Sauté onions in skillet until golden.

Add meat mixture, pepper, salt, and dill. Brown and mix about 5 minutes. Let cool.

Wash and core peppers. Fill peppers with meat mixture and place open side up in Dutch oven.

Combine chicken stock and tomato paste and pour over peppers.

Cover and cook in oven at 375 degrees until peppers are done.

When serving add generous amounts of sour cream.

TOTAL GRAMS 84.4
GRAMS PER SERVING 10.6

Beef Stroganoff

4 servings

2 tablespoons chopped parsley
1 cup finely chopped onion
3 cups mushroom caps, sliced
2 pounds sirloin, cut into strips
1 ½ tablespoons powdered mustard
½ cup sour cream
3 tablespoons unsweetened ketchup
3 tablespoons oil
freshly ground white pepper
salt to taste

Combine mustard powder, ketchup, and enough hot water to form thick paste.

Sauté onions and mushrooms in 2 tablespoons of oil until golden and soft. Remove with slotted spoon to preheated Dutch oven.

Add remaining oil to skillet and sauté meat strips in batches (quickly, like in stir-frying). Transfer meat to Dutch oven.

Put mustard paste and sour cream in skillet with any remaining juices. Stir gently all ingredients until smoothly mixed.

Pour over meat and onions and mix well. Gently simmer until hot. Sprinkle with parsley, salt, and freshly ground white pepper and serve immediately.

TOTAL GRAMS 45.3
GRAMS PER SERVING 11.3

Blackened Beef with a Basil and Parsley Cream

6 servings

1 ½ pounds of beef tenderloin, trimmed

Marinade:
1 stick clarified butter
4 cloves garlic, crushed
1 tablespoon ground black pepper
1 tablespoon paprika
1 teaspoon grated horseradish or cold horseradish sauce
1 tablespoon soy sauce
1 tablespoon mixed herbs (basil, thyme, parsley, marjoram), chopped

Sauce:
2 cups heavy cream
1 tablespoon parsley, chopped
1 tablespoon basil, chopped
2 cloves garlic, crushed
1 cup white wine
1 tablespoon butter

Blend together the ingredients for the marinade in a food processor.

Cut the beef into 8 medallions.

Cover the beef with the marinade and allow it to rest overnight in the refrigerator.

Next day:

To make the sauce, melt the butter in a warm saucepan. Gently sauté the garlic, parsley, and basil, occasionally stirring.

Add the white wine and then simmer uncovered to reduce by ½.

Add the heavy cream and simmer for 5 minutes until the cream thickens. Season according to taste.

To cook the beef, place a skillet on the heat until it is very hot, then place the marinated beef medallions into the pan (the mixture must remain on the beef). Cook for 1 minute. Then turn the medallions and cook for 1 more minute.

TOTAL GRAMS 37.9
GRAMS PER SERVING 6.3

Chipped Beef Balls

12 balls

8 ounces cream cheese, room temperature
¼ teaspoon sage
¼ teaspoon onion juice
¼ teaspoon Worcestershire sauce*
dash of lemon juice, dash of Tabasco sauce
5 ounces chipped or dried beef, chopped

Mix together all ingredients except chipped beef.

Chill for at least 1 hour.

Shape into small balls and roll in chipped beef. Refrigerate. Serve on toothpicks.

TOTAL GRAMS 10.0
GRAMS PER SERVING 0.8

*We have used Lea & Perrin's because it is the lowest in carbohydrate grams—1 tablespoon has a trace.

Sauerkraut with Variety of Cooked Meats

6 servings

3 cups sauerkraut
1 pound cooked chicken
1 pound roast pork (or ham hocks)
1 pound sausage
4 tablespoons lard
¼ cup beef broth
3 tablespoons unsweetened tomato puree
2 cups chopped onions
1 cup vodka
½ cup white wine
bouquet garni of peppercorns, allspice, laurel leaf, juniper berries

Preheat oven to 350 degrees.

Wash sauerkraut. Blanch and drain.

Heat lard in heavy skillet. Add chopped onions, sauté until golden. Add beef stock, vodka, wine and tomato puree. Mix well and simmer for 5 minutes.

Put layer of sauerkraut in heavy casserole. Place some meats on top. Repeat this until all sauerkraut and meats have been used. Pour beef stock, vodka, etc. mixture on top of sauerkraut and meat. Insert bouquet garni. Cover and bake at 350 degrees for about 2 hours.

TOTAL GRAMS 61.8
GRAMS PER SERVING 10.3

Stuffed Veal Chops with Wild Mushrooms

4 servings

4 double veal chops
    (have butcher cut a pocket into each chop)
½ cup minced shallots
2 cups cooked spinach
3 cups mushroom caps, thinly sliced
1 cup dried porcini mushrooms
½ cup chicken broth
3 tablespoons butter
½ cup white wine
2 tablespoons cognac
1 teaspoon ground white pepper
1 teaspoon salt

½ cup heavy cream
2 tablespoons oil

Preheat oven to 400 degrees.

Sauté shallots and mushroom caps in 1 tablespoon butter and 1 tablespoon oil until golden. Add chopped spinach, white pepper, and salt and cook until spinach is wilted. Set aside. Let cool.

Soak Porcini mushrooms in hot chicken stock while preparing stuffing. Stuff each chop with mixture. Close opening with toothpicks.

Heat remaining butter and oil in skillet and thoroughly brown stuffed chops on both sides. Place into Dutch oven.

Mix chicken stock and Porcini mushrooms with cognac, white wine, and heavy cream. Pour over chops and bake at 400 degrees 45 minutes to 1 hour. Turn chops once after 30 minutes. Remove chops, sprinkle with fresh pepper, and serve.

TOTAL GRAMS 45.6
GRAMS PER SERVING 11.4

Veal Stew

6 servings

1 stalk celery, diced
1 carrot, diced
1 bay leaf
3 pounds stewing veal
¾ cups white wine
1 pound pearl onions
1 ½ pounds mushroom caps, sliced
5 egg yolks
1 cup heavy cream
salt to taste

In Dutch oven, bring first seven ingredients to a slow boil. Cover and simmer an additional 30 minutes.

In bowl, stir egg yolks and cream. Dribble in cup of broth, stirring continuously. Stir in egg-cream mixture into veal until sauce thickens.

TOTAL GRAMS 73.6
GRAMS PER SERVING 12.3

Escalopes of Veal Stuffed with Puree of Mushrooms

4 servings

4 thin slices loin or tenderloin veal

Filling:
1½ cups mushrooms
1 cup chopped onion
1 cup ruby port

Coating:
4 ounces Parmesan cheese, grated
2 eggs, whipped

3 separate tablespoons butter
1 eggplant, peeled and diced
6 cups good veal stock
½ pint red wine
minced parsley

Puree:
Melt the butter in a warm saucepan. Sauté the onions until tender, then add the mushrooms and cook for a further 5 minutes. Add the ruby port and simmer the mixture until most of the moisture has evaporated. Occasionally stir to prevent burning. Remove from heat and allow to cool.

Puree the mixture in a food processor.

Flatten veal until very thin. Place a spoonful of the mixture on top of each veal escalope, then fold it in half, sealing the edges.

Dip each escalope into the whipped egg and then into the Parmesan cheese. Repeat this procedure once more.

Sauce:
Reduce the veal stock and red wine together by simmering uncovered until you are left with ⅔ cup. Season with salt and pepper. If the reduction is thin, it can be thickened with a little arrowroot and water mixture.

Garnish:
Fry the eggplant in a little butter until golden brown.

To serve:
Melt a little butter in a skillet and fry the veal escalopes on both sides until golden brown. Place onto a warm plate and surround with a little sauce. Sprinkle the fried eggplant around the garnish with minced parsley.

TOTAL GRAMS 72.5
GRAMS PER SERVING 18.1

Roast Leg of Lamb

10 servings

10- to 12-pound leg of lamb
5 cloves garlic
2 tablespoons rosemary
1 teaspoon salt

Preheat oven to 500 degrees.

Make slits all over lamb and insert slivers of garlic. Rub salt and rosemary over lamb.

Place lamb fat side up on rack in open roasting pan. Roast at 500 degrees for 15 minutes. Reduce heat to 350 degrees and roast 2 to 2½ hours more.

TOTAL GRAMS 5.0
GRAMS PER SERVING 0.5

Medallions of Lamb with Green Lentils and Bacon

2 servings

2 medallions lamb, noisette from the best end
½ cup small French green lentils
6 slices of smoked bacon
Lamb drippings with garlic
vegetables to garnish (onion, celery, leek), 1 ounce of each
clarified butter
2 cloves garlic, minced

To cook the lentils, finely chop onion, celery, leek and garlic. Steam it in clarified butter. Add the lentils, then lamb stock, and cook until the lentils are tender.

Seal the medallions of lamb, place some cooked lentils on top of each piece, and wrap it in smoked bacon. Skewer the bacon to hold it in place. While this is cooking, cook the noisettes in a hot pan.

Place a bed of lentils onto the plate. Place the lamb on top of the lentils and napee with a lamb garlic-flavored jus. Arrange vegetables around the lamb.

Choice vegetables would be fine green beans.

TOTAL GRAMS 30.1
GRAMS PER SERVING 15.1

Lamb Jus with Garlic

2 servings

lamb trimmings, no fat
6 shallots, sliced
4 cloves garlic, crushed
3 slices smoked bacon
1 pint lamb stock
1 cup dry white wine

Sauté the lamb trimmings until brown, tip off any excess fat. Add the shallots and crushed garlic and smoked bacon. Sauté for a further 2 minutes. Add the white wine and simmer uncovered to reduce. Then add the lamb stock and reduce. When the sauce has reduced by one-half, strain it through a fine strainer. Correct the seasoning and finish with a little unsalted butter.

TOTAL GRAMS 22.1
GRAMS PER SERVING 11.1

Cassolette of Shrimp Flavored with Vegetables and Bay Leaves

4 servings

16 good-sized shrimp, peeled and deveined
½ cup parsnip, finely chopped
1 medium leek, finely chopped
2 stalks of celery, finely chopped
½ cup dry white wine
1 cup heavy cream
2 bay leaves
1 tomato, skinned, seeds removed, and diced
1 tablespoon chives, snipped
1 tablespoon butter
salt and pepper (optional)

Melt the butter in a warm saucepan. Sauté the vegetables and bay leaves in the butter for 2 minutes. Add the shrimp and cook for 1 more minute.

Add the white wine and reduce the liquid by half. Then add the heavy cream and simmer for approximately 3 minutes.

Season according to taste with salt and pepper.

Divide into 4 soup bowls and garnish with the chopped tomato and snipped chives.

TOTAL GRAMS 34.7
GRAMS PER SERVING 8.7

Warm Avocados and Lobster Glazed with Béarnaise Sauce

4 servings

2 medium-sized ripe California avocados
8 ounces cooked lobster meat, cut into chunks
¾ cup mushrooms, sliced
1 cup finely chopped onion
½ cup dry white wine
1 cup Béarnaise sauce (see recipe, page 298)
1 tablespoon butter

Cut the avocados in half and remove the stones. Scoop out the pump, leaving the outer shell intact. Cut the pulp into bite-sized chunks.

Melt the butter in a warm saucepan. Sauté the chopped onions and sliced mushrooms for approximately 1 minute. Add the lobster and avocado chunks and give the mixture a stir. Add the white wine. Simmer for 3 to 4 minutes.

Place the mixture into the empty avocado shells. Coat each one with the Bearnaise sauce.

Glaze under a hot salamander or grill until golden brown.

Serve immediately.

TOTAL GRAMS 48.6
GRAMS PER SERVING 9.7

Poached Salmon with Béarnaise Sauce

4 servings

4 thick salmon steaks
1 cup chicken stock
1 cup white wine
1 bay leaf
1½ cups Béarnaise sauce (see recipe, page 298)
fresh dill

Put salmon into deep skillet. Combine remaining ingredients and pour over salmon. Cover and simmer gently 10 to 15 minutes. Sprinkle with dill and serve.

TOTAL GRAMS 12.2
GRAMS PER SERVING 3.1

Béarnaise Sauce

1½ cups

3 egg yolks
1 cup warm clarified butter
1 tablespoon tarragon, chopped
3 tablespoons dry white Chablis
1 tablespoon tarragon or distilled vinegar
6 black peppercorns
1 shallot, chopped

Place the last four ingredients into a pan and simmer uncovered until only 1 tablespoon of liquid remains. Allow it to cool, then strain the liquid.

Place the egg yolks into a bowl with strained liquid and whip them over a gentle heat (bain-marie) until it acquires a ribbon texture. Add the melted butter slowly. Keep whipping the mixture until all the butter has been incorporated.

Remove the pan from the heat and mix in the chopped tarragon.

Serve with fish or meats.

TOTAL GRAMS 3.3

Chilled Marinated Oysters with a Dressing of Sour Cream and Cucumber

For a Main Course you will need 12 oysters per person
For an Appetizer you will need 6 oysters per person
¾ cup cooked spinach
½ cucumber
2 cups sour cream
freshly chopped dill
1 lime, freshly squeezed
Tabasco sauce
Cayenne pepper
salt and pepper
black caviar (optional)

Oysters
Open and clean the oysters. Retain the juice and the shells.

Place the oysters in a bowl with the juice and add a dash of Tabasco, 2 tablespoons lime juice, and a little freshly chopped dill. Allow them to marinate for 1 hour.

Cook 4 cups of spinach in boiling water, then refresh it in ice water. Squeeze out any excess water. Season the spinach with a little salt and pepper and place a little of the spinach in each oyster shell.

Dressing
Peel and dress ½ a cucumber, then dice.

Add to the cucumber 2 cups of sour cream, 1 teaspoon freshly chopped dill, and a pinch of Cayenne pepper.

To serve, place the oysters on top of the spinach in the shells. Coat each oyster with a little dressing and sprinkle a little Cayenne pepper on top.

Garnish the top with black caviar (optional).

Serve the oysters on a bed of crushed ice.

GRAMS PER SERVING (APPETIZER) 12.1
GRAMS PER SERVING (MAIN COURSE) 24.2

Fried Fillet of Sea Bass with Leeks and Tomatoes in an Olive Oil Dressing

4 servings

4 nice-sized fillets of sea bass
2 medium leeks, cut into small strips
2 large firm tomatoes, skinned, seeds removed, and chopped
1 tablespoon shredded basil
1 tablespoon balsamic vinegar
4 tablespoons virgin olive oil
1 tablespoon butter
freshly milled black pepper

Fry the sea bass in a tablespoon of olive oil in a skillet until golden brown on each side. Then remove from the pan and keep warm.

Add the butter to the same pan and gently sauté the leeks until tender. Add the balsamic vinegar, shaking the pan. Slowly add the 3 tablespoons of olive oil to make a sauce. Remove from the heat and add the chopped tomatoes, the shredded basil, and the milled black pepper.

Place the mixture onto a plate and sit the fillets of fish on top.

TOTAL GRAMS 25.8
GRAMS PER SERVING 6.5

Mousseline of Queen Scallops with Saffron Sauce

4 servings

Mousse:
1 tablespoom chives, chopped
6 ounces queen scallops
2 ounces Dover sole fillets
1 cup heavy cream
1 egg white
Cayenne pepper
salt and pepper

Garnish:
4 large spinach leaves, blanched
4 queen scallops per person

Sauce:
½ cup dry white wine
bones of 3 Dover soles
¼ cup shallots, sliced
⅓ cup mushroom parings
1 teaspoon saffron stamens
1 cup heavy cream
2 tablespoons butter

Line 4 buttered single-serving-sized baking dishes with the blanched spinach leaves.

Blend the scallops and Dover sole fillets in a food processor with the egg white. Place the fish puree through a fine sieve and place it in a bowl on ice to allow it to cool.

Slowly beat in the heavy cream. Season with salt and pepper and cayenne pepper and add the finely chopped chives. Place the mousseline into the lined baking dishes and cover them with buttered foil.

Place in a bain-marie and cook in a low oven at 350 degrees for 10 minutes.

Place all ingredients except heavy cream in a sauce pan. Reduce the ingredients for the sauce by simmering uncovered to approximately 1 tablespoon with a syrupy consistency and add the cream. Bring to a boil.

Whisk in 2 tablespoons of butter and correct seasoning.

To serve:
Place the baking dishes on a warm plate turned over. Around it place a little sauce, on top of which you sprinkle the warm blanched saffron and garnish with 4 slightly steamed queen scallops.

TOTAL GRAMS 34.7
GRAMS PER SERVING 8.7

Salads &
Dressings

Warm Lobster Salad with a Tarragon Butter Dressing

4 servings

1 pound cooked lobster, chopped into large pieces
1 cup chopped raw onion
1 head Romaine or Iceberg lettuce
½ cup fresh tarragon, ½ chopped, ½ for garnish
½ cup heavy cream
1 stick unsalted butter
1 tablespoon tarragon vinegar
1 pinch Cayenne pepper

Dressing:
Place the chopped tarragon and vinegar in a saucepan and bring to a boil. Add the heavy cream. Simmer for approximately 2 minutes. Remove the pan from heat and whisk the butter into the cream. Add a pinch of Cayenne pepper.

To serve:
Wash and dry the lettuce thoroughly. Break it into bite-sized pieces and arrange on a plate.

Place the lobster and chopped onion into the warm dressing until the lobster has become lukewarm. Place the lobster mixture on top of the Iceberg lettuce and decorate with leaves of fresh-picked tarragon.

TOTAL GRAMS 40.8
GRAMS PER SERVING 10.2

Salmon Salad in a Hurry

1 serving

1 7-ounce can salmon
2 tablespoons chopped scallions
½ stalk celery, diced
3 tablespoons Roquefort dressing (see below)

Remove bone and skin of salmon. Break in chunks in bowl. Mix scallions and celery with salmon. Turn into salad bowl and pour dressing over. This can also be served on lettuce leaves.

TOTAL GRAMS 2.9

Our Favorite Roquefort Dressing

1 cup

¼ cup tarragon vinegar
¼ teaspoon seasoned salt
3 turns of pepper mill
6 tablespoons olive oil
2 tablespoons heavy cream
½ teaspoon lemon juice
¼ cup crumbled Roquefort cheese

Beat all ingredients together except cheese. Stir in cheese.

TOTAL GRAMS 6.0

Mushroom Salad

6 servings

8 slices bacon, diced
⅓ cup minced onion
2 tablespoons butter, melted
3 tablespoons lemon juice
2 tablespoons parsley
3 cups white mushrooms, thinly sliced
2 tablespoons grated Parmesan cheese

Fry bacon until transparent. Add minced onion; continue frying until bacon is crisp and onion is golden. Pour off bacon fat.

Add butter, lemon juice, and parsley. Bring to boil.

Pour over mushrooms, and garnish with Parmesan cheese to taste.

TOTAL GRAMS 28.0
GRAMS PER SERVING 4.6

Basic French Dressing

½ cup

3 tablespoons tarragon vinegar
1 tablespoon lemon juice
½ teaspoon seasoned salt
3 turns of pepper mill
6 tablespoons olive oil
2 tablespoons vegetable oil
½ teaspoon Dijon mustard
¼ teaspoon dry mustard

Beat all ingredients together until well blended.

TOTAL GRAMS 4.2

Avocado Dressing

24 tablespoons

1 ripe medium avocado, cubed
½ cup lemon juice
¼ cup mayonnaise
1 teaspoon-equivalent sugar substitute
¼ teaspoon salt
¼ teaspoon paprika

Blend all ingredients at high speed until smooth.

TOTAL GRAMS 22.8
GRAMS PER TABLESPOON 1.0

Russian Dressing

20 tablespoons

½ cup mayonnaise
½ cup sour cream
1 tablespoon Dijon mustard
1 tablespoon Worcestershire sauce
2 tablespoons tomato sauce
½ teaspoon grated onion
⅛ teaspoon garlic powder

Combine ingredients. Mix well.

TOTAL GRAMS 8.1
GRAMS PER TABLESPOON 0.4

Cucumbers in Sour Cream

4 servings

2 cups thinly sliced cucumber
½ teaspoon salt
½ cup sour cream
½ teaspoon-equivalent sugar substitute
1 tablespoon vinegar
½ teaspoon dill

In a shallow bowl place cucumber, and sprinkle with salt.
    Allow to set for ½ hour. Drain.
    Add remaining ingredients. Mix well. Chill.

TOTAL GRAMS 12.1
GRAMS PER SERVING 3.0

Warm Beef, Mushroom and Watercress Salad Flavored with Horseradish

👑 4 servings

16 ounces cooked beef, shredded
8 ounces raw mushrooms, sliced
2 bunches fresh watercress
1 tablespoon freshly grated horseradish
2 egg yolks
1 tablespoon wine vinegar
4 tablespoons sesame oil
1 tablespoon toasted sesame seeds

Wash the watercress and dry thoroughly.

Mix the vinegar and sesame oil. Pour over the watercress and toss. Arrange the watercress on a cold plate.

Mix the shredded beef, mushrooms, and grated horseradish and egg yolks together. Place the mixture on top of the watercress and sprinkle with the toasted sesame seeds.

TOTAL GRAMS 10.3
GRAMS PER SERVING 2.6

Cold Salad of Scrambled Egg and Cottage Cheese with Asparagus

👑 4 servings

6 eggs, lightly scrambled and allowed to cool
1 cup cottage cheese
1 tablespoon chives, chopped
12 asparagus spears, peeled
3 cups iceberg lettuce, endive, radicchio, baby spinach leaves;
*   washed and picked*
1 tablespoon wine vinegar
4 tablespoons olive oil
salt and pepper

Scramble the eggs until quite soft. Allow them to cool. Mix them together with the cottage cheese and chives. Add the salt and pepper to taste.

Cook the asparagus spears by plunging them into boiling water and cooking them for 5 minutes. Cool the spears by placing them into ice water.

Mix the vinegar and olive oil together. Pour this over the lettuce and toss. Place the lettuce onto a cold plate. Arrange the egg and cheese mixture on top and decorate with the asparagus spears.

TOTAL GRAMS 23.4
GRAMS PER SERVING 5.9

Chicken Salad

6 servings

2 *large chicken breasts, cooked*
2 *large dill pickles, chopped*
3 *hard-boiled eggs, chopped*
3 *scallions, trimmed, washed, and chopped*
½ *teaspoon freshly ground pepper*
⅓ *cup sugar-free mayonnaise*
⅓ *cup sour cream*
2 *tablespoons drained capers*
3 *tablespoons fresh dill, chopped*
½ *cup pecan halves*

Cut chicken meat into strips. Combine all other ingredients. Add chicken and toss well.

TOTAL GRAMS 33.3
GRAMS PER SERVING 5.6

Vegetarian Dishes

String Beans with Walnut Sauce

6 servings

3 cups fresh string beans, trimmed
½ cup chicken broth
2 cloves garlic, minced
1 cup finely chopped onion
¼ cup balsamic vinegar
3 tablespoons dill, finely chopped
⅓ cup walnut oil
¼ pound walnuts, coarsely chopped

Bring 3 quarts of salted water to a rapid boil. Add string beans and boil uncovered for about 10 minutes or until they are *al dente*. Drain beans.

Combine all the remaining ingredients. Add cooked beans and toss until beans are well covered.

Serve hot or cold.

TOTAL GRAMS 68.1
GRAMS PER SERVING 11.4

Celery Root Salad

2 servings

1 celery root
2 tablespoons sour cream
2 tablespoons sugar-free mayonnaise
1 teaspoon soy sauce

Grate celery. Combine with the rest of the ingredients. Mix well and serve.

TOTAL GRAMS 13.6
GRAMS PER SERVING 6.8

Spinach Egg Pie

4 servings

2 cups cooked spinach
1 cup grated onion
3 cloves garlic, crushed
½ cup butter
½ teaspoon salt

freshly ground pepper to taste
½ teaspoon nutmeg
6 eggs
1 teaspoon baking soda

Preheat oven to 350 degrees.

Defrost spinach and sauté in 3 tablespoons butter for 5 minutes.

Put eggs into large bowl. Add pepper, salt, and baking soda and beat until fluffy. Add cooled sautéed spinach, grated onion, nutmeg, and crushed garlic and mix thoroughly.

Grease baking pan thoroughly with remaining butter and place in 350-degree oven. When butter is melted, remove from oven and pour in egg-spinach mixture. Return dish to oven and bake about 45 minutes or until golden on top.

TOTAL GRAMS 40.0
GRAMS PER SERVING 10.0

Baked Spinach Flavored with Basil and Ricotta Cheese

4 servings

2 cups cooked spinach
1 tablespoon fresh basil, chopped
2 tablespoons ricotta cheese
2 egg yolks
2 cups heavy cream
1 tablespoon grated Parmesan cheese
salt, pepper, and grated nutmeg

Preheat oven to 450 degrees.

Cook the spinach by placing in boiling water for 1 minute. Cool the spinach in ice water. Squeeze out any excess water from the cooked spinach and place into a food processor with the basil, ricotta cheese, egg yolks, a pinch of salt, a little ground pepper, and grated nutmeg.

Puree the whole mixture. Place the mixture into an ovenproof dish.

Simmer cream uncovered to reduce cream by ½ and pour it over the puree mixture. Sprinkle with Parmesan cheese and bake at 450 degrees until golden brown.

TOTAL GRAMS 31.1
GRAMS PER SERVING 7.8

Brussels Sprouts Crisps

2 servings

1 cup Brussels sprouts
3 tablespoons olive oil
½ teaspoon salt

Preheat oven to 375 degrees.

Cut end of each floret and separate all leaves.

Put leaves into baking pan, sprinkle with olive oil and salt, and roast at 375 degrees for 40 minutes. Stir occasionally.

TOTAL GRAMS 9.9
GRAMS PER SERVING 5.0

Eggplant Balls

8 servings

4 medium eggplants
2 tablespoons soy flour (defatted)
1 large egg
½ teaspoon white pepper
1 small Italian pepper
1 cup vegetable oil
salt to taste

Peel eggplants, quarter, and boil in salted water until tender.

Combine all ingredients except vegetable oil in food processor until smooth paste is formed.

Heat vegetable oil in heavy pot and drop in eggplant paste a spoonful at a time. Fry until golden. Salt to taste. Drain on paper towels.

TOTAL GRAMS 72.2
GRAMS PER SERVING 9.0

Stuffed Fried Mushrooms with Goat Cheese

4 servings

16 medium-sized fresh mushroom caps
8 ounces goat cheese
1 clove garlic
1 teaspoon oregano
1 egg, beaten
1 cup ground almonds
salt and pepper

Clean mushroom caps with a clean cloth.

Place the goat cheese, garlic, and oregano into a food processor and puree. Add salt and pepper to taste.

Place the mixture into the mushroom caps, then roll the caps in beaten egg and then into the ground almonds. Repeat this process and then fry the mushrooms in hot fat until crispy.

Drain on a paper towel and serve immediately.

TOTAL GRAMS 29.6
GRAMS PER SERVING 7.4

Snacks

Swiss Snack

1 serving

¼ pound Swiss cheese, cut into cubes
4 slices bacon
oil

Wrap each cube of cheese in ½ slice bacon. Deep fry in very hot oil for 30 seconds.

TOTAL GRAMS 3.0

Sweet Cheese Snack

18 snacks

4 ounces cream cheese, room temperature
2 eggs, separated
9 packets white sugar substitute

Preheat oven to 350 degrees.

Cream the cheese with egg yolks until smooth. Add sugar substitute. Beat egg whites until stiff, but not dry. Fold cheese mixture into stiff whites. Be careful not to break down egg whites.

Grease° cookie sheet. Drop mixture by teaspoonfuls onto cookie sheet and bake in 350 degree oven for 10 minutes.

TOTAL GRAMS 6.3
GRAMS PER SERVING 0.4

°We use Pam.

Guacamole

4 servings

1 ripe California avocado, cubed
2 medium tomatoes, cubed
¾ cup minced onion
2 to 3 tablespoons chopped cilantro
1 teaspoon sea salt
1 teaspoon fresh lemon juice

Chop all ingredients together. Chill and serve.

TOTAL GRAMS 36.9
GRAMS PER SERVING 9.2

Breads,
Pancakes,
Muffins

Basic Protein Bread

1 loaf

1 cup Atkins Diet Bake Mix
2 eggs
½ cup heavy cream
¼ cup seltzer
butter for greasing pan

Preheat oven to 375 degrees. Butter loaf pan (8½ x 4½ x 2½ inches). Whisk together all ingredients in a large bowl. Pour the batter into the prepared pan and bake for 25 minutes. Let cool for 5 minutes. Serve immediately or store, wrapped well, in the refrigerator for up to 5 days.

TOTAL GRAMS 17.0

French Toast

1 tablespoon butter
1 tablespoon canola oil
¼ cup cream
1 egg
½ teaspoon vanilla extract
½ teaspoon maple extract
powdered cinnamon sweetened with saccharine and aspartame
dash of salt
1 loaf protein bread, sliced

Heat butter and canola oil in skillet. Place egg, cream, and vanilla and maple extracts in small bowl and beat gently with fork. Dip bread in bowl and drop in skillet until golden brown. Sprinkle powdered cinnamon to taste.

3.7 GRAMS PER SLICE

Basic Pancakes

6 servings

½ cup soy flour or Atkins Diet Bake Mix
3 eggs
½ cup seltzer
¼ teaspoon salt
cooking oil

Combine first 4 ingredients in a blender.

Heat 8-inch omelet pan or skillet covered with oil. When oil is piping hot, add 3 tablespoons of batter. Spread evenly in pan. Sauté quickly one side, then the other. Put pancake on platter and finish batter.

These pancakes can be used as a base for cannelloni, lasagna, blintzes, even pizza.

TOTAL GRAMS 15.1 (7.5 WITH ATKINS DIET BAKE MIX)
GRAMS PER SERVING 2.5 (1.3 WITH ATKINS DIET BAKE MIX)

Pizza

2 servings

4 pancakes (see preceding recipe)
2 tablespoons unsweetened tomato sauce
2 medium tomatoes
¾ cup shredded mozzarella
½ cup grated Parmesan cheese

Put one pancake on top of the other. Spread tomato sauce. Place mozzarella on top of sauce. Place thinly sliced tomatoes on mozzarella. Sprinkle with Parmesan cheese. Broil until Parmesan is golden.

You can make any pizza you like by adding your favorite things to the basic recipe.

TOTAL GRAMS 28.2 (23.2 WITH ATKINS DIET BAKE MIX)
GRAMS PER SERVING 14.1 (11.6 WITH ATKINS DIET BAKE MIX)

Small Pancakes

2 servings

½ cup soy flour or Atkins Diet Bake Mix
¼ cup designer whey protein
3 eggs
½ cup seltzer
¼ cup heavy cream
¼ teaspoon salt
½ cup cooking oil
1 cup sour cream

Mix all ingredients except cooking oil and sour cream in food processor. The batter should be liquid enough to pour.

Heat heavy skillet or griddle. Add 2 tablespoons oil. When oil is hot, add batter by the spoonful. Let it spread naturally. Sauté on one side for about 2 minutes. Turn and sauté other side.

When ready, put onto a plate and keep warm in oven or serve immediately with lots of sour cream.

TOTAL GRAMS 31.5 (22.1 WITH ATKINS DIET BAKE MIX)
GRAMS PER SERVING 15.8 (11.1 WITH ATKINS DIET BAKE MIX)

Bran-Soy Muffins

6 servings

3 eggs, separated, room temperature
3 tablespoons sour cream
½ cup soy flour or Atkins Diet Bake Mix
⅛ cup wheat bran
¼ cup walnuts
1½ teaspoons baking powder

Preheat oven to 350 degrees.

Mix egg yolks with the rest of ingredients. Beat egg whites until stiff. Fold in carefully. Place in buttered muffin tins and bake at 350 degrees until done.

TOTAL GRAMS 23.7 (16.1 WITH ATKINS DIET BAKE MIX)
GRAMS PER SERVING 4.0 (2.7 WITH ATKINS DIET BAKE MIX)

Desserts

Rum Truffles

10 servings

2 cups heavy cream
12 ounces baker's unsweetened chocolate
5 packages each of Sweet 'N' Low, Equal, and Sweet One
3 tablespoons rum or cognac
½ cup crushed pecans

Bring cream to a boil. Add rum or cognac and simmer about 5 minutes. Add chocolate and melt, stirring continuously for about 2 to 3 minutes. Add nuts. Blend in well. Turn off heat. Let cool for 10 minutes, then add sweeteners. Mix well.

Line baking sheet with wax paper. Spread chocolate mixture evenly on sheet. Cover with foil and put in refrigerator. Let set for several hours or overnight.

When ready to serve, cut chocolate spread into squares and put in tin container.

TOTAL GRAMS 134.9
GRAMS PER SERVING 13.5

Lemon Mousse

12 servings

7 eggs, separated, room temperature
1½ cups heavy cream
juice from 3 large lemons
1 envelope unsweetened gelatin
3 tablespoons orange cordial
6 to 10 packets (according to taste) of as many different sugar substitutes you can find

Cream sweeteners and egg yolks.

In a double boiler, combine lemon juice with gelatin and melt. When melted, dribble in sweetened egg yolks, stirring constantly. Add cordial and set aside.

Whip heavy cream. When stiff, fold in egg-gelatin mixture.

Beat egg whites until peaks form. Fold into cream.

Adjust sweetness.

Cover with foil and let it set in refrigerator for several hours.

TOTAL GRAMS 46.7
GRAMS PER SERVING 3.9

Chocolate Truffles

10 servings

12 ounces unsweetened baker's chocolate
3 cups heavy cream
2 egg yolks
3 tablespoons rum
10 packages mixed sweeteners
½ cup roasted almonds

Simmer cream for about 5 minutes.

Cream egg yolks and sweeteners. Add rum. Set aside.

Melt chocolate in cream. Turn off heat and very slowly dribble in egg yolks while stirring continuously. Add nuts and mix.

Spread chocolate mixture in wax-paper-coated baking pan and let set in refrigerator for several hours.

TOTAL GRAMS 140.8
GRAMS PER SERVING 14.1

Walnut Butter Cookies

12 servings

1 cup ground walnuts
1 tablespoon sugar substitute (or according to taste)
3 tablespoons rum
2 eggs, separated, room temperature
¾ stick butter
1 heaping tablespoon soy protein isolate (available in most health food stores)
⅓ cup walnuts, coarsely chopped

Preheat oven to 350 degrees.

Cream egg yolks with sugar substitute.

Beat egg whites until stiff and set aside.

Cream together all ingredients except coarsely chopped walnuts and fold in egg whites.

Put dough (1 tablespoon at a time) on buttered cookie sheet, place walnuts on top, and bake for about 40 minutes or until golden.

TOTAL GRAMS 21.2
GRAMS PER SERVING 1.8

Italian Sponge Cake

8 servings

5 eggs, separated, at room temperature
4½ packets sugar substitute
1 tablespoon and 1 teaspoon vanilla
½ teaspoon grated lemon rind
3 tablespoons soy flour or Atkins Diet Bake Mix
4 tablespoons heavy cream
½ teaspoon cream of tartar

Preheat oven to 325 degrees.

Grease a layer cake pan with butter or oil.

Place egg yolks and sugar substitute in bowl. Beat with electric hand mixer until well blended. Add vanilla and lemon rind. Continue to beat and add soya powder 1 tablespoon at a time. Beat until well blended. Add heavy cream.

Beat egg whites with cream of tartar until stiff. Fold yolk mixture into whites with an under-and-over movement. Be careful not to break down egg whites.

Turn into layer cake pan and bake in 325 degree oven until done (about ½ hour).

TOTAL GRAMS 24.0 (22.2 WITH ATKINS DIET BAKE MIX)
GRAMS PER SERVING 3.0 (2.9 WITH ATKINS DIET BAKE MIX)

Zabaglione

6 servings

1 cup heavy cream
3 eggs, separated
1½ tablespoon-equivalents sugar substitute
¼ cup sherry
2 cups strawberries, washed and hulled

Scald heavy cream (do not boil). Beat egg yolks with 1 tablespoon sugar substitute. Pour cream over egg yolks and beat with wire whisk until well blended.

Cook mixture in top of double boiler, beating constantly with hand mixer or rotary beater until it begins to thicken. Cool.

Remove from heat and stir in sherry. Beat egg whites with remaining artificial sweetener until stiff. Fold into cream mixture carefully so that egg whites do not break down.

Refrigerate and serve with whole or sliced strawberries.

TOTAL GRAMS 44.5
GRAMS PER SERVING 7.4

Fruit Mold

8 servings

2 envelopes sugar-free raspberry gelatin
½ cup sliced strawberries
½ cup heavy cream, whipped

Prepare 1 package gelatin according to package directions. Add strawberries. Pour into mold. Chill until firm.

Prepare second package of gelatin without cold water. Cool. Fold in whipped cream.

Place on top of strawberry gelatin. Refrigerate for at least two hours.

To unmold: Run a wet knife along edge. Dip bottom of mold in warm water. Turn over onto wet plate.

TOTAL GRAMS 10.3
GRAMS PER SERVING 1.3

Blueberry Ice Cream

9 servings (½ cup each)

5 egg yolks
3 teaspoons vanilla extract
2 tablespoon-equivalents sugar substitute
¼ cup water
½ cup unsweetened frozen blueberries, drained well
2 cups heavy cream, whipped

Place yolks, vanilla extract, sugar substitute, and water in blender. Blend at medium speed for 30 seconds. Add blueberries. Blend for 10 more seconds.

Fold yolk mixture into whipped cream. Blend lightly until you have marbled effect. Pour into freezer container. Freeze.

TOTAL GRAMS 41.8
GRAMS PER SERVING 4.6

Vanilla Ice Cream

1 quart or 8 servings (½ cup each)

5 egg yolks
3 teaspoons vanilla extract
2 tablespoon-equivalents sugar substitute
¼ cup water
2 cups heavy cream, whipped

Place yolks, vanilla extract, sugar substitute, and water in blender. Blend at medium speed for 30 seconds.

Fold yolk mixture into whipped cream. Blend well, being careful not to break down volume of whipped cream. Empty into refrigerator tray. Freeze for 2 hours.

TOTAL GRAMS 30.4
GRAMS PER SERVING 3.8

Flan

4 servings

5 eggs
1 cup heavy cream
1 cup water
5 packets of Equal or equivalent
1 capful almond extract
dash nutmeg or dash cinnamon

Preheat oven to 350 degrees. Whip first five ingredients in blender for 3 to 4 minutes. Pour into large baking dish or individual dishes and sprinkle top with nutmeg or cinnamon. In oven set in larger pan half-filled with water. Bake for 40 minutes or until set at 350 degrees.

TOTAL GRAMS 15.5
GRAMS PER SERVING 3.9

Carbohydrate Gram Counter

Foods	*Grams of Carbohydrate*

Milk Products

Milk (whole, 1 cup)	11.0
Half and half (1 tbs.)	0.7
Cream (light, 1 tbs.)	0.6
(sour, 2 tbs.)	1.0
(heavy, 1 tbs.)	0.5
Soy milk (unsweetened, 1 cup)	13.0
Plain yogurt (skim, 1 cup)	13.0
(whole, 1 cup)	12.0

Cheese

Cheddar (1 oz.)	0.6
Swiss (1 oz.)	0.5
American (1 oz.)	0.5
Cottage (fat-free, 1 cup)	10.0
(whole, 1 cup)	8.0
Cream cheese (2 tbs.)	1.0
Camembert (1 oz.)	0.5
Feta (1 oz.)	1.0
Muenster (1 oz.)	1.0
Provolone (1 oz.)	1.0

Nuts

Almond Paste (1 oz.)	14.5
Almonds (1 oz.)	5.5
Brazil (1 oz.)	3.1
Cashews (1 oz.)	8.3
Coconut (1 oz.)	4.3
Hazelnuts (filberts) (1 oz.)	4.7
Macadamia (1 oz.)	4.5
Peanuts (1 oz.)	5.4
Peanut Butter (1 tbs.)	3.0
Pecans (1 oz.)	4.1
Pignolia (1 oz.)	3.3
Pistachio (1 oz.)	5.4
Pumpkin Seeds (1 oz.)	4.2
Sesame Seeds (1 tbs.)	1.4
Soybeans (½ cup)	6.0
Sunflower Seeds (1 oz.)	5.6
Walnuts (1 oz.)	4.2

Grains

Pumpernickel bread (1 slice)	17.0
Whole-wheat bread (1 slice)	11.0
Bagel (1)	30.0
Corn muffin	20.0
Pancake (using dry mix)	17.4
Frozen waffle	29.0
Rice: cooked (1 cup)	49.6
puffed (1 cup)	11.5
Noodles (1 cup cooked)	37.3
Oatmeal (1 cup cooked)	27.0
Farina (1 cup)	22.0
Popcorn (popped, 1 cup)	5.0

Soups

Chicken Consommé (1 cup)	1.9
Cream of Chicken (1 cup)	14.5

Chicken Gumbo (1 cup)	7.4
Cream of Mushroom (1 cup)	16.2
Turkey Rice (1 cup)	10.0

Herbs

Allspice (1 tsp.)	1.4
Basil (1 tsp.)	0.9
Caraway (1 tsp.)	1.1
Celery (1 tsp.)	0.6
Cinnamon (1 tsp.)	1.8
Coriander leaf (1 tsp.)	0.3
Dill Seed (1 tsp.)	1.2
Garlic Clove (1)	0.9
Saffron (1 tsp.)	0.5
Thyme (1 tsp.)	0.9
Tarragon (1 tsp.)	0.8
Vanilla (double strength, 1 tsp.)	3.0
Ginger Root (fresh, 1 oz.)	3.6
Ginger Root (ground, 1 tsp.)	1.3

Vegetables

Asparagus (4 spears)	2.2
Beans, green (boiled, 1 cup)	6.8
Beans, yellow or wax (boiled, 1 cup)	5.8
Broccoli (1 cup)	8.5
Brussels sprouts (1 cup)	9.9
Cabbage (1 cup)	6.2
Carrot (7 in.)	7.0
Cauliflower (1 cup)	5.1
Celery (1 stalk)	1.6
Collards (1 cup)	9.8
Corn (1 ear, 5 in.)	16.2
Coleslaw (1 cup)	8.5
Cucumber (sliced, 1 cup)	3.6
Dandelion (1 cup)	6.7
Endive (1 cup)	2.1
Kale (1 cup)	6.7
Kohlrabi (1 cup)	8.7
Lettuce: Romaine (1 cup)	1.9

Lettuce: Boston (1 cup)	1.4
Iceberg (1 cup)	1.6
Mushrooms (1 cup)	3.1
Mustard greens (1 cup)	5.6
Okra (1 cup)	9.6
Onion (1 cup)	14.8
Parsley (1 tbs.)	0.3
Parsnips (1 cup)	23.1
Peas, cooked (1 cup)	19.4
Peppers: green (1 cup)	7.2
red (dried, 1 tsp.)	1.4
Potato (baked, 1)	32.8
Potato Salad (1 cup)	33.5
Pumpkin (3½ oz.)	7.0
Radish (large, 10)	2.9
Spinach (1 cup)	6.5
Squash: summer (1 cup)	6.5
winter (1 cup)	25.5
Sweet Potato (baked, 1)	37.0
Tomato: raw (2½ in.)	5.8
cooked (1 cup)	13.3
Juice (1 cup)	10.4
Turnips: cooked (1 cup)	11.3
greens (1 cup)	5.2

Protein (fat or lean, without breading)

Fish, poultry, meat, or eggs	0–trace amts.

Fats/oils

Olive, canola, safflower, etc.	0–trace amts.

Beans (cooked)

Navy (1 cup)	40.3
Black-eyed (1 cup)	38.0
Split peas (1 cup)	41.6
Lima (1 cup)	33.7
Red Kidney (1 cup)	39.6
Soybeans (cooked, 1 cup)	19.4

Tofu/bean curd (2-in. cube)   2.9

Fruit

Apple (1 medium, 2¾ in.)	20.0
Applesauce (unsweetened, 1 cup)	26.4
Apricots (3 fresh)	13.7
Avocado (California)	13.0
Avocado (Florida)	27.0
Banana (1)	26.4
Blackberries (1 cup)	18.6
Blueberries (1 cup)	22.2
Raspberries (1 cup)	21.0
Strawberries (1 cup)	12.5
Cantaloupe (½ melon, 5 in.)	20.4
Cherries (1 cup)	20.4
Grapefruit (pink, ½)	10.3
Grapes (10)	9.0
Lemon	6.0
Lemon juice (1 cup)	19.5
Olive (green, pitted)	2.5
Peach (2 ½ in.)	9.7
Pear (3 ½ in.)	31.0
Pineapple (1 cup)	21.2
Plum (1 medium)	17.8
Prunes (1)	5.6
Honeydew (1 cup)	13.1
Kiwi (1, medium)	9.0
Papaya (1, medium)	30.4
Mango (1 cup)	27.7
Orange (1, medium)	16.0
Rhubarb (cooked with sugar, 1 cup)	97.2

Samples of Carbohydrate "Fattening" Items

Banana Split	91
Shake (medium)	90
Bean Burrito	48
Cheeseburger (¼ pounder)	33
Popsicle	17

Toaster pastry (frosted, blueberry)	34
Waffles (plain homemade, 1)	28
Apple Pie (homemade, 1 slice)	61
Ice Cream Soda (1 cup)	49
Cornbread stuffing (½ cup)	69
Onion Rings (fast food order)	33
Tapioca, Cream (½ cup)	22
Apple Turnover	30
Pecan Pie (homemade, 1 piece)	41
Devil Dog	30
Hot Dog with Bun (1)	24
French Toast (2 slices)	34
Macaroni with Cheese (1 cup)	40
Pizza (1 piece)	24
Egg Roll (1)	30
Sherbet (lemon, ½ cup)	45
White sugar (1 oz.)	28
Peanut brittle (1 oz.)	23
Honey (1 oz.)	34
Rolled oats (1 cup, cooked)	23
Saltines (1)	2
Soda crackers (1)	4
Graham crackers (1)	5
chocolate covered (1)	8
Hard candy, gum drops, jelly beans (1 oz.)	25
Whaler	64
Chicken salad sandwich	27

References

Chapter 1

1. Yudkin, J., and Carey, M. "The treatment of obesity by the 'high-fat' diet. The inevitability of calories," *Lancet* 2 (1960), pp. 939–941.

Chapter 2

1. Putnam, J. J., and Allshouse, J. E. *Food Consumption, Prices, and Expenditures, 1968–89*, United States Department of Agriculture, Statistical Bulletin No. 825, 1991, p. 61.

Chapter 3

1. Putnam, J. J., and Allshouse, J. E., op. cit., p. 61.
2. See especially the bibliography to Shafrir, E., "Effect of sucrose and fructose on carbohydrate and lipid metabolism and the resulting consequences," in Reitner, R., ed., *Regulation of Carbohydrate Metabolism*, vol. II, Boca Raton, Florida, CRC Press, 1985.
3. Dolnick, E. "Le Paradoxe Francais," *Hippocrates* May/June 1990, pp. 37–43.
4. Beasley, Joseph, M.D., et al. *The Kellogg Report*, 1989. Annandale-on-Hudson, N.Y., 144

Chapter 4

1. Bernstein, Richard K. *Diabetes Type II* (New York: Prentice Hall Press, 1980), pp. 32–33.
Also: Ferrannini, E., et al. "Essential hypertension: an insulin resistance state," *Journal of Cardiovascular Pharmacology* 1990, 15 (supplement 5), pp. S18–S25.

Chapter 5

1. Cahill, G., and Aoki, T.T. *Medical Times* 98 (1970).
2. Grey, N. J., and Kipnis, D. M. "Effect of diet composition on the

hyperinsulinism of obesity," *New England Journal of Medicine* 1971, 285, p. 827.
Also: Pfeiffer, E.F., and Laube, H. *Advances in Metabolic Disorders* 1974, vol. 7.
Also: Muller, W.A., et al. "The influence of the antecedent diet upon glucagon and insulin secretion, *New England Journal of Medicine* 285(26) 1971, 1450–54.

3. Chalmers, T.M., Kekwick, A., Pawan, G.L.S., and Smith, I. "On the fat-mobilising activity of human urine," *Lancet* 1 (1958), p. 866.
See also: Pawan, G.L.S., and Kekwick, A. "Fat-mobilising and ketogenic activity of urine extracts: relation to cortilcotrophin and growth hormone," *Lancet* 2 (1960), p. 6.

Chapter 6

1. Council on Foods and Nutrition, "A critique of low-carbohydrate ketogenic weight reduction regimens," *Journal of the American Medical Association* 224:10 (June 4, 1973), pp. 1415–1419.

2. Kekwick, A., and Pawan, G. L. S. "Calorie intake in relation to body weight changes in the obese," *Lancet* 2:155 (1956).

3. Kekwick, A., and Pawan, G. L. S. "Metabolic study in human obesity with isocaloric diets high in fat, protein or carbohydrate," *Metabolism* 6 (1957), pp. 447–460.

4. Pilkington, T. R. E., et al. "Diet and weight reduction in the obese," *Lancet* 1 (1960), pp. 856–858.

5. Kekwick, A., and Pawan, G. L. S. "The effect of high fat and high carbohydrate diets on rates of weight loss in mice," *Metabolism* 13:1 (1964), pp. 87–97.

6. Stevenson, J. A. F., et al. "A fat mobilising and anorectic substance in the urine of fasting rats," *Proceedings of the Society for Experimental Biological Medicine* 115 (1964), p. 424.
See also Braun, T., et al. "Factor in human urine inhibiting lipid metabolism," *Experientia* 19 (1963), p. 319.
Also: Friesen, H., et al. "Metabolic effects of two peptides from the anterior pituitary gland," *Endocrinology* 70 (1962), p. 579.
Also: Li, C. H. "Lipotropin, a new active peptide from pituitary glands," *Nature* 201 (1964), p. 924.

7. Olesen, E.S., and Quaade, F. "Fatty foods and obesity," *Lancet* 1 (1960), pp. 1048–1051.
Also: Werner, S.C. "Comparison between weight reduction on a high calorie, high fat diet and on an isocaloric regimen high in carbohydrate," *New England Journal of Medicine* 252 (1955), pp. 661–665.

8. Benoit, F., et al. "Changes in body composition during weight reduction in obesity," *Archives of Internal Medicine* 63:4 (1965), pp. 604–612.

9. Grande, F. "Energy balance and body composition changes: a critical study of three recent publications," *Annals of Internal Medicine* 68 (1968), pp. 467–480.

10. Krehl, W. A., et al. "Some metabolic changes induced by low carbohydrate diets," *The American Journal of Clinical Nutrition* 20:2 (1967), pp. 139–148.

11. Young, C. M., et al. "Effect on body composition and other parameters in young men of carbohydrate level of reduction diet," *American Journal of Clinical Nutrition* 24 (1971), pp. 290–296.

12. Rabast, U., et al. "Comparative studies in obese subjects fed carbohydrate-

restricted and high carbohydrate 1,000 calorie formula diets," *Nutritional Metabolism* 22 (1978), pp. 269–277.

13. Kasper, H., et al. "Response of body weight to a low carbohydrate, high fat diet in normal and obese subjects," *The American Journal of Clinical Nutrition* 26 (1973), pp. 197–204.

Also: Rabast, U., et al. "Therapy of adiposity using reduced-carbohydrate and high-carbohydrate isocaloric formula diets (comparative studies)," *Verhandlungen Der Deutschen Gesellschaft fur Innere Medizin* 81 (1975), p. 1400–1402.

Also: Rabast, U., et al. "Dietetic treatment of obesity with low and high carbohydrate diets," *International Journal of Obesity* 3(3) 1979, pp. 201–211.

Also: Rabast, Reigler, E. "Weight reduction by a high protein, low carbohydrate diet," *Medizinische Klinik* 71(24) 1976, pp. 1051-1056.

Also: Rabast, U., et al. "Loss of weight, sodium, and water in obese persons consuming a high or low carbohydrate diet," *Annals of Nutrition and Metabolism* 26(6) 1981, pp. 341–349.

Chapter 12

1. Ricketts, H. T., et al. "Biochemical studies of pre-diabetes," *Diabetes* 15(12) 1966, pp. 880-888.

2. Ezrin, Calvin, and Kowalski, Robert. *The Endocrine Control Diet.* (New York: Harper and Row, 1990).

3. DeFronzo, R,. et al., *Diabetes Care* 1992: 15(3):318–368.

4. Muller, W. A., et al. "The influence of the antecedent diet upon glucagon and insulin secretion," *New England Journal of Medicine* 285 (1971), pp. 1450–1454.

5. Cohen, A. M. Senate Hearings, April 30, 1973.

6. Jarrett, R. J., et al. "Glucose tolerance and blood pressure in two population samples: their relation to diabetes mellitus and hypertension," *International Journal of Epidemiology* 7 (1978), pp. 15–24.

Also: Wright, D. W., et al. "Sucrose-induced insulin resistance in the rat: modulation by exercise and diet," *The American Journal of Clinical Nutrition* 38 (1983), pp. 879–883.

Also: Reaven, G. M., et al. "Characterization of a model of dietary-induced hypertriglyceridemia in young, non-obese rats," *Journal of Lipid Research* 20 (1970), pp. 371–378.

Also: Zavaroni, I., et al. "Effect of fructose feeding on insulin secretion and insulin action in the rat," *Metabolism* 29 (1980), pp. 970–973.

Also: Hwang, I. S., et al. "Fructose-induced insulin and hypertension in rats," *Hypertension* 10 (1987), pp. 512–516.

Also: Reaven, G. M. "Insulin independent diabetes mellitus: metabolic characteristics," *Metabolism* 29 (1980), pp. 445–454.

7. Freund, H., et al. "Chromium deficiency during total parenteral nutrition," *Journal of the American Medical Association* 241(5) 1979, pp. 496–498.

Also: Liu, V. J., and Abernathy, R. P. "Chromium and insulin in young subjects with normal glucose tolerance," *American Journal of Clinical Nutrition* 25(4) 1982, pp. 661–667.

8. Brichard, S., et al., *Trends in Pharmacological Science* 1995; 16(8):265–270.

9. Solomon, S. J., and King, J. C. "Effect of low zinc intake on carbohydrate and fat metabolism in men," *Federal Proc* 42 (1983), p. 391.

Also: Tauri, S. "Studies of zinc metabolism: III. Effect of the diabetic state on zinc metabolism: A clinical aspect." *Endocrinol. Japam* 10 (1963), pp. 9–15.

10. Coggeshall, J.C., et al. "Biotin status and plasma glucose in diabetics," *Annals of New York Academy of Science* 447 (1985), pp. 389–392.

Chapter 13

1. Crook, W. G. *The Yeast Connection.* Jackson, Tenn.: Professional Books, 1985.

2. Svare, C. W., et al. "The effect of dental amalgams on mercury levels in expired air," *Journal of Dental Research* 60(9) 1981, pp. 1668–1671.

Chapter 14

1. Egger, J., et al. "Is migraine food allergy? A double-blind controlled trial of oligoantigenic diet treatment," *Lancet* (October 29, 1984), pp. 719–721.

Chapter 15

1. Council on Foods and Nutrition, "A critique of low-carbohydrate ketogenic weight reduction regimens," *Journal of the American Medical Association* 224(10) 1973, pp. 1415–1419.

2. Tolstoi, E. "The effect of an exclusive meat diet on the chemical constituents of the blood," *Journal of Biological Chemistry* 83 (1929), pp. 753–758.

3. Reissel, P. K., et al. "Treatment of hypertriglyceridemia," *American Journal of Clinical Nutrition* 19 (1966), pp. 84–98.

4. Krehl, W. A., et al. "Some metabolic changes induced by low carbohydrate diets," *The American Journal of Clinical Nutrition* 20(2) 1967, pp. 139–148.

5. Rabast, U., et al. "Outpatient treatment of obesity using a low-carbohydrate diet," *Medizinische Klinik* 73(2) 1978, pp. 55–59.

6. Riegler, E. "Weight reduction by a high protein, low carbohydrate diet," *Medizinische Klinik* 71(24), 1976, pp. 1051–1045.

7. Rickman, F., et al. "Changes in serum cholesterol during the Stillman diet," *Journal of the American Medical Association* 228 (1974), p. 54.

8. Phinney, S. D., et al. "The transient hypercholesterolemia of major weight loss," *The American Journal of Clinical Nutrition* 53 (1991), pp. 1404–1410.

9. Newbold, H. L. "Reducing the serum cholesterol level with a diet high in animal fats," *Southern Medical Journal* 81 (1988).

10. Kaplan, N. M. "The deadly quartet: upper-body obesity, glucose intolerance, hypertriglyceridemia, and hypertension," *Archives of Internal Medicine* 149 (1989), pp. 1514–1520.

11. Lichtenstein, M. J., et al. "Sex hormones, insulin, lipids, and prevalent ischemic heart disease," *American Journal of Epidemiology* 126 (1987), pp. 647–657.

Also: Pyorala, K. "Relationship of glucose tolerance and plasma insulin to the incidence of coronary heart disease: results from two population studies in Finland," *Diabetes Care* 701 (1985), pp. 38–52.

Also: Fontbonne, A., et al. "Coronary heart disease mortality risk: plasma insulin level is a more sensitive market than hypertension or abnormal glucose tolerance in overweight males: the Paris prospective study," *International Journal of Obesity* 12 (1988), pp. 557–565.

12. Manninen, V. "Joint effects of serum triglycerides and LDL cholesterol and HDL cholesterol on coronary heart disease in the Helsinki Heart Study. Implications for treatment," *Circulation* 85(1) 1992, pp. 365–367.

13. Assmann, G., et al., *American Journal of Cardiology* 1992: 70(7):733–737.

14. *Medical Tribune* 33(2), January 30, 1992.

15. Reiser, S., et al. "Serum insulin and glucose in hyperinsulinemic subjects fed three different levels of sucrose," *The American Journal of Clinical Nutrition* 34 (1981), pp. 2348–2358.

16. Reaven, G. M., et al. "Role of insulin in endogenous hypertriglyceridemia," *Journal of Clinical Investigation* 46 (1967), pp. 1756–1767.
See also: Coulston, A. M., et al. "Deleterious metabolic effects of high-carbohydrate, sucrose-containing diets in patients with non-insulin-dependent diabetes mellitus," *American Journal of Medicine* 82 (1987), pp. 213–220.

17. See 37 references in Coulston, A. M., et al. "Original articles: Persistence of hypertriglyceridemic effect of low-fat high-carbohydrate diets in NIDDM patients," *Diabetes Care* 12(2) 1989, pp. 94–101.

18. Reaven, G. M., et al. "Hypertension as a Disease of Carbohydrate and Lipoprotein Metabolism," *The American Journal of Medicine* 87 (suppl. 6A) 1989, pp. 6A-2S–6A-6S.

19. Reaven, G. M. "The role of insulin resistance in human disease," *Diabetes* 37 (1988), pp. 1595–1607.

20. Stout, R. W. "Hyperinsulinaemia—a possible risk factor for cardiovascular disease in diabetes mellitus, *Hormone and Metabolic Research* 15 (1985), pp. 37–41.

21. Rocchini, A. P. "Proceedings of the council for high blood pressure research, 1990: insulin resistance and blood pressure regulation in obese and nonobese subjects: special lecture," *Hypertension* Supplement 1, 17(6) 1991, pp. 837–842.

22. Childs, M. T., et al. "The contrasting effects of a dietary soya-lecithin product and corn oil on lipoprotein lipids in normolipidemic and familial hypercholesterolemic subjects," *Athersclerosis* 38 (1981), pp. 217–228.

23. Horrobin, D. F. "The importance of gamma-linolenic acid and prostaglandin E_1 in human nutrition and medicine," *Journal of Holistic Medicine* 3 (1981), pp. 118–139.

24. Saynor, R. "Effects of omega-3 fatty acids on serum lipids," *Lancet* 2 (1984), pp. 696–697.

25. Railes, R., and Albrink, M. J. "Effect of chromium chloride supplementation on glucose tolerance and serum lipids including high density lipoprotein of adult men," *American Journal of Clinical Nutrition* 34 (1981), pp. 2670–2678.

26. Cattin, L., et al. "Treatment of hypercholesterolemia with pantethine and fenofibrate: An open randomized study on 43 subjects," *Current Therapeutic Research* 38(3) 1985, pp. 386–395.
See also: "Pantethine treatment of hyperlipidemia," *Clinical Therapy* 8 (1986), p. 537.

27. Grundy, S. M., et al. "Influence of nicotinic acid on metabolism of cholesterol and triglycerides in man," *Journal of Lipid Research* 22 (1981), pp. 24–36.

28. Bordia, A. "Effect of garlic on blood lipids in patients with coronary heart disease," *The American Journal of Clinical Nutrition* 34 (1981), pp. 100–103.
Also: Ernst, E., et al. "Garlic and blood lipids," *British Medical Journal* 291 (1985), pp. 139.

29. Ferrari, R., et al. "The metabolical effects of L-carnitine in angina pectoris," *International Journal of Cardiology* 5 (1984), p. 213.

30. Simons, L. A., et al. "Long-term treatment of hypercholesterolaemia with a new palatable formulation of sugar gum," *Atherosclerosis* 45(1) 1982, pp. 101–108. Also: Kay, R. M., and Truswell, A. S. "Effect of citric pectin in blood lipids and fecal steroid excretion," *The American Journal of Clinical Nutrition* 30(2), 1977, pp. 171–175.

Chapter 16

1. Tremblay, A., et al. "Nutritional determinants of the increase in energy intake associated with a high-fat diet," *The American Journal of Clinical Nutrition* 53 (1991), pp. 1134–1137.

2. Cleave, T .L. *The Saccharine Disease*. New Canaan, CT: Keats, 1978.

3. Masironi, P. *Bulletin of World Health Organization* 42 (1970).

4. McGill, Jr., H. C. "The relationship of dietary cholesterol to serum cholesterol concentration and to atherosclerosis in man," *The American Journal of Clinical Nutrition* 32 (1979), pp. 2664–2702.

5. Masironi, op. cit.

6. Herrick, J. B. "Clinical features of sudden obstruction of the coronary arteries," *Journal of the American Medical Association*, 1912, LIX, p. 2105.

7. Willett, W. C., et al. "Relation of meat, fat, and fiber to the risk of colon cancer in a prospective study among women," *The New England Journal of Medicine* 323(24) 1990, pp. 1664–1672.

8. Willett, W. C., et al. "Original article: dietary fat and the risk of breast cancer," *The New England Journal of Medicine* 316(1) 1987, pp. 22–28.

9. Macquart-Moulin, G., et al. "Case-control study on colorectal cancer and diet in Marseilles," *International Journal of Cancer* 38(2) 1986, pp. 183–191. Also: Berta, J. L., et al. "Diet and rectocolonic cancers. Results of a case-control study," *Gastroenterologie Clinique et Biologique* 9(4) 1985, pp. 348–353. Also: Haenszel, W., et al. "A case-control study of large bowel cancer in Japan," *Journal of the National Cancer Institute* 64(1) 1980, pp. 17–22. Also: Tuyns, A. J., et al. "Colorectal cancer and the intake of nutrients: oligosaccharides are a risk factor, fats are not. A case-control study in Belgium," *Nutrition and Cancer* 10(4) 1987, pp. 181–196.

10. Warburg, O. *The Metabolism of Tumors*. London: Constable and Co., 1930.

11. Dilman, V. M. "Pathogenic approach to prevention of age associated increase of cancer incidence," *Annals of the New York Academy of Science* 621 (1991), pp. 385–400.

12. *Federal Register.* Department of Agriculture Document, 56 (no. 229), November 27, 1991, pp. 60764–60824.

Chapter 21

1. Tuominen, J. A. *Clinical Physiology* 1997: 17:19–30.

Chapter 22

1. Evan, G. W. "The effects of chromium picolinate on insulin controlled parameters in humans," *International Journal of Biosocial Medical Research* 11 (1989), pp. 163–180.

2. Cattin, L. op. cit.

3. McNeill, J. H. op. cit.

4. Coggeshall, J. C. op. cit.

5. Naylor, G. J., et al. "A double-blind placebo controlled trial of ascorbic acid in obesity," *Nutrition and Health* 1985, p. 425.

6. Ferrari, R. op. cit.

7. Van Gall, L., et al. "Exploratory study of coenzyme Q_{10} in obesity," in Folkers, K., and Yamamura, Y., eds. *Biomedical and Clinical Aspects of Coenzyme Q*, vol. 4. Amsterdam: Elsevier Science Publishers, 1984, pp. 369-373.

8. Clinical use of glutamine at the Atkins Center for Complementary Medicine.

9. Clinical results obtained at the Atkins Center for Complementary Medicine.

10. Azuma, J., et al. "Therapeutic effect of taurine in congestive heart failure: a double blind crossover trial," *Clinical Cardiology* 8 (1985), pp. 276–282.

11. Ellis, F. R., and Nasser, S. "A pilot study of vitamin B_{12} in the treatment of tiredness," *British Journal of Nutrition* 30 (1973), pp. 277–283.

12. Atkins, R. C. *Dr. Atkins' Health Revolution*. Boston: Houghton Mifflin, 1988.

13. Mohler, H., et al. "Nicotinamide is a brain constituent with benzodiazepine-like actions," *Nature* 278 (1979), pp. 563–565.
Also: Yogman, M., and Zeisel, S. "Diet and sleep patterns in newborn infants," *The New England Journal of Medicine* 309(19) 1983, p. 1147.

14. Anderson, R. A., et al. "Chromium supplementation of humans with hypoglycemia," *Federal Proc.* 43 (1984), p. 471.
Also: Curry, D. L., et al. "Magnesium modulation of glucose induced insulin secretion by the perfused rat pancreas," *Endocrinology* 101 (1977), p. 203.

15. Coggeshall, J. C. op. cit.
Also: Liu, V. J., and Abernathy, R. P. "Chromium and insulin in young subjects with normal glucose tolerance," *The American Journal of Clinical Nutrition* 25(4) 1982, pp. 661–667.
Also: Ceriello, A., et al. "Hypomagnesemia in relation to diabetic retinopathy," *Diabetes Care* 5 (1982), pp. 558–559.
Also: Shigeta, Y., at al. "Effect of coenzyme Q_7 treatment on blood sugar and ketone bodies of diabetics," *Journal of Vitaminology* 12 (1966), p. 293.

16. Childs, op. cit.
Also: Horrobin, op. cit.; Saynor, op. cit.; Railes and Albrink, op. cit.; Cattin, op. cit.; Grundy, op. cit.; Bordia, op. cit.; Ernst, op. cit.; Simons, op. cit.; Day and Trueswell, op. cit.

17. Jamal, C. A., et al. "Gamma-linolenic acid in diabetic neuropathy," *Lancet* 1 1986), p. 1098.
See also: Ceriello, A., et al. "Hypomagnesemia in relation to diabetic retinopathy," *Diabetes Care* 5 (1982), pp. 558–559.

18. Cohen, L. "Magnesium and hypertension," *Magnesium Bulletin* 8 (1986), pp. 1847–1849.
Also: Azuma, J., op. cit. Also: Norris, P. G., et al. "Effect of dietary supplementation with fish oil on systolic blood pressure in mild essential hypertension," *British Medical Journal* 293 (1986), p. 104.

19. Kosolcharoen, P., et al. "Improved exercise tolerance after administration of carnitine," *Current Therapeutic Research,* November 1981, pp. 753–764.

Also: Haeger, K. "Long-time treatment of intermittent claudication with vitamin E," *American Journal of Clinical Nutrition* 27(10) 1974, pp. 1179–1181.

Also: Kamikawa, T., et al. "Effects of coenzyme Q_{10} on exercise tolerance in chronic stable angina pectoris," *American Journal of Cardiology* 56 (1985), p. 247.

Also: Taussig, S. J., and Nieper, H. A. "Bromelain: its use in prevention and treatment of cardiovascular disease: Present status," *Journal of International Academy of Preventive Medicine* 6(1) 1979.

Also: Bordia, op. cit.

20. Goebel, K. M., et al. "Intrasynovial orgotein therapy in rheumatoid arthritis," *Lancet* 1 (1981), pp. 1015–1017.

Also: Barton-Wright, E.C., and Elliot, W. A. "The pantothenic acid metabolism of rheumatoid arthritis, *Lancet* 2 (1963), pp. 862–863.

Also: Roberts, P., et al. "Vitamin C and inflammation," *Medical Biology* 62 (1984), p. 88.

Also: Sorenson, J., in *The Anti-Inflammatory Activities of Copper Complexes, Metal Ions and Biological Systems*. Marcel Dekker, 1982, pp. 77–125.

Chapter 24

1. Willett, W., et al., "Is Dietary Fat a Major Determinant of Body Fat?" *American Journal of Clinical Nutrition* 1998: 67: 556S-562S

Chapter 25

1. *European Journal of Applied Physiology and Occupational Physiology* 1994: 69(4): 287–93.

Chapter 26

1. Cahill, G. and Aoki, T. T. *Medical Times* 98 (1970).

2. Spirt, B. A., et al., "Gallstone formation in obese women treated by a low-calorie diet," *International Journal of Obesity* 1995: 19: 595–595.

3. Spencer, H., et al., *American Journal of Clinical Nutrition* June 1983: 37(6): 924–929.

4. Giovannucci, E., et al., "Alcohol, low-methionine–low-folate diets, and risk of colon cancer in men," *Journal of the National Cancer Institute* 1995: 87(4): 265–273.

5. Skog, K., et al., "Effect of cooking temperature on the formation of heterocyclic amines in fried meat products and pan residues," *Carcinogenesis* 1995: 16(4): 861–867.

6. Franceschi, S., et al., "Food Groups and Risk of Colorectal Cancer in Italy," *International Journal of Cancer* 1997: 72: 56–61.

7. Gilman, Matthew, *JAMA* 1997: 278(24): 2145–2150.

Index

Dr. Atkins' *New* Diet Cookbook

Contents

1 | *Introduction*

You have all seen diet cookbooks, but for the past 20 years I suspect you haven't seen one like this. This isn't a copycat cookbook. It doesn't attempt to refurbish and bring to life the tired and repetitious diet styles of the recent past. in fact, if you start leafing through the recipes, you'll be in for the shock of your life. *Where's the diet?* you'll say. What happened to the austerity? No austerity, no diet, right? *Wrong!*

What sort of diet is this, then? Just glance at the wonderful, mouth-watering recipes Fran Gare has prepared for this book. Yes, they appear nondietetic because they're *not* fat-restricted. You quickly notice that oil, butter, and mayonnaise appear in them. *Why, Dr. Atkins, this is not the food of weight loss!* You tremble. Don't! This is the food of weight loss, and you can become slim eating it. (And, better yet, healthy.) But, I have to tell you that if you're relying on fat restriction to get you slim, this cookbook is certainly not for you.

On the other hand, if, like so many of the people I meet, you've been trying fat restriction and getting nowhere, I'll hazard a guess that this cookbook and the diet principles that go with it are exactly what you need.

You need a new start; new principles; a diet that works.

The success I promise is not done by magic. Low-carbohydrate dieting is the answer, and that means the application of well-attested facts about overweight that you've probably never heard about. Quite simply, since the late 1970s a simplistic theory of weight loss that focuses obsessively on dietary fat and by implication teaches the old, stale doctrine that gaining or losing weight is just a matter of calorie consumption has ruled the roost.

To know how simplistic it is to look at overweight that way, you only have to consider the different people you know, their different body types, and their different levels of appetite. Right away you'll see that there's no necessary connection between how much you eat and how heavy you are or between eating a lot of fat and being fat. You've surely noticed that folks who eat bacon and eggs for breakfast aren't consistently overweight. Nor folks who eat steaks or butter. Yet the restriction of fat has become the basis of a whole new weight-loss industry. Weight Watchers and its many imitators wage the battle of the bulge. Low-fat tips crowd the pages of women's magazines, and dire warnings resound from medical authorities on high.

And, as a result, we as a nation are without question and by all statistical measures eating less fat. The American public must be getting slimmer. Is it? That's a question I can easily answer. NHANES, the major government survey that tracks the weight patterns of the nation, found just last year that from 1980 to 1990, the percentage of overweight American adults went up from 26 percent of the population to 34 percent—a truly massive and astonishing 30 percent jump. If pudge-proneness is a virus, then tens of millions of us caught it even as we struggled to obey our antifat mentors.

Food for thought here. I know I haven't shocked you enough, so let me talk about eating. After all, this is a book that promises to be a source of the richest and most diverse dining pleasure. Disguise it though they may, most diet cookbook authors want to teach you how you can like carrot sticks and granola, skim milk and skinless chicken, celery stalks and butterless toast. They set a hard task for themselves. In their attempt to deploy a few delicious salads (though no more delicious than the ones our own Fran Gare will reveal to you), they are fundamentally working from poverty. Good cuisine has always rooted itself firmly in luxurious fat. That's why I feel confident you're going to relate to a diet and a cookbook that allows you New England Clam Chowder and Spicy Spareribs, Steak Au Poivre, Pâté and Roast Chicken, Duck in Red Wine, and desserts like Cheesecake and Chunky Chocolate Ice Cream.

I can see your mouth has fallen open, partly from appetite and partly from disbelief. *Dr. Atkins,* you're saying, *I heard you mention the merits of low carbohydrate dieting and I was perfectly willing to suspend my disbelief, but this is beyond the beyond. I've been reading magazine articles for the past dozen years trying to wean me from these delights. You're not serious!*

COULDN'T BE MORE SERIOUS, MY FRIEND

So, what gives? I'll tell you frankly out of my experience in advising overweight patients for a quarter of a century. In spite of all the hoopla and hysteria of the preceding years, most overweight men and women are *not* particularly sensitive to dietary fat.

What makes them fat and keeps them fat is a disorder of their *carbohydrate* metabolism. The foods they can't handle are *carbohydrate* foods. Trying to lose weight by fat restriction is torture for them because it doesn't address the *carbohydrate* basis of their problem.

Many of our major health problems and most of our weight problems are indeed nutritional, but they spring from eating the refined, processed, and devitalized food of the modern world, not from eating too many steaks or chicken breasts. I'd like to assure you that the health-problem foods that are really waiting to ambush you are sugar and sweeteners, hydrogenated oils and white flour, margarine and soda pop.

Do you realize that if you're overweight, there's a better than 90 percent chance that you have a problem with blood sugar and insulin levels? There's a very good chance that you are or will become diabetic. You're putting yourself at risk for heart disease. You probably suffer from fatigue and irritability that's totally curable if you eat a low-carbohydrate diet. And there's sound scientific evidence for what I'm telling you now that is largely being ignored.

I'd like to see you on the Atkins diet not just because it will slim you down remarkably, not just because it's delightful to imagine eating the delicious recipes Fran has prepared for you, but because you deserve to be a healthy person. The Atkins diet is a diet that reverses hypertension, controls diabetes, ends fatigue, corrects many eating and digestive disorders, and greatly reduces allergies.

Low-carbohydrate diets have often gotten a bum rap in the press and for that reason I hope that before you go on the Atkins diet you'll begin by having blood tests and measuring your blood pressure. After you've been on the diet for a few weeks, have these numbers checked again. Then, if your family or friends criticize you for doing something so unorthodox as ignoring the low-fat dogmas prevalent now, you'll be able to point to the irrefutable, numerical improvements in such health indicators as cholesterol and triglyceride levels and blood pressure. There's nothing like showing people that you're getting healthy even while they're watching you get slim.

INSULIN, OVERWEIGHT, AND YOU

If—as is most likely—you're among the overweight to whom my description of carbohydrate sensitivity applies, then your weight problem is caused by a problem with insulin, the hormone produced in the pancreas that we cannot live without. This is a scientific fact never mentioned in the weight-loss manuals of the antifat brigades.

Yet obesity is almost always found together with an excessive release of insulin after eating, the medical term for which is hyperinsulinism. When you eat, your body produces blood sugar (glucose). If you eat carbohydrate food, especially the refined carbohydrates I mentioned above, the glucose level goes up rapidly. Insulin is released to lower it. The insulin enables some of that glucose to be used for energy and stores the rest as . . . fat.

In fact, one wise scientist referred to insulin as "the fat-producing hormone."

Now if you want to lose weight, I've just told you the secret. Simply restrict the foods that stimulate excessive insulin release. Carbohydrates provide that kind of stimulation. Fats and proteins don't.

You simply need to severely restrict your consumption of carbohydrates (down to one or two small salads a day to start with), and you're on a weight-loss plan that has an unparalleled record of success.

And success doesn't stop when the pounds are off. I know you don't just want to lose weight, you want to keep it off.

Weight regain is the demon that bedevils dieters. They put time and effort and high hopes into adhering to a diet, and they lose 20 or 30, or perhaps 60 or 70 pounds, and then, presto, six months or eight months or a year after the diet is done they're back up where they were before. It's almost worse than never having lost.

No need for that on this diet plan. The Atkins maintenance diet is a natural transition from the initial weight-loss diet, and on it the vast majority of my dieters maintain their slimness. The lifetime diet you can move into once you're at your ideal weight is a healthy omnivorous diet that includes meats, fish, fowl, vegetables, nuts, seeds, grains, and fruits and starches in moderation.

THIS IS WHAT YOU CAN EXPECT

Let me mention just a few things—besides good food—that you can expect to experience on the Atkins diet. Those of you who want to do the diet would be well advised to obtain *Dr. Atkins' New Diet Revolution* and learn step-by-step the essentials of successful low-carbohydrate dieting. I know many of you already have and now you're turning to this cookbook to make your diet experience more enjoyable. For those of you who are newcomers to the Atkins diet, this chapter aims to make it possible for you to begin the diet and carry it through with success. The final pages of this chapter will explain the four stages of the Atkins lifetime-diet plan.

By following the simple rules, you'll find yourself on a weight-loss program that has the following surprising characteristics. Study them carefully for very few diets can claim even one of them.

This is a diet that:

- Sets no limit on the amount of food you can eat.
- Completely excludes hunger from the dieting experience.
- Includes rich and luxurious foods that you've never associated with dieting before.
- Reduces your appetite by a perfectly natural function of the body.
- Gives you a metabolic edge so significant that the whole concept of watching calories will become absurd to you.
- Produces steady weight loss, even if you have experienced dramatic failures on other diets.
- Is so perfectly adapted to use as a lifetime diet that, unlike most diets, the lost weight won't come back.
- Consistently produced improvements in most of the health problems that accompany overweight.

I'm sure you wonder how all this is possible. Why does the diet work? How will my appetite be reduced? What's all this talk of a metabolic edge? Those were all the questions I hoped you'd ask. Listen.

KETOSIS/LIPOLYSIS

On the Atkins diet, you'll lose weight without hunger. To most dieters that's the miraculous part. No more counting calories, skimping on portions, rising from the table with an ache of appetite still present and unaccounted for. I not only tell my dieters, *Well, if you're hungry, eat!* but I take pleasure in the fact that low-carbohydrate dieting suppresses appetite. Most of you will find that the change in your appetite level is one of the most astonishing experiences of your dieting life.

You see, your body was designed to suppress hunger during

periods of food deprivation. If any of you have fasted or watched other people fast, you'll have noticed that after the first two days hunger disappears. Carbohydrate restriction produces the same phenomenon.

What does the body of a faster or a low-carbohydrate dieter do to provide energy? It burns off its own stored fat. In the case of a fast you'll also burn off muscle tissue, which is not advisable and can even be dangerous. On a low-carbohydrate diet, you burn off *nothing but fat.*

In the metabolic pecking order, the first fuel that the body uses for energy—glucose—is derived from carbohydrate food. But when you drastically restrict carbohydrate intake, very little glucose is produced in your bloodstream after you've eaten. Your crafty metabolism appraises the alternatives and for two days after the diet begins it turns to stored carbohydrate (called glycogen) to power its operations. Once that is gone, your body moves down the pecking order. It turns to its own fat for fuel. Presto! you've begun to lose weight.

You enter a state called ketosis because among the by-products of fat burning are compounds called ketone bodies. They're your new-found source of energy. Be assured, your body is just as happy using them as it was using glucose. Another name for the whole process is lipolysis, which means "the dissolving of fat."

As you go into ketosis/lipolysis, the appetite suppression I just mentioned occurs. Because this usually results in a decrease in your intake of calories, your rate of weight loss is accelerated. But if you continue to eat as many calories as you did before the diet started, you will generally lose weight anyway only at a slower pace.

YOUR METABOLIC ADVANTAGE

This "extra" weight loss is the result of a very exciting side benefit of low-carbohydrate dieting called a metabolic advantage. Very simply—and this has been repeatedly demonstrated in scientific studies—*a person who's eating a strict low-carbohydrate diet loses more weight at whatever his or her level of caloric intake is than he or she would be losing if eating the same number of calories on any other type of diet.* Startling, but at least ten studies conducted in the '60s, '70s, and '80s demonstrated that effect. A low-carbohydrate diet is a calorically wasteful diet. More calories are burned off by your metabolism than on any other diet.

I'm sure I don't need to tell you what an advantage this is. You don't need to concentrate on restricting calories; all you need to do is keep your intake of carbohydrate at such a level that you're in ketosis and enjoying the metabolic advantage nature has provided for you. From that there automatically follows appetite suppression and accelerated rate of weight loss per unit of caloric intake.

Let me emphasize one simple fact: Your body *wants* you to use up your fat stores. It elaborates all sorts of messenger chemicals to facilitate the burning of your stored fat—they're called fat mobilizers. The fat mobilizers redirect your metabolic processes so that you comfortably switch from your normal sugar-burning pathway to the alternative pathway where fat is your body's—and your brain's—primary fuel.

Ketosis/lipolysis is the happiest condition a dieter can be in. Not only does it work, but it requires no willpower, no hunger, and no suffering of any kind. After two or three days of adjustment to the diet, most of you will feel better and more energetic than you've felt in years.

Being on the Atkins diet is a great convincer, but you have to bring some degree of resolution and commitment to your nutritional changeover. A halfhearted low-carbohydrate diet may make you feel physically better, but it probably won't produce much weight loss. Smooth, consistent weight loss is a consequence of so severely restricting carbohydrate intake that you do go into ketosis and begin to burn your own fat for fuel.

To do this you must initally cut down your carbohydrates to one or two small salads or a salad and a helping of vegetables per day. Bread, pasta, sugar, and starchy foods in general will not be allowed while you're in the weight-loss phase of your diet plan. Once you've reached your ideal weight you'll be able to cautiously increase your intake of carbohydrate foods.

OTHER ESSENTIALS OF THE ATKINS DIET

Knowing whether you're in ketosis/lipolysis or not is obviously crucial to your success. Some people play it by ear (or ounce). If they're losing weight they know they're following the game plan. I think it's more effective to get Bioketone testing strips, which you can put in your urine once a day (preferably in the evening). If the strips turn purple, you know you're in ketosis.

Another crucial aspect of dietary success is nutritional supplementation. In the strict early phase of the diet, which I call the Induction phase, you'll need vitamins and minerals to keep you at a healthy level for all nutrients. Even when you're at the advanced and more liberalized levels of the diet I strongly advise supplementation because it's good for you. See "Nutritional Supplementation" in the appendices for a description of what your basic multivitamin formula should include.

BE PREPARED

My other advice for the beginning Atkins dieter is in the area of preparation. Prepare your relatives and prepare your kitchen. Qualitatively speaking, this is a strict diet. There's no room for cheating. I can already hear your spouse saying, "Just this one little piece of cake won't hurt you." It will. You can't do the diet that way.

So start by telling the folks you live with just what you intend to do. Tell them that you take your diet seriously, and you'd appreciate their doing the same. If they question the wisdom of a high-protein diet that isn't interested in fat restriction, tell them to watch and wait. When they see how terrific you feel and how good you look, their temptation to criticize will start to fade away. Be diplomatic and gentle but firm. Eating is a very emotional habit, and changes in the way you eat affect everyone around you. Nonetheless, this is your diet, not your relatives'.

As for your kitchen, if you live alone it will be easy. Invite some friends over to finish off the ice cream, and give all your forbidden goods away to friends and neighbors. If there are others in the house, and they're not going to be on this diet, then simply see that there are separate portions of such forbidden foods as bread, potatoes, and sugar-laden desserts for them. The main course, the salads, and the vegetables will be suitable for everyone.

Now, before you turn to the wonderful part of this book (the food!), look at the next chapter and make sure you know how you'll do the series of diets that together comprise the Atkins diet. This is going to be your gateway to a lifetime of eating pleasure and dieting success.

2 | *Four Diets in One*

This chapter is designed for those of you who haven't read *Dr. Atkins' New Diet Revolution*. It will give, I hope, a simple and effective description of the Atkins diet in its four stages.

These are:

1. The Induction Diet
2. The Ongoing Weight-Loss Diet
3. The Premaintenance Diet
4. The Maintenance Diet

These four stages are an effective way of breaking up and explaining what—for you—will be one continuous lifetime diet. The Induction diet gets you into weight loss with a bang; the Ongoing Weight-Loss diet carries you through the weeks or months of weight loss needed to get you close to your ideal weight; the Premaintenance diet takes you the final few steps and eases your transition to what is perhaps the most important diet of all; and that is the Maintenance diet—your lifetime ticket to health and slimness. Let's take them in order.

GETTING STARTED

The Induction diet—your start-up diet—is very strict in its limitation of carbohydrates. *Because of its rigor, this phase of the diet is not appropriate for pregnant women and people with severe kidney disease.* You'll only be eating 15 to 20 grams of carbohydrates on it, which might be two medium salads and a helping of vegetables. The purpose of this strictness is to ensure that your body does indeed go into ketosis/lipolysis, does begin releasing fat-mobilizing hormones that will suppress your appetite, and does, after the first two or three days, begin to consume your own fat. This is what you're working toward initially, and your success is pretty well assured.

Once you're in ketosis, your body has made a transition from burning carbohydrate (glucose) for fuel to employing its alternative metabolic pathway that was evolved millions of years ago to enable you to survive periods of famine. You now break down fat, and the by-products of this fat breakdown—ketone bodies—are consumed for energy.

This is the basic Atkins diet, so let me explain it in full. The other three diets are careful, gradual liberalizations of the Induction diet, and they'll be easy to explain once you're grounded in the Induction diet.

THE RULES OF THE INDUCTION DIET

1. *Your diet must contain no more than 20 grams of carbohydrates a day.* For most people, induction of ketosis/lipolysis can be achieved on this intake. This allows for approximately 3 cups of salad vegetables (loosely packed) or 2 cups of salad plus ⅔ cup of cooked vegetables in the below 10 percent carbohydrate category.

2. You are no longer on a quantitative diet. Therefore you should adjust the quantities to your appetite. When hungry, eat the amount that makes you feel satisfied but not stuffed. When not hungry, eat nothing or just a small protein snack to accompany your vitamins.

3. You are, however, on a qualitative diet. This means that if the food is not on your diet, you are to have absolutely none of it. Your "just this one taste won't hurt" rationalization is the kiss of death on this diet. Addicts will find this rule builds character in a hurry.

4. Your diet will consist of pure proteins (not many of those in nature, however), pure fats (this means butter, olive oil, and mayonnaise are permitted), and combinations of protein and fat (this is the mainstay of your diet). Foods that are protein-and-carbohydrate or fat-and-carbohydrate are *not* on this diet, because carbohydrate is not on this diet.

5. Using a carbohydrate gram counter, one could find other combinations totaling less than 20 grams of carbohydrate. One would be using foods like nuts, seeds, olives, avocados,

cheeses, cream and sour cream, lemon and lime juices, and low-carbohydrate diet foods. Don't assume these foods are low, unless you absolutely know the carbohydrate content of the portion you are eating. In the Carbohydrate Gram Counter on page 230, I will include the carbohydrate content in grams of the foods you may include on this 14-day *Induction* diet as well as on more liberal levels of the diet that you will be doing as your lifetime diet plan.

FREE FOODS:

MEAT	FISH	FOWL
Beef	Tuna	Chicken
Pork	Salmon	Turkey
Lamb	Sole	Duck
Bacon	Trout	Goose
Veal	Flounder	Cornish Hen
Ham	Sardines	Quail
Venison	Herring	Pheasant
in fact, all meat	*in fact, all fish*	*in fact, all fowl*

SHELLFISH	EGGS	CHEESE
Oysters	Scrambled	Aged and fresh
Mussels	Fried	Cow and goat
Clams	Poached	Cream cheese
Squid	Soft Boiled	Cottage cheese
Shrimp	Hard Boiled	Swiss
Lobster	Deviled	Cheddar
Crabmeat	Omelets	Mozzarella
in fact, all shellfish	*in fact, all eggs*	*in fact, almost** *all cheeses*

Exceptions: 1) luncheon meats with nitrites or sugar added
2) products that are not exclusively meat, fish, or fowl, such as imitation fish

---

*All cheeses have some carbohydrate content, and quantities are governed by that. (See Carbohydrate Gram Counter.) No diet cheese, cheese spreads, or whey cheeses. Those with a known yeast infection, dairy allergy, or cheese intolerance must avoid cheese. Imitation cheese products are not allowed, except for Tofu (soy cheese)—but check carbohydrate content.

OTHER INDUCTION DIET FOODS:

Vegetables of 10 Percent Carbohydrate or Less

SALAD VEGETABLES:

Alfalfa Sprouts	Endive	Parsley
Arugula	Escarole	Peppers
Bok Choy	Fennel	Posse Pied
Boston Lettuce	Jicama	Radicchio
Celery	Mache	Radishes
Chicory	Morels	Romaine
Chives	Mushrooms	Sorrel
Cucumber	Olives	

SALAD HERBS:

Basil	Dill	Rosemary
Cilantro	Oregano	Thyme

For salad dressing use the desired oil plus vinegar or lemon juice and spices. Grated cheese, chopped eggs, bacon, or fried pork rinds may be added.

VEGETABLES IN ADDITION TO SALAD VEGETABLES:

Artichoke Hearts	Christophene	Sauerkraut
Asparagus	Collard Greens	Scallions
Avocado	Dandelion Greens	Snow Pea Pods
Bamboo Shoots	Eggplant	Spaghetti Squash
Bean Sprouts	Hearts of Palm	Spinach
Beet Greens	Kale	String or Wax Beans
Broccoli	Kohlrabi	Summer Squash
Brussels Sprouts	Leeks	Tomato
Cabbage	Okra	Turnips
Cauliflower	Onion	Water Chestnuts
Celery Root (celeriac)	Pumpkin	Zucchini Squash
Chard	Rhubarb	

SALAD GARNISHES:

Anchovies	Minced Hard-Boiled Egg Yolk
Crumbled Crisp Bacon	Minced Sautéed Mushrooms
Grated Cheese	Sour Cream

SPICES:

All spices to taste, but make sure sugar is not in the seasoning.

BEVERAGES:

Water

Mineral Water

Essence Flavored Seltzer
(must say "No Calories")

Decaffeinated coffee or tea

Diet Soda (read label)

Iced tea with artificial sweetener

Cream (heavy or light);
note carbohydrate content

Natural and artificial orange
soda products have some
carbohydrate—they may be
one of your options for a few
grams

Spring Water

Club Soda

Herb Tea
(no barley, dates, figs, sugar)

Caffeine is not allowed

Carbohydrate-free, artificially
sweetened powder for making
fruit-flavored drinks

Clear broth/bouillon (not all
brands)

Grain Beverages (i.e., imitation
coffee substitutes) are not
allowed

FATS AND OILS:

Many fats, especially certain oils, are essential to good nutrition. Include a source of GLA (gamma-linolenic acid) and omega-3 oils (EPA, salmon oil, linseed oil). Olive oil (monounsaturated) is valuable. All vegetable oils are allowed. The best are canola, walnut, soybean, sesame, sunflower, and safflower oils, especially if they are labeled "cold pressed." Butter is allowed; margarine is not. Margarine should be avoided not because of its carbohydrate content but because it is a potential health hazard. Mayonnaise is permitted unless you are on a yeast restriction. The fat that is part of the meat or fowl you eat is permitted.

Avoid the seeming paradox provided by today's "diet foods." Understand why cream is allowed but not skim milk, why sour cream can be used but not yogurt, why low-fat chicken breading is not allowed even though chicken may be pan-fried. The answer common to all of these seeming inconsistencies lies in the higher carbohydrate content of the low-fat dieter's foods.

ARTIFICIAL SWEETENERS:

Dieters must determine which artificial sweeteners agree with them, but the following are allowed: saccharine, aspartame, acesulfame-K.

Sweeteners such as sorbitol, mannitol, and other hexitols are not allowed, nor are any natural sweeteners ending in the letters -ose, such as maltose, fructose, and so on.

COMMON MISTAKES TO AVOID:

1. Note that the 14-day diet contains no fruit, bread, grains, starchy vegetables, dairy products other than cheese, cream, or butter.
2. Avoid diet products unless they specifically state "no carbohydrates." Most dietetic foods are for fat-restricted, not carbohydrate-restricted, diets.
3. The word sugarless is not sufficient. The product must state the carbohydrate content, and that's what you go by.
4. Many products you do not normally think of as foods such as chewing gum, cough syrups, and cough drops are filled with sugar and other caloric sweeteners and must be avoided.

THE ONGOING WEIGHT-LOSS DIET

You won't need to do the Induction diet for more than a couple of weeks. By that time, I feel confident that you'll not only be losing weight but feeling healthier than you have in years. Most people feel energized by a low-carbohydrate diet. On the weight-loss front, most of you will have seen five to ten pounds disappear, and that means you can now liberalize your intake of carbohydrate slightly. You've begun the Ongoing Weight-Loss diet, which will carry you pleasantly along for as many weeks or months as it takes to get you very close to your ideal weight.

This minor liberalization of carbohydrate is, of course, not an invitation to go back to eating the way you did before. What, in fact, you'll be doing is increasing the daily amount of carbohydrate by 5 grams at a time. You'll do this very gradually because you don't want to fall out of ketosis/lipolysis. I suggest that each week you increase your daily carbohydrate consumption by 5 grams. Typical 5-gram increments are 10 Brazil nuts or 20 macadamias, or half of an avocado or half a tomato, or 3 ounces of plain, unflavored yogurt, or $2/3$ of a cup of string beans or broccoli or $2\frac{1}{2}$ wafers of GG Bran Crispbread.

Those of you who have been chafing at the absolute restriction of alcohol on the induction diet might now add 4 ounces of dry wine or 6 ounces of a light beer, or 1 ounce of whiskey or gin daily.

Yeast Infections

I have to tell you a little bit about yeast infections because—if you have them—they could derail your diet and blight your predestined success.

In my experience, more than a quarter of the patients I see have an overgrowth of one particular yeast, which is known as *Candida albicans.* *Candida* is a normal part of your body, one of four hundred species of bacteria resident in the human intestinal tract. In healthy competition with your other intestinal flora, *Candida* serves you well performing yeasty bacterial mission in your gut. But when some disturbance upsets the bacterial equilibrium in your body, a yeast infection can ensue. *Candida* overgrows, suppresses less aggressive bacteria, and causes a multitude of symptoms.

A short list of the problems a yeast infection can cause include lethargy; fatigue; depression; inability to concentrate; headaches; gastrointestinal disorders, including constipation, abdominal pain, gas, diarrhea, and bloating; respiratory ailments; and disorders of the urinary tract and reproductive organs. The most specific symptom is bloating—gas in the lower abdomen.

Let me repeat: A *Candida albicans* yeast infection will also make it very difficult to lose weight.

The four most common contributing causes to a yeast infection are:

1. A diet high in sugar and refined carbohydrates.
2. Antibiotics (more than 20 weeks in a lifetime would make *Candida* overgrowth a probability).
3. The mercury in silver dental fillings.
4. Birth control pills, prednisone, and other steroids.

This is an embarrassing list for medicine since the last three provokers of yeast overgrowth are all related to medical care. Perhaps that explains why *Candida* hasn't received nearly the attention it deserves.

If you think you have a yeast infection, you may need to see a physician who's experienced in treating them. In *Dr. Atkins' New Diet Revolution* I devote a chapter to *Candida* and its treatments. For now, let me simply say that whatever therapies your doctor proposes, he will certainly also tell you that you need to make alterations in the way you eat. Fermented and yeast-containing foods are inappropriate for a person who's suffering from yeast overgrowth. Please turn to the section on the yeast-free diet for further information on this dietary problem.

Of course, as you increase your carbohydrate consumption, you will see a gradual decrease in your rate of weight loss. That's fine. The purpose of this diet is not to lose weight in a hurry, but to get it off and *keep it off.* By slowing down your rate of loss, you go gradually toward your ultimate diet.

THE PREMAINTENANCE DIET

The Premaintenance diet is a further extension of the diet liberalization that you went toward on the Ongoing Weight-Loss diet. When you're getting fairly close to your ultimate goal weight, it's very important that you lose weight slowly. Many of you are such determined dieters that this will be psychologically burdensome. You've got that final five or six pounds to go, you know you can do it in two weeks, why postpone success? Sorry, folks, that's not the best way to proceed. I think you should carve off those final pounds over the course of two or three months. Here's why.

The biggest problem with weight control is not the losing but the maintenance. How many celebrity dieters have you heard of who lost their weight in a crash program and then gained it back faster than they lost it? What you should do is just the opposite. Lose those final pounds with excruciating slowness so that by the time you say, "I'm there!" you'll be virtually eating your lifetime diet.

As for doing Premaintenance, it's simple. Either add another 10 grams of carbohydrate a day to what you've been eating on Ongoing Weight-Loss, or give yourself a 20-gram carbohydrate treat two or three times a week. You can even touch some forbidden starches. A bagel, a baked potato, some French toast, a slice of pizza, a side dish of lasagna. Or else add some of your favorite fruits—apples, oranges, grapefruits, peaches, bananas. As long as you don't start gaining weight but continue to lose at an almost imperceptible rate, you're doing fine.

GOING ON YOUR LIFETIME MAINTENANCE DIET

Now that you've arrived, offer yourself some well-deserved self-congratulation, and prepare for a slim lifetime.

As you already know, there's no shortage of delicious food for you to eat. The one scientific fact of importance that you must be aware of, however, is that once you've totally stopped your weight loss, your appetite will increase toward its normal level. For this reason, your lifetime maintenance diet will still be fairly restrictive of carbohydrate foods.

You'll need to find your own level, and that level will be what I call your Critical Carbohydrate Level for Maintenance. This is the level *above* which you *gain* weight. At this level, you will have enough carbohydrate restriction to keep *some* curbing of your appetite, and, for most of you, this will range between 40 and 90 grams of carbohydrate a day. Still considerably less than the average American consumption of 300 grams a day!

Here are my final suggestions for you happy dieters who have now reached your ideal weight.

1. Be food aware—meat, fish, fowl, nuts, seeds, vegetables, and occasional fruits and starches are the foods nature designed you to eat. Avoid processed foods. Eat fresh and natural to the best of your ability.
2. Avoid sugar and corn syrup and white flour and cornstarch like the plague. For most people these are the foods of overweight and ill health.
3. Individualize your diet. Try new foods. Create the diet that's right for you.
4. Consider the program of vitamin and mineral supplementation that's explained in Appendix 1 and that you've been using while you were on the weight-loss portion of the diet.
5. Use caffeine and alcohol in moderation.
6. If you regain more than five pounds of weight go right back to the Induction diet. Within two weeks you should find yourself back at your ideal weight.
7. Please do exercise. Though there isn't time to talk about it here, it's wonderful for health and very helpful in maintaining slimness.

Now for a final word about eating. . . .

ARE YOU READY TO BE HAPPY?

I can't guarantee that I'll make you wealthy and wise, but I have every intention of making you happy in your body. That doesn't just mean slim, it also means healthy and thrilled by the food you eat. It's simply essential that your foods thrill you. If they don't, how can I fulfill my promise that for you the Atkins diet will be a lifetime diet?

I want your new meals to provide you with every bit as much emotional satisfaction and eating happiness as your normal pre-Atkins way of eating did. Hopefully more. If we succeed at this, then there will be no reason for you to return to your old way of eating—the way that didn't work.

If you follow the suggestions that that ever-so-talented food wizard, Fran Gare, has prepared for you in this book, you will probably end up much better at cooking than you were before. This is no small advantage. Add to that the fact that on the Atkins maintenance diet, you will be eating sufficient fat to produce satiety and avoid disruptive blood sugar patterns, and I think you're an odds-on favorite to succeed.

Let me give you a dieting tip. One of the advantages of fat in your diet is that it buffers your changing blood sugar levels, it prevents swift, disturbing changes, and it thereby suppresses the craving for sweets. The successful effort to lower the amount of fat in the American diet over the past two decades has been bought at a crippling price. During this same period the American consumption of sugar has increased by 20 pounds yearly. That's not only a catastrophe for dieters but a catastrophe for health.

You may have heard of the French paradox. The French consume more fat than Americans (including four times as much butter and twice as much cheese), but they have less than half our heart attack rate. How can this be? It demands an answer, and the theorists of low fat have done a spectacularly ineffectual job of providing one. But the true answer is evident. We eat three times as much sugar as the French, and the research linking sugar to excess insulin production to heart disease is strong and growing stronger.

So don't be afraid of fat. Not only can you use it for weight loss, you can eat it in good health. The Atkins diet is not a high-fat diet since many of the junk food sources of fat are not permitted on it, but it is a diet that's unafraid of fat. The lifetime maintenance diet that will keep you slim is natural for human beings and well suited to the improvement of your health.

As you succeed on the Atkins diet and eat the scrumptious recipes Fran Gare has prepared for you, there will be one final question you'll have to ask yourself: Am I happier eating this way than I was before? Personally, I think nothing compares with smelling a delectable main course sizzling in the frying pan and experiencing appetite combined with the sure and certain knowledge that appetite is shortly to be gratified.

On many other diets people are asked, "Are you satisfied with the food?" and often they'll reply, "Oh, yes, I'm satisfied." All too often, these responses fail the acid test of dieting: The hopeful dieters who made them end up gaining their weight back and resuming their former eating patterns.

But so seldom does that happen with the diet you're committed to trying now. So very seldom. And, of course, that's because dieters are happier eating the Atkins way. Most of them feel better than they've felt in years, all of them look better, and, far from feeling deprived, they're luxuriating in a whole new world of delicious foods.

And now that I've said the magic words, *delicious foods,* please proceed to the rest of the book. I leave you in the capable hands of Fran Gare.

3 | *Meal Plans*

The Induction Diet

DAY 1

Breakfast

> 2–3 Eggs, *Poached, *Hard or Soft Boiled
> 4 slices no-nitrate bacon
> 1 ounce Cheddar cheese
> Tea or decaffeinated coffee with 1 tablespoon cream and sugar substitute

Lunch

> *Chicken Salad Ham Rolls
> *Orange Cooler

Dinner

> *Spicy Cocktail
> *Luscious Lamb
> Tossed green salad with *Vinaigrette Cream Dressing

Snack

> *Snappy Raspberries and Lemons

---

*Those dishes noted with an asterisk are found in Chapter 4, Recipes.

DAY 2

Breakfast

*Scrambled or *Sunny-Side-Up and Over Easy eggs
2 slices smoked ham wrapped around a celery stick stuffed with
1 tablespoon of cream cheese
Tea or decaffeinated coffee with 1 tablespoon cream and sugar
substitute

Lunch

*¡Ole! Burger
½ cucumber, sliced, sprinkled with cayenne pepper

Dinner

*Salami and Parmesan
*Fabulous Flounder
Tossed green salad with *Lime Dill Dressing
Tea or decaffeinated coffee with 1 tablespoon cream and sugar
substitute

Snack

*Hot Mint Chocolate Nog

DAY 3

Breakfast

> *Cheese-Baked Eggs
> 2 sausage patties
> Tea or decaffeinated coffee with 1 tablespoon cream and sugar substitute

Lunch

> *Chicken Croquettes on a bed of lettuce
> *Orange Cooler

Dinner

> *Sour Cream Clam Dip with fried pork rinds
> *Fennel Red Snapper
> Tossed green salad with *Dressing of the House
> Tea or decaffeinated coffee with 1 tablespoon cream and sugar substitute

Snack

> *Vanilla Ice Cream

DAY 4

Breakfast

> *Mocha Drink
> *Herb Omelet

Lunch

> *Sardine snack on lettuce leaves
> Sliced celery and olives
> Tea or decaffeinated coffee with 1 tablespoon cream and sugar substitute

Dinner

> *Tomato Lemon Jell-O
> *Lemon-Basted Roast Chicken
> *Ricotta Sauce for Chicken

Tea or decaffeinated coffee with 1 tablespoon cream and sugar substitute

Snack

*Sweet Lemonade with Lecithin

DAY 5

Breakfast

4 *Deviled-Salmon Egg halves
2 1-gram crisp breads (GG is an example)
*Spiced Iced Decaf Coffee

Lunch

*Fresh Tuna and Avocado Salad
*Spice Cocktail

Dinner

*Japanese Egg Custard Soup
*Oriental Shrimp
Tea or decaffeinated coffee with 1 tablespoon cream and sugar substitute

Snack

*Raspberry Jell-O Cream

DAY 6

Breakfast

*Spicy Sausage Omelet
Tea or decaffeinated coffee with 1 tablespoon cream and sugar substitute

Lunch

*U.S. Hamburgers
Tossed green salad with *Our Favorite Roquefort Dressing
Diet soda or diet iced tea

Dinner

*Gourmet Game Hens
*Crispy White Radish
Tea or decaffeinated coffee with 1 tablespoon cream and sugar substitute

Snack

*Vanilla Ice Cream

DAY 7

Breakfast

Steak and *Scrambled Eggs with 2 tablespoons *Cheese Sauce
Tea or decaffeinated coffee with 1 tablespoon cream and sugar substitute

Lunch

*Cold Avocado Soup
Tuna in olive oil with lemon wedge
1/2 cucumber, sliced
2 tablespoons *Mustard Vinaigrette
Tea or decaffeinated coffee with 1 tablespoon cream and sugar substitute

Dinner

    *Shrimp Parmesan
Tossed salad with *Tomato Dressing

Snack

    *Mocha Drink

The Ongoing Weight-Loss Diet

DAY 1

Breakfast

>   *Two-Cheese Omelet
> 3 strips no-nitrate bacon
> 1 slice *4 Grain and Seed Bread
> Tea or decaffeinated coffee with 1 tablespoon cream and sugar substitute

Lunch

>   *Eggplant Parmigiana
> Tossed green salad with *Italian Dressing
> *Orange Cooler

Dinner

>   *Caribbean Crabmeat
> *Halibut Roll-Ups
> *Broccoli in Cheese Sauce
> Tea or decaffeinated coffee with 1 tablespoon cream and sugar substitute

Snack

> 2 squares of *Chocolate Fudge
> Diet soda

DAY 2

Breakfast

>   *Poached Eggs on ham with 2 tablespoons *Hollandaise Sauce
> 2 slices *4 Grain and Seed Bread
> Tea or decaffeinated coffee with 1 tablespoon cream and sugar substitute

Lunch

>   *Chicken Salad
> 6 fried pork rinds

Diet soda or diet iced tea

Dinner

   *Enchiladas
   Tossed green salad with *Dressing of the House
   *Baked Cream
   Tea or decaffeinated coffee with 1 tablespoon cream and sugar
   substitute

Snack

   *Spiced Iced Decaf Coffee
   2 *Peanut Butter Cookies

DAY 3

Breakfast

   *Crabmeat and Mushroom Omelet
   2 slices *Rye Bread with cream cheese
   Tea or decaffeinated coffee with 1 tablespoon cream and sugar
   substitute

Lunch

   *Dr. Atkins' Fromage Burger
   ½ tomato, sliced
   ¼ cucumber, sliced
   Diet soda

Dinner

   *New England Fish Chowder
   *Broiled Tarragon Lobster Tails
   *Porcini Mushrooms
   *Raspberry Cream Jell-O
   Tea or decaffeinated coffee with 1 tablespoon cream and sugar
   substitute

Snack

   2 *Almond Ball Cookies

DAY 4

Breakfast

>*Rye Bread, smoked salmon and cream cheese
2 slices onion
Tea or decaffeinated coffee with 1 tablespoon cream and sugar substitute

Lunch

>*Ham and Artichoke Omelet
Tossed green salad with *Basic French Dressing
1 slice *Cheese Cake
Iced decaffeinated coffee with cream

Dinner

>*Fran's Special Pâté
Roast Beef with *Frozen Horseradish Cream
Endive with *Parmesan Caesar Dressing
Tea or decaffeinated coffee with 1 tablespoon cream and sugar substitute

Snack

>½ cup *Decaf-Coffee Ice Cream

DAY 5

Breakfast

>*Two-Cheese Omelet
4 slices crisp no-nitrate bacon
2 slices *4 Grain and Seed Bread

Lunch

>*Vegetable Stock with *Dumplings
*Zucchini Stuffed with Cream Sauce
Romaine Lettuce with *Mustard Vinaigrette
Diet soda

Dinner

>*Sardine Snack stuffed into celery sticks

*Fennel Red Snapper
*Chic Asparagus
Tea or decaffeinated coffee with 1 tablespoon cream and sugar substitute

Snack

2 *Brownie Squares

DAY 6

Breakfast

*Cappuccino
*Scrambled Eggs with ham and *Mustard Sauce
1 slice *Rye Bread with cream cheese
Tea or decaffeinated coffee with 1 tablespoon cream and sugar substitute

Lunch

*Salad Niçoise with Fresh Tuna
*Orange Cooler

Dinner

*Tricolor Salad with Three Cheeses
*Chicken à la Firenze
$\frac{1}{2}$ small tomato, sliced
Tea or decaffeinated coffee with 1 tablespoon cream and sugar substitute

Snack

Diet Jell-O with 1 tablespoon of whipped cream

DAY 7

Breakfast

Smoked whitefish with scallion cream cheese on 2 slices *Rye Bread
*Scrambled Eggs
Tea or decaffeinated coffee with 1 tablespoon cream and sugar substitute

Lunch

*U.S. Hamburgers with 1 slice of onion and lettuce
*Chocolate Shake

Dinner

*Cream of Shiitake Mushroom Soup
*Chicken Croquettes served on spaghetti squash
Tossed green salad with *Dill Vinaigrette Dressing

Snack

*Butter Pecan Ice Cream
Diet soda

The Premaintenance Diet

DAY 1

Breakfast

  *Turkey Sausage
  Scrambled Eggs
  2 slices *Zucchini Bread

Lunch

  *Crunchy Seafood Salad
  *Vanilla Ice Cream
  Diet soda

Dinner

  ¼ Cantaloupe with lemon slice
  *Stuffed Steak
  *Ratatouille
  *Lemon-Lime Mousse
  Tea or decaffeinated coffee with 1 tablespoon cream and sugar substitute

Snack

  2 ounces (20) macadamia nuts or
  ½ cup *Coconut Macadamia Ice Cream

DAY 2

Breakfast

> *Eggplant and Cheddar Omelet
> ¼ pound grilled ham
> 2 slices *Rye Bread

Lunch

> *Fresh Tuna and Avocado Salad
> 3 1-gram crisp breads (GG is an example)
> *Fresh Lemonade with Lecithin

Dinner

> *Manicotti
> *Green Bean Chokes
> *Tomato Lemon Jell-O on lettuce leaves
> Tea or decaffeinated coffee with 1 tablespoon cream and sugar
> substitute

Snack

> 2 ounces almonds

DAY 3

Breakfast

> French toast made with 4 slices *4 Grain and Seed Bread dipped
> into a beaten egg and fried in butter
> 4 slices of crisp no-nitrate bacon
> Tea or decaffeinated coffee with 1 tablespoon cream and sugar
> substitute

Lunch

> *Hot Beef Salad
> *Orange Cooler

Dinner

> *Cannelloni
> 1 cup steamed broccoli
> Tossed salad with *Tomato Mayonnaise

*Italian Rum Cake
Tea or decaffeinated coffee with 1 tablespoon cream and sugar substitute

Snack

¼ cup fresh raspberries and 2 tablespoons whipped cream

DAY 4

Breakfast

Your favorite cut of steak, sliced
*Scrambled Eggs with *Hot Barbecue Sauce
Tea or decaffeinated coffee with 1 tablespoon cream and sugar substitute

Lunch

*Salad Niçoise With Fresh Tuna
2 slices *Rye Bread and butter
Diet soda
*Lemon Jell-O Cream

Dinner

*Enchiladas
Tossed green salad with *Creamy Celery Dressing
*The Most Delicious Cucumbers
Tea or decaffeinated coffee with 1 tablespoon cream and sugar substitute

Snack

½ cup *Decaf-Coffee Ice Cream

DAY 5

Breakfast

Smoked salmon, onion, and eggs scrambled
2 slices *Zucchini Bread with scallion cream cheese
Tea or decaffeinated coffee with 1 tablespoon cream and sugar
substitute

Lunch

*Eggplant Little Shoes
Tossed green salad with *Italian Dressing
Tea or decaffeinated coffee with 1 tablespoon cream and sugar
substitute

Dinner

*Fish Stock with *Dumplings
*Sun Luck Scallops
*Chic Asparagus
Tea or decaffeinated coffee with 1 tablespoon cream and sugar
substitute

Snack

3 *Almond Ball Cookies

DAY 6

Breakfast

*Shrimp and Goat Cheese Omelet
2 slices *4 Grain and Seed Bread
Tea or decaffeinated coffee with 1 tablespoon cream and sugar
substitute

Lunch

*Poached Salmon Salad
3 1-gram crisp breads (GG is an example)
Tea or decaffeinated coffee with 1 tablespoon cream and sugar
substitute

Dinner

*Cauliflower Soup with Dill and Caraway
*Gourmet Pork Chops
*String Beans Almandine
*Crispy White Radish
Tea or decaffeinated coffee with 1 tablespoon cream and sugar substitute

Snack

1/2 cup *Maple Walnut Ice Cream

DAY 7

Breakfast

*Peaches and Cream Omelet
*Hot Chocolate

Lunch

1/2 cantaloupe stuffed with *A Mold of Roquefort
*Tuna Loaf
Iced tea or iced decaf coffee

Dinner

*Roast Turkey With Almond Stuffing
*Baked Spinach
1/2 cup *Peach Melba Frozen Yogurt
Tea or decaffeinated coffee with 1 tablespoon cream and sugar substitute

Snack

2 ounces pecans (about 20)

The Yeast-Free Diet

The Yeast-Free Diet has food restrictions that the other diets do not have. Therefore, it is necessary to begin with a list of yeast no-no's. To learn more about how yeast affects your body, see page 15.

DO NOT EAT OR DRINK

Alcoholic beverages
Barbecue sauce
Bread or hamburger buns
Buttermilk
Cake
Cashews
Catsup
Cheeses (except fresh)
Chili peppers
Citric acid
Dried roasted nuts
Fruit (especially dried and cured)
Horseradish
Mayonnaise
Malted products
Milk
Mincemeat
Mushrooms
Pastry
Peanuts
Pickles
Pistachios
Pretzels
Rolls
Root beer
Sauerkraut
Smoked foods
Sour cream
Soy sauce
Sugars of any type
Tomato sauce
Vitamins in a yeast base

This list may seem overwhelming. It is not! As you will see, this book is filled with wonderful recipes that will delight the taste buds and give a feeling of well-being.

Happily being faithful to this diet has very positive results. You will be able to overcome (with the help of supplements) your yeast sensitivity and once again enjoy—in moderation—foods containing yeast.

DAY 1

Breakfast

2–3 Eggs *Poached, *Hard or Soft Boiled
6 cooked shrimp
*Lemon Barbecue Sauce
Tea or decaffeinated coffee with 1 tablespoon cream and sugar substitute

Lunch

*Gazpacho
Tuna fish with *Vinegar-Free Mayonnaise
2 1-gram crisp breads (GG is an example)
*Orange Cooler

Dinner

*Spicy Spareribs
Hearts of lettuce salad with *Tomato Mayonnaise Dressing
Sugar-free Jell-O

Snack

*Vanilla Ice Cream

DAY 2

Breakfast

> *Scrambled or *Sunny-Side-Up and Over Easy eggs
> 3 slices boiled ham wrapped around a celery stick that is stuffed with cream cheese
> Tea or decaffeinated coffee with 1 tablespoon cream and sugar substitute

Lunch

> *Brit Burger
> ½ cucumber, sliced, with minced fresh basil
> *Shape-Up Shake

Dinner

> *Broiled Lobster Tails with Tarragon
> *Crispy White Radish
> Tossed green salad with *Creamy Celery Seed Dressing made with *Vinegar-Free Mayonnaise
> Tea or decaffeinated coffee with 1 tablespoon cream and sugar substitute

Snack

> *Hot Mint Chocolate Nog

DAY 3

Breakfast

> Sliced steak sautéed in garlic butter
> ½ small onion, raw or sautéed in butter
> 2 slices *4 Grain and Seed Bread
> Tea or decaffeinated coffee with 1 tablespoon cream and sugar substitute

Lunch

> *Luncheon Omelet
> *Mocha Drink

Dinner

> *Sardine Snack on lettuce leaves
> *Lemon-Basted Roast Chicken
> Endive with *Lime Dill Dressing

Snack

> *Black and White Ice Cream Soda

DAY 4

Breakfast

> *Herb Omelet
> 2 slices *4 Grain and Seed Bread with cream cheese
> *Cappuccino

Lunch

> *Chicken Salad Ham Roll made with fresh ham (always use *Vinegar-Free Mayonnaise)
> *Blender-Thick Raspberry Shake

Dinner

> *Japanese Egg Custard Soup (exclude mushrooms)
> *Oriental Shrimp
> *Raspberry Jell-O Cream
> Tea or decaffeinated coffee with 1 tablespoon cream and sugar substitute

Snack

> *Lemon Cream Jell-O

DAY 5

Breakfast

>4 *Deviled-Salmon Egg halves
>2 slices *Rye Bread with butter
>*Spiced Iced Decaf Coffee

Lunch

>*U.S. Hamburgers with *Tomato Mayonnaise
>*Mock Potato Salad (exclude pickle)
>Diet soda

Dinner

>*Chicken Stock with *Dumplings
>*Gourmet Game Hens
>Tossed green salad with *Basic Vinegar-Free Salad Dressing
>Tea or decaffeinated coffee with 1 tablespoon cream and sugar substitute

Snack

>*The 'Pop' Pop

DAY 6

Breakfast

>*Ham and Artichoke Omelet
>2 slices *Rye Bread
>Tea or decaffeinated coffee with 1 tablespoon cream and sugar substitute

Lunch

>*Chicken Croquettes
>Tossed green salad with *Tomato Mayonnaise
>*Raspberry Cream Jell-O
>Diet soda

Dinner

>*Klara's Eggplant Appetizer on celery rounds
>*Curried Crabmeat

Steamed broccoli
*Baked Cream
Tea or decaffeinated coffee with 1 tablespoon cream and sugar
substitute

Snack

Two *Brownie squares
Diet soda

DAY 7

Breakfast

*Salmon Soufflé
2 slices *4 Grain and Seed Bread
Tea or decaffeinated coffee with 1 tablespoon cream and sugar
substitute

Lunch

*Curry Burgers
Tossed green salad with *Lime Dill Dressing
2 *Almond Ball Cookies
Diet soda

Dinner

*Chicken Cacciatore with spaghetti squash
*String Beans Almandine
*Lemon-Lime Mousse
Tea or decaffeinated coffee with 1 tablespoon cream and sugar
substitute

Snack

½ cup *Decaf-Coffee Ice Cream

The Maintenance Diet

When you have reached your ideal weight, you will begin Maintenance. At this level you may choose freely from any recipe in the book. And you may add back dried beans; all vegetables, including carrots, peas, beets, potatoes, sweet potatoes; all the sweet winter squash and plaintains. Grains are permitted on the Maintenance Level. Actually you will be eating a very healthy diet. That is the good news.

Sugars of all types are excluded from all of our diets. Although some of you may think they taste good, sugars are destructive to your health. Therefore, sugars—including honey, molasses, maple sugar and syrup, fructose, beet sugar, barley malt sugar, glucose, maltose, dextrose, corn syrup, sorbitol, mannitol, and hexitol—still are and will always be the bad news.

We encourage you to eat more protein than carbohydrates, unless the condition of your health does not permit it. Please drink 6 to 8 glasses of water a day and see a nutritionist who can help you with a vitamin program specific to your needs. When this becomes your lifestyle, you will be the slim, healthy, and energetic person that you always aspired to be.

The Yeast-Free Maintenance Diet

This diet is much the same as the Maintenance Diet. However, on this diet you will restrict cheeses, vinegars, and all fermented foods as well as sugar. In addition, you may wish to ask for yeast-free products at your health food store.

4 | *Recipes*

Eggs

Eggs are the perfect protein and we recommend them, especially **free range, organic eggs** (available in health food stores). In the New York area, these high-quality eggs are in supermarkets. The chickens that lay these eggs have not been injected with antibiotics or hormones and have not been fed chemicals. Always check the date on the box to ensure that the eggs are fresh.

You know that I don't have to tell you how to cook eggs. You have been cooking them for years. But I'd like to share some hints that have helped me. With any luck they may make your egg dishes even better than your usual great!

Separating An Egg:

Egg white will not beat stiff if one drop of yolk gets mixed with the white when you separate the eggs. You can remove a small drop of yolk from white by using the cracked egg shell. Just dip it into the white and remove the yolk.

Beating Egg Whites:

To get the most volume from egg whites, bring them to room temperature before beating. They may be beaten with a wire whisk in a large metal bowl, a rotary beater, or an electric mixer. The electric mixer is most practical. Since egg whites lose volume quickly, beat them just before you need them.

Adding a pinch of cream of tartar to the unbeaten whites will help them sustain stiffness.

When adding beaten whites to a recipe, fold them in with a rubber spatula being careful not to break them down.

Using Egg Yolks as Thickeners:

This book uses egg yolks to thicken sauces, ice creams, and soufflés. Two egg yolks are equal to 1 tablespoon of flour or thickener. Beat eggs in a separate bowl and add ¼ cup of sauce to be thickened to the bowl. Beat together well. When eggs are blended with sauce, add egg mixture to sauce—stirring constantly over a low flame until sauce thickens. Do not boil sauce or egg yolk will scramble and sauce will become lumpy.

Soft-Boiled Eggs

1 serving

2 large eggs at room temperature
cold water to cover

Purchase a device called an "egg pricker" and put a small hole in the large end of the egg. This keeps eggs from cracking during cooking. Place eggs in water and bring to a boil. Boil for 3 minutes for loose eggs, 4 minutes for runny yolks and firmed whites, and 5 minutes for firmed yolks and whites. Run under cold water to stop cooking. Crack open tops and serve in egg cups.

GRAMS PER SERVING 1.2

Hard-Boiled Eggs

1 serving

2 large eggs at room temperature
cold water to cover
Prick broad side of the egg. Place eggs in water. Bring water to a boil. Cover egg pan and turn off heat. Allow eggs to remain in water for 20 minutes. Refrigerate to cool.

GRAMS PER SERVING 1.2

How to Tell if an Egg Is Hard Boiled:
    Hard-boiled eggs will spin in their shells. Eggs that have not been cooked will not spin.

Scrambled Eggs

1 serving

2 eggs
1 tablespoon heavy cream
1 tablespoon sweet butter
salt and pepper to taste

Break eggs into a small bowl. Add cream and beat well with a wire whisk. Melt butter in a nonstick skillet, then add eggs. Cook on a low heat until eggs set. Season with salt and pepper (you may add other seasonings). When eggs set, "scramble" them with a fork. Slide out of skillet and enjoy.
Variation: Sprinkle grated cheese over set eggs before scrambling.

GRAMS PER SERVING 1.6

Sunny-Side-Up and Over Easy

1 serving

2 eggs
1 tablespoon sweet butter
salt and pepper to taste

Melt butter in nonstick skillet. Break eggs, one at a time, into a flat saucer and slide them into the pan. Cook on a low heat until whites become solidly white and center is runny. If Sunny-Side-Up is your preference, remove from pan to plate after about 2½ minutes. For Over Easy use a spatula and carefully flip eggs over. Cook for 30 seconds more. Salt and pepper to taste.

GRAMS PER SERVING 1.2

Poached Eggs

1 serving

2 eggs at room temperature
salt and pepper to taste

Fill a skillet or saucepan halfway with water and heat to a simmer. Break eggs one at a time into a flat saucer. Slide into the simmering water, one at a time. Allow to simmer for 3 minutes until whites are no longer transparent. Remove from water with a slotted spoon. Place on a plate, season with salt and pepper and enjoy.

GRAMS PER SERVING 1.2

Cheese-Baked Eggs

1 serving

2 eggs at room temperature
2 tablespoons grated Parmesan cheese
2 teaspoons sweet butter
2 tablespoons heavy cream
salt and pepper to taste

Preheat oven to 375° F.

Fill a baking dish halfway with boiling water. Place 1 teaspoon butter each in the bottom of 2 custard cups. Carefully break an egg into each cup. Place 1 tablespoon of cream over each egg. Top with remaining cheese. Place custard cups in water bath in baking pan and set in the oven. Bake for 10 minutes. Salt and pepper to taste.

GRAMS PER SERVING 2.4

Basic Omelet

2 servings

2 tablespoons butter
4 eggs
1 tablespoon heavy cream
½ teaspoon seasoned salt
freshly cracked pepper to taste

Melt butter in a nonstick skillet or omelet pan. Tilt pan to cover well with butter.

Beat eggs with cream, salt, and pepper. Pour into pan and tilt pan to spread eggs to edges of pan.

Cook over a low flame until eggs begin to set. Loosen eggs from sides of pan with a spatula. Tilt pan again to allow uncooked eggs to run to the sides. Carefully fold outer edges of omelet into the center to resemble a flat cone. Slide omelet out of pan and serve.

When filling omelet, spoon mixture onto center of omelet before folding edges into the center.

TOTAL GRAMS 2.8
GRAMS PER SERVING 1.4

Bacon and Onion Omelet

2 servings

9 strips bacon
¼ cup diced onion
1 Basic Omelet recipe

Cut bacon into small pieces. Fry in small skillet until crisp. Add onion and sauté until translucent. Pour off fat. Follow recipe for *Basic Omelet,* above.

Place bacon and onion in center of omelet before folding over. Fold over and cook 1 minute. Serve immediately.

TOTAL GRAMS 6.0
GRAMS PER SERVING 3.0

Cheese-Tease Omelet

4 servings

8 eggs
½ cup creamed cottage cheese
½ cup cream cheese, softened
pinch salt
2 packets sugar substitute
1 teaspoon vanilla
½ teaspoon cinnamon
¼ cup heavy cream
3 tablespoons butter
2 tablespoons sour cream (optional)

Combine all ingredients except butter and sour cream in a bowl and beat with a wire whisk or mixer until smooth.

Melt butter in a large nonstick omelet pan. Follow recipe for *Basic Omelet.*

Slide out of pan and serve plain or garnished with sour cream.

Total Grams 19.8
Grams per Serving 5.0

Peaches and Cream Omelet

4 servings

1 8-ounce package cream cheese, softened
8 eggs
pinch salt
¼ cup heavy cream
1 packet Equal
2 tablespoons butter
⅓ cup Stewed Peaches (p. 214), chopped

Combine all ingredients except butter and chopped peaches in a bowl and beat until smooth.

Cook according to directions for *Basic Omelet* (p. 49).

When center is firm, spoon peaches onto the center, fold over sides. Slide out of pan and serve.

TOTAL GRAMS 18.7
GRAMS PER SERVING 4.7

Eggplant and Cheddar Omelet

4 servings

1 cup eggplant, peeled and cubed
4 tablespoons virgin olive oil
1 clove garlic, chopped (or ¼ teaspoon garlic powder)
½ cup tomato sauce
8 eggs, beaten
½ teaspoon seasoned salt
½ cup cheddar cheese, grated

Soak the eggplant in a bowl of cold water for ½ hour. Dry eggplant well.

Place 3 tablespoons of olive oil into skillet. Add eggplant and garlic or garlic powder. Sauté until eggplant begins to brown. Add tomato sauce and heat through. Set aside.

Heat remaining 1 tablespoon oil in large skillet. Add eggs, salt and cheese. Continue to cook over low heat until they set.

Spoon eggplant mixture onto center of omelet, fold over sides.

TOTAL GRAMS 19.4
GRAMS PER SERVING 4.8

Herb Omelet

2 servings

4 eggs
1 tablespoon chopped chives
1 tablespoon minced dill
2 tablespoons mascarpone cheese
2 tablespoons butter
seasoned salt to taste

Combine all ingredients; beat until smooth and thoroughly combined. Cook according to directions for *Basic Omelet.*

TOTAL GRAMS 4.1
GRAMS PER SERVING 2.0

Eggs Florentine

6 servings

2 cups fresh spinach (or 1 10-ounce package frozen spinach)
6 eggs
seasoned salt to taste
1 recipe Cheese Sauce *(p. 183)*

Preheat oven to 350° F.

Cook spinach in a medium saucepan over low heat. Drain well. Chop fine.

Place hot spinach in shallow baking dish.

Make a depression for each egg in spinach. Break one egg into each depression. Salt to taste.

Prepare cheese sauce. Pour over eggs and spinach. Bake for 25 minutes.

TOTAL GRAMS 29.7
GRAMS PER SERVING 5.0

Salmon Soufflé

6 servings

2 tablespoons butter
3 tablespoons soy flour
1 teaspoon seasoned salt
1 cup heavy cream, heated
1 cup salmon, poached or canned, boned and drained
seasoned salt and cayenne pepper to taste
3 eggs, separated
1⅓ tablespoons lemon juice

Preheat oven to 400° F.

Prepare soufflé dish by greasing bottom and sides with 1 tablespoon of butter. Place in refrigerator until ready to use.

Melt remaining butter over low heat and stir in flour and salt. Whisk vigorously for 1 full minute to avoid floury taste. Add heated cream and continue cooking, whisking constantly until thickened. Remove from heat and cool.

Add salmon, salt, and cayenne. Beat egg yolks, and blend them into the sauce mixture.

Fold in stiffened beaten egg whites and lemon juice. Pour mixture into soufflé dish.

Set in a pan filled with 3 inches of hot water, and bake about 35 minutes until firm and puffed. Serve immediately.

TOTAL GRAMS 14.9
GRAMS PER SERVING 2.5

Spicy Sausage Bake

4 servings

½ pound spicy sausage, cut in bite-size pieces
1 clove garlic, minced
¼ cup olive oil
1 teaspoon seasoned salt
1 teaspoon caraway seeds
1 tablespoon tomato paste
2 drops Tabasco sauce, or to taste
6 eggs, beaten
1 tablespoon grated Parmesan cheese

Preheat oven to 325° F.

Sauté sausage and garlic in olive oil until sausage is well browned. Drain off fat. Add salt, caraway seeds, tomato paste, and Tabasco sauce. Stir well. Cool. Combine eggs and Parmesan cheese. Spoon meat mixture into baking dish and cover with eggs. Bake for 45 minutes or until set.

TOTAL GRAMS 11.4
GRAMS PER SERVING 2.9

Luncheon Omelet

4 servings

2 tablespoons olive oil
6 shiitake mushrooms, thinly sliced
4 scallions, minced
12 snap peas, trimmed
2 slices sun-dried tomatoes, diced
6 eggs
2 tablespoons heavy cream
1 tablespoon fresh dill, minced (½ tablespoon dried)
2 tablespoons sweet butter
2 ounces herbed goat cheese
salt and pepper to taste

Heat olive oil in a skillet over medium heat. Sauté mushrooms and scallions for 2 minutes. Add snap peas and sun-dried tomatoes. Cook for 3 minutes (snap peas will remain crunchy).

Whisk eggs with cream and dill; pour carefully over vegetables. Dot center of omelet with goat cheese and butter. Fold over sides. Season with salt and pepper.

TOTAL GRAMS 34.6
GRAMS PER SERVING 8.7

Two-Cheese Omelet

2 servings

2 tablespoons sweet butter
2 tablespoons onion, minced
4 eggs
2 tablespoons heavy cream
½ cup each of two cheeses, grated
1 tablespoon chopped parsley

This omelet is delicious when you choose one hard and one soft cheese such as cream cheese and Cheddar or Camembert and Parmesan. Use the soft cheese to mix with the egg mixture and the hard cheese in the center of the omelet.

Heat butter in a nonstick skillet over medium heat. Add onion and cook until transparent. Beat eggs with heavy cream and soft cheese. Pour into pan. Spread egg mixture by tilting pan. Cook until eggs set. Sprinkle grated hard cheese in pan. Cook 1 minute. Slice egg pancake in two. Fold each semicircle in half. Flip over to melt cheese and brown both sides. Serve hot and crisp. Garnish with parsley.

TOTAL GRAMS 7.2
GRAMS PER SERVING 3.6

Crabmeat and Mushroom Omelet

6 servings

2 tablespoons butter
6 shiitake mushrooms, thinly sliced
2 tablespoons white onions, chopped
½ cup lump crabmeat
1 tablespoon sherry
6 eggs
3 tablespoons heavy cream

Melt butter in nonstick skillet. Add mushrooms and onion and sauté until light brown. Stir in crabmeat.

Simmer for 3 minutes. Add sherry and simmer 1 minute more. Reserve one half crab mixture.

Beat eggs and cream together. Pour carefully over crab mixture in pan. Cook until set.

Place remaining mixture over top of omelet after it has been folded.

TOTAL GRAMS 21.8
GRAMS PER SERVING 3.6

Ham and Artichoke Omelet

4 servings

1 6-ounce jar marinated artichoke hearts, drained
2 tablespoons grated Parmesan cheese
8 eggs
3 tablespoons mascarpone cheese
seasoned salt and pepper to taste
¼ pound ham, thinly sliced

Use a large nonstick omelet pan.

Place artichoke hearts on paper towel and pat oil off. Roll hearts in Parmesan cheese; set aside. Beat eggs, mascarpone cheese, and salt and pepper together in a bowl until smooth. Follow the *Basic Omelet* instructions for cooking on page 49. When egg mixture is set, cover surface with ham slices. Place artichoke hearts into center and fold sides over. Slice in four pieces before removing from pan, and serve.

TOTAL GRAMS 18.7
GRAMS PER SERVING 9.4

Shrimp and Goat Cheese Omelet

2 servings

8 raw shrimp, shelled, cleaned, and butterflied
4 tablespoons garlic oil
2 tablespoons sweet butter
4 eggs
2 ounces herbed goat cheese, crumbled
4 sun-dried tomato halves softened in olive oil, minced

Use a 9-inch nonstick skillet or omelet pan.

Butterfly shrimp by cutting ³/₄ of the way through—along the back vein. Open shrimp to resemble a butterfly.

Sear the shrimp in hot garlic oil (about 2 minutes on each side). Remove to paper toweling. Wipe oil from pan with paper towel.

Add butter to pan. Beat eggs with goat cheese and follow the *Basic Omelet* instructions for cooking on page 49.

When eggs are set, place shrimp and sun-dried tomatoes on egg pancake and fold over.

TOTAL GRAMS 15.4
GRAMS PER SERVING 7.7

Appetizers

Marbleized Tea Eggs From China

12 egg halves

6 eggs
2 tablespoons soy sauce
2 tablespoons salt
3 tablespoons black tea
1 tablespoon anise extract

Cover eggs with cold water and bring to a boil. Reduce heat and simmer 10 minutes.

Remove eggs, cool, and crack the shells in several places, but do not peel.

Bring 4 cups of water to a boil. Add remaining ingredients and eggs. Simmer for one hour. Cool.

Place eggs, still in the water in the refrigerator. Leave overnight.

To serve, shell eggs and cut in half. They are very attractive on the hors d'oeuvres tray.

TOTAL GRAMS 5.2
GRAMS PER SERVING 0.4

Deviled-Salmon Eggs

12 egg halves

6 eggs
3 tablespoons mayonnaise
½ cup boned and flaked salmon, canned or smoked
½ teaspoon lemon juice
1 teaspoon prepared mustard
1 teaspoon Worcestershire sauce
½ teaspoon salt
dash of pepper

Cover eggs with cold water and bring to a boil. Reduce heat and simmer gently for 15 minutes, turning often to help keep yolks in center. Run eggs under cold water and remove shells. Slice eggs in half lengthwise. Remove yolks.

Mash yolks and mayonnaise together until smooth. Add remaining ingredients and mix well.

Spoon mixture into egg whites.

Garnish with additional pieces of salmon if desired. Refrigerate for at least ½ hour before serving.

TOTAL GRAMS 5.7
GRAMS PER SERVING 0.5

Swedish Meatballs

8 meatballs

¼ cup heavy cream
¼ cup water
¼ cup fried sugar-free pork rinds, crushed
¼ pound beef, ground
¼ pound pork, ground
¼ pound veal, ground
1 large onion, chopped fine
3 tablespoons butter
2 teaspoons seasoned salt
1 recipe Cream Sauce *(page 177)*
½ teaspoon nutmeg
1 teaspoon caraway seeds

Mix heavy cream and water together in a small bowl. Add crushed pork rinds and allow to soak until softened, about 10 minutes. Combine beef, pork, and veal.

Mix cream mixture, meats, and onion together. Add seasoned salt. Shape into small balls, and brown in butter in a medium skillet over medium heat.

Remove balls to chafing dish and keep warm.

Make *Cream Sauce* and pour over meatballs. Garnish with nutmeg and caraway seeds.

TOTAL GRAMS 7.0
GRAMS PER SERVING 0.9

Turkey Meatballs

8 meatballs

2 tablespoons butter
1 small onion, minced
1 medium stalk of celery, minced
1 clove garlic, minced
½ pound turkey, ground

1 teaspoon seasoned salt
¼ teaspoon grated Parmesan cheese
½ teaspoon thyme
1 egg
¼ teaspoon curry powder

Heat butter in a medium skillet. Sauté onion, celery, and garlic until golden brown.

Place turkey in a bowl, add onion mixture and remaining ingredients. Mix well with a fork. Shape into 1-inch balls and sauté until well-browned.

TOTAL GRAMS 10.4
GRAMS PER SERVING 1.3

Salami and Parmesan

8 cubes

½ pound salami, cut into eight cubes
2 eggs, beaten
8 tablespoons grated Parmesan cheese
walnut oil for frying

Dip salami cubes into beaten eggs. Roll in Parmesan cheese until coated.

Repeat.

Deep fry in hot oil for 30 seconds, until lightly browned.

TOTAL GRAMS 7.0
GRAMS PER SERVING 0.9

Heavenly Wings

Hors d'oeuvres for 6

1½ pounds chicken wings, about twelve
1 cup Tamari soy sauce
4 packets sugar substitute
¼ cup white wine
2 cloves garlic, mashed
¼ cup sesame oil
½ teaspoon ground ginger

Wash wings and pat dry. Cut into pieces at joints. Discard wing tips. Combine remaining ingredients.

Spread wings in shallow baking dish. Do not overlap. Pour sauce over wings. Marinate overnight in refrigerator. Preheat oven to 325° F. Bake in marinade for 1½ hours.

TOTAL GRAMS 19.9
GRAMS PER SERVING 3.3

Sardine Snack

3 snacks

1 3-ounce can skinless and boneless sardines, drained
½ teaspoon dried parsley
¼ teaspoon dried dill weed
3 hard-boiled eggs, mashed
¼ teaspoon salt
6 ounces cream cheese, softened
2 tablespoons chopped onion
¾ teaspoon lemon juice

Combine all ingredients in a blender or food processor. Blend until smooth. Serve, well chilled, on bed of lettuce leaves.

TOTAL GRAMS 7.1
GRAMS PER SERVING 2.4

Sour Cream Clam Dip

8 servings

1 cup sour cream
1 7-ounce can minced clams, drained, reserving 1 tablespoon juice
1 tablespoon grated onion
1 teaspoon celery seed
¼ cup mayonnaise
1 tablespoon lemon juice
seasoned salt and pepper to taste
1 tablespoon Worcestershire sauce

Mix all ingredients together well. Refrigerate for at least 1 hour. Serve with fried pork rinds.

TOTAL GRAMS 30.2
GRAMS PER SERVING 3.8

Guacamole

8 ¼-cup servings

1 avocado, peeled and chopped
½ cup onion, chopped
1 tomato, chopped
½ cucumber, peeled and chopped
½ teaspoon paprika
½ teaspoon seasoned salt
1 jalapeño pepper, minced
⅛ teaspoon hot chili pepper, dried
1 tablespoon sour cream
1 tablespoon chopped parsley

Place avocado, onion, tomato, and cucumber in the work bowl of a food processor and process 10 seconds. Season with paprika, salt, and peppers. Add sour cream and parsley. Process 5 seconds. Refrigerate. Use as dip with sliced cucumbers.

TOTAL GRAMS 34.6
GRAMS PER SERVING 4.3

Fran's Special Pâté

20 slices

4 slices no-nitrate bacon
1 pound chicken livers
½ chicken breast, skinless and boned, pounded flat
4 teaspoons seasoned salt
3 tablespoons bacon fat
2 tablespoons butter
2 tablespoons white wine
½ 8-ounce can water chestnuts, drained
2 hard-boiled eggs
1 Boursin cheese, about 3 ounces
3 tablespoons sweet basil
freshly ground black pepper

Preheat oven to 275° F.

Cook bacon until crisp. Reserve fat.

Place 2 tablespoons of bacon fat in frying pan. Sauté chicken livers about 5 minutes over medium heat. Remove from pan and set aside.

Add butter to pan and melt over medium heat; add chicken breast and sauté in butter for 3 minutes on each side. Add wine and simmer for 3 minutes.

Place cooked bacon, chicken livers, chicken breast, water chestnuts, and eggs into a large wooden chopping bowl or food processor and chop fine.

Add seasoned salt, reserved bacon fat, Boursin cheese, basil, and pepper. Mix well. Pack into a large buttered loaf pan. Place a heavy weight on top to keep pâté from rising.

Bake for 2 hours. Turn oven off and allow pâté to remain undisturbed until oven is cold. Remove from oven and refrigerate. Unmold and cut into slices.

TOTAL GRAMS 29.6
GRAMS PER SERVING 1.5

Cheesy Ham Snack

6 servings

1 tablespoon mayonnaise
1 tablespoon grated Parmesan cheese
6 slices Black Forest ham
1 small tomato, sliced thin
6 thin slices Swiss cheese

Mix mayonnaise with Parmesan cheese.

Spread mixture on slice of ham, top with tomato slices. Roll up. Place ham roll on a thin slice of Swiss cheese and roll again. Fasten with toothpick.

TOTAL GRAMS 9.4
GRAMS PER SERVING 1.6

Caribbean Crabmeat

30 canapés

2 tablespoons butter
2 tablespoons onion
1 clove garlic, minced
½ cup grated coconut, unsweetened
2 cups lump crabmeat, fresh or canned
1 egg
2 tablespoons cream
2 teaspoons curry powder
1 teaspoon salt
½ cup fried sugar-free pork rinds, crushed
½ cup oil

Melt 2 tablespoons butter in medium skillet over medium heat. Sauté onion and garlic until transparent.

Add coconut to skillet and sauté until light brown. Remove from heat and cool.

In a separate bowl, combine crabmeat, egg, cream, curry powder, and salt. Add onion and garlic mixture and coconut. Mix well.

Shape into 1-inch balls. Roll in pork rinds. Heat oil in skillet. Brown crabmeat balls in hot oil. Drain thoroughly on absorbent paper. Serve on toothpicks.

TOTAL GRAMS 20.3
GRAMS PER SERVING 0.7

Klara's Eggplant Appetizer

6 servings

1 medium eggplant
1 medium onion, sliced
1 tablespoon extra-virgin olive oil
1 teaspoon balsamic vinegar
¼ teaspoon seasoned salt
pepper to taste

Preheat oven to 350° F. Bake eggplant for 1 hour until soft. Cool and peel. Mash eggplant until smooth and combine with remaining ingredients.

TOTAL GRAMS 38.3
GRAMS PER SERVING 7.0

Toasted Nuts

½ cup toasted nuts

1 teaspoon butter
½ cup nuts of your choice

Melt butter in non-stick pan. Stir in nuts and sauté until lightly browned.
Place on paper toweling to absorb excess oil
If you like them salty, use seasoned salt to taste.
If you like them sweet, use a sugar substitute to taste.
If you like them spicy, use chili powder to taste.

TOTAL GRAMS FOR TOASTED ALMONDS 5.8
TOTAL GRAMS FOR TOASTED WALNUTS 10.4
TOTAL GRAMS FOR TOASTED PECANS 5.2
TOTAL GRAMS FOR TOASTED PINE NUTS 8.0

Soups

These four stocks are important to many of the recipes in this book. They freeze easily and safely. I freeze them in small containers (no more than two cups) so they can be defrosted quickly. Once you've tried these stocks, their value will be apparent. Every recipe will taste much more zesty and flavorful as a result of using them.

Chicken Stock

10 1-cup servings

1 4–5 pound chicken, cleaned and washed
3 quarts cold water
1 teaspoon seasoned salt
2 stalks celery , chopped
1 tablespoon parsley, chopped
1 small onion, chopped
1 parsnip, diced
1 bay leaf
½ teaspoon dried thyme
1 Knorr chicken bouillon cube

Place cleaned chicken in cold water in a large saucepan. Bring to a boil over medium heat. Skim foam that form on top of water, as the chicken cooks.

Add remaining ingredients, cover and simmer chicken until it is tender (about 1½ hours).

Cool. Remove chicken and strain stock. Chill the stock in a covered container in refrigerator.

Remove layer of fat that will rise to the top when thoroughly chilled.

Heat stock for soup and sauces. Or use it cold to make an aspic or jellied soup.

The chicken and vegetables may be returned to stock for a chicken soup meal or use chicken to make *Chicken Salad,* pages 84–85.

TOTAL GRAMS 19.8
GRAMS PER SERVING 2.0

Cream of Chicken Soup

1 serving

1 cup Chicken Stock *(page 68)*
2 tablespoons heavy cream
1 egg yolk (for thickening)
Whisk cream and yolk into hot stock. Simmer 1 minute. Do not boil!

TOTAL GRAMS 3.3

Vegetable Stock

8 1-cup servings

2 tablespoons butter
2 sprigs fresh parsley (or 1 teaspoon dried parsley flakes)
1 large onion, sliced
1 large carrot, sliced
3 stalks celery, sliced
2 quarts water
6 whole peppercorns
2 whole cloves
1 bay leaf
2 tablespoons wine vinegar (optional)

Melt butter in deep saucepan over medium flame. Add vegetables and sauté for 5 minutes. Add water and seasonings, cover tightly, and simmer for 30 minutes.

Strain and use as directed in recipes.

TOTAL GRAMS 20.1
GRAMS PER SERVING 2.5

Beef Stock

10 1-cup servings

2 pounds beef stew meat
1 teaspoon salt
3 quarts cold water
¼ teaspoon pepper
½ cup onion, diced
½ cup carrot, diced
½ cup celery, diced
½ cup tomato, diced
1 teaspoon parsley, chopped
1 tablespoon green pepper, chopped

Place meat and salt in cold water, and bring to a boil over low heat. Skim bubbles off the top. Cover and simmer for 2½ hours.

Add the vegetables, seasonings, and pepper and cook slowly for an additional 1½ hours.

Remove meat and serve with horseradish or mustard sauce. Strain stock and use as directed in recipes.

TOTAL GRAMS 15.3
GRAMS PER SERVING 1.5

Fish Stock

8 1-cup servings

2 pounds fish
2 quarts water
2 cloves
½ teaspoon mace
3 stalks celery, with tops, diced
1 sprig parsley, chopped
1 bay leaf
5 peppercorns
1 tablespoon salt

Place all ingredients in deep saucepan. Cover tightly and bring to a boil. Lower flame and simmer gently for 45 minutes. Strain, cool, and store in refrigerator. Use as directed in recipes.

TOTAL GRAMS 5.4
GRAMS PER SERVING 0.7

Dumpling Soup

4 servings

1 tablespoon soft butter
1 egg plus 1 yolk
½ cup heavy cream
pinch of nutmeg
4 cups Chicken Stock *(page 68)*

Grease bottom and sides of the top of a double boiler with butter.

Beat egg, egg yolk, heavy cream, salt, and nutmeg together with fork. Pour into top of double boiler.

Cook over hot (not boiling) water for 45 minutes, or until set and firm. Turn out onto waxed paper and cool. Slice into cubes. Add to clear hot stock. Serve immediately.

TOTAL GRAMS 13.3
GRAMS PER SERVING 3.3

Cream of Shiitake Mushroom Soup

10 servings

½ pound shiitake mushrooms, sliced thin
½ medium onion, minced
¼ pound butter
1 quart Chicken Stock *(page 68)*
1 quart Beef Stock *(page 70)*
2 tablespoons toasted sesame seeds
½ teaspoon seasoned salt
1 cup heavy cream
1 tablespoon chives, minced

Sauté mushrooms and onions in half the butter for 5 minutes over medium heat. Mix the stocks; add mushrooms and onions.

Add crushed sesame seeds and remaining butter; heat stirring until butter melts.

Add salt. Cook over low heat for 10 minutes. Cool slightly. Stir in heavy cream until well blended. Do not allow to boil.

Serve warm or cold, garnished with chives.

TOTAL GRAMS 44.6
GRAMS PER SERVING 4.5

Creamy Ricotta Soup

6 servings

1 onion, chopped fine
1 stalk celery, chopped
2 green peppers, chopped
3 tablespoons butter
3 cups Vegetable Stock *(page 69)*
1½ teaspoon seasoned salt
½ teaspoon paprika
2 cups ricotta cheese, sieved
4 sprigs parsley, minced
3 strips bacon, fried crisp and crumbled

Sauté onion, celery, and peppers in butter in a deep saucepan. Add vegetable stock, seasoned salt, and paprika.

Cover and simmer gently for 1 hour over low heat.

Add ricotta cheese and blend well. If greater smoothness is desired, put mixture in blender; blend at medium speed until smooth.

Garnish with minced parsley and bacon pieces. Serve hot.

TOTAL GRAMS 40.2
GRAMS PER SERVING 6.7

Gazpacho

6 servings

¼ teaspoon garlic powder
1 onion, chopped
4 sprigs parsley, chopped
2 tablespoons wine vinegar
3 tablespoons olive oil
¼ teaspoon cayenne pepper
¼ teaspoon seasoned salt
1½ cups Chicken Stock *(page 68)*
4 large tomatoes, peeled and chopped
½ cucumber, peeled, seeded, and diced
2 tablespoons sugar-free fried pork rinds, crushed

Place all ingredients in blender or food processor. Blend until smooth. Chill overnight. Serve in chilled bowls. Garnish each with additional cucumber, pepper, and crushed pork rinds, as desired.

TOTAL GRAMS 43.2
GRAMS PER SERVING 7.2

Cold Avocado Soup

6 servings

1½ cups avocado, peeled and diced
3 tablespoons lime juice
½ teaspoon salt
dash pepper
dash nutmeg
3 cups Chicken Stock *(page 68)*
¼ cup heavy cream, whipped

Place avocado, lime juice, salt, pepper, and nutmeg in a blender. Add ½ cup *Chicken Stock*. Blend 30 seconds at high speed. Pour into bowl.
 Whisk in remaining broth and chill until icy cold.
 Serve garnished with a spoonful of whipped cream and a sprinkle of nutmeg.

TOTAL GRAMS 31.3
GRAMS PER SERVING 5.2

Japanese Egg Custard Soup

6 servings

1 cup julienne-cut cooked chicken or diced raw, peeled shrimp
3 water chestnuts, diced
6 mushrooms, diced
2 scallions, chopped
1 tablespoon sherry
4 eggs, beaten
1 teaspoon salt
3 cups Beef Stock *(page 70)*
12 spinach or lettuce leaves

Preheat oven to 300° F.
 Combine chicken or shrimp, water chestnuts, mushrooms, scallions, and sherry.
 Divide mixture evenly among 6 custard cups.

Beat eggs, salt, and stock together. Pour into custard cups. Cover with spinach or lettuce leaves.

Place in large pan with 3 inches boiling water. Cover pan and bake for 30 minutes or until mixture is set.

TOTAL GRAMS 16.5
GRAMS PER SERVING 2.8

New England Fish Chowder

6 servings

2 pounds cod fillets
4 slices bacon, diced
1 small onion, diced
2 tablespoons parsley, chopped
2 cups Fish Stock *(page 71)*
1 bay leaf
1 teaspoon seasoned salt
pepper to taste
2 cups heavy cream

Cut fish fillets into 1-inch cubes. Place bacon in deep saucepan over low heat and sauté until golden brown. Add onions and sauté until transparent. Add parsley and cook 1 minute more.

Add stock, bay leaf, salt, and pepper. Cover and cook for a few minutes to combine flavors. Add fish, and simmer for 10 minutes. Add cream and heat just until heated through. Do not boil. Serve immediately.

TOTAL GRAMS 20.4
GRAMS PER SERVING 3.4

New England Clam Chowder

6 servings

Wash 3 dozen clams thoroughly. Steam in covered pot in 4–6 inches of boiling water until shells open (no longer than 5 minutes). Strain clam stock and use as part of water in recipe. Chop clams coarsely and substitute for cod fillets in *New England Fish Chowder,* page 75.

TOTAL GRAMS 33.6
GRAMS PER SERVING 5.6

Baked Scallop and Fish Soup

4 servings

1 ounce sweet butter
1 large fish fillet, any variety
2 cloves garlic, minced
3 small ripe tomatoes, peeled and chopped
½ medium onion, chopped
10 shiitake mushrooms or any mushrooms, sliced thin
½ cup pine nuts
1 pound sea scallops
¼ cup white wine
1 tablespoon fresh dill, minced (or 2 teaspoons dried dill)

Preheat oven to 350° F.

Melt butter on bottom of a deep-sided baking dish.

Place fish in dish and top with garlic. Add tomato, onion, mushrooms, nuts, and scallops. Sprinkle with wine. Cover and bake for 20 minutes. Remove cover and cook 10 minutes more. Place in soup bowls. Garnish with dill.

TOTAL GRAMS 58.0
GRAMS PER SERVING 14.5

Cauliflower Soup with Dill and Caraway

6 servings

2 tablespoons sweet butter
3 leeks (white part only), chopped
1/2 medium cauliflower, chopped
3 cups Chicken Stock (page 68)
1 chicken bouillon cube
1 cup heavy cream
2 tablespoons dill, minced
2 tablespoons caraway seeds
seasoned salt to taste
6 tablespoons mascarpone cheese
6 tablespoons grated Parmesan cheese

Melt butter in a medium-sized saucepan. Add leek and cauliflower and sauté for 3 minutes. Stir in *Chicken Stock* and bouillon cube. Cook over medium heat for 1/2 hour. Remove from heat. Cool. Place in food processor and blend. Add cream and blend 10 seconds more. Return to pan. Stir in fresh dill and caraway seeds. Warm to desired heat. Place in individual bowls. Top each with 1 tablespoon mascarpone and 1 tablespoon Parmesan. Serve hot.

TOTAL GRAMS 66.9
GRAMS PER SERVING 11.2

Salads

Chicken Salad Ham Rolls

4 servings

1 cup cooked chicken, diced
¼ cup mayonnaise
¼ cup chopped parsley
¼ cup chopped celery leaves
1 teaspoon seasoned salt
6 black olives, diced
4 tablespoons minced fresh green pepper
8 slices boiled ham
lettuce leaves

Combine all ingredients except ham and lettuce. Spread mixture on ham slices and roll each one up, insert toothpick and place them seam side down on bed of lettuce leaves.

TOTAL GRAMS 6.8
GRAMS PER SERVING 1.7

Fresh Tuna and Avocado Salad

6 servings

1 large avocado, pitted, peeled, and cubed
2 stalks celery, chopped
6 radishes, sliced
2 tablespoons lemon juice
2 tablespoons tarragon vinegar
½ small onion, chopped
¼ teaspoon cayenne pepper
seasoned salt to taste
1½ pounds fresh tuna fish, grilled

Toss all ingredients together well, except fish. Divide into 6 portions.
Cut fish in strips and place across top of each serving.
Serve with *Dill Vinaigrette* (page 97).

TOTAL GRAMS 29.7
GRAMS PER SERVING 5.0

Cole Slaw

6 ½-cup servings

¼ cup Dijon mustard
¼ cup mayonnaise
½ packet sugar substitute
1 tablespoon lemon juice
½ teaspoon salt
1 medium cabbage, shredded (3 cups)

Mix mustard, mayonnaise, sugar substitute, lemon juice, and salt
together. Add cabbage and toss well.

TOTAL GRAMS 41.4
GRAMS PER SERVING 6.9

(A Mold of) Roquefort Spread

12 servings

1 envelope unflavored gelatin
¼ cup cold water
6 ounces Roquefort cheese
6 ounces cream cheese, softened
½ cup heavy cream
4 scallions, minced
2 tablespoons pine nuts
4 black olives, chopped
seasoned salt to taste

Sprinkle gelatin over water.

Push Roquefort cheese through strainer. Add cream cheese and heavy cream to Roquefort cheese. Mix well. Add gelatin, scallions, pine nuts, olives, and salt to cheese mixture. Mix well.

Pour into 3-cup ring mold that has been sprayed with oil substitute. Chill until set.

TOTAL GRAMS 25.9
GRAMS PER SERVING 2.2

Mock Potato Salad

8 ½-cup servings

1 medium rutabaga
½ packet sugar substitute
1 tablespoon lemon juice
½ cup finely chopped scallions
1 medium dill pickle, chopped
1 cup minced celery with leaves
1½ teaspoon salt
dash of paprika
¾ cup mayonnaise
4 hard-boiled eggs, chopped

Pare rutabaga, and cut into 4 pieces. Drop into boiling water and boil until tender (about ½ hour). Drain well. Cool.

After rutabaga has cooled, dice (should be approximately 2½ cups), and place in salad bowl. Sprinkle with sugar substitute and lemon juice. Add scallions, pickle, celery, salt, paprika, and mayonnaise.

Toss well. Fold in eggs. Chill before serving.

TOTAL GRAMS 48.0
GRAMS PER SERVING 6.0

Tossed Salad with Tomato Dressing

12 servings

2 heads lettuce (any variety)
2 tomatoes, peeled and seeded
6 scallions, minced
1 tablespoon dry mustard
½ teaspoon garlic powder
1 tablespoon Dijon mustard
1 teaspoon seasoned salt
2 tablespoons olive oil
2 tablespoons tarragon vinegar
4 tablespoons vegetable oil
1 tablespoon mayonnaise

Wash lettuce, dry thoroughly, and tear into bite-size pieces.
Refrigerate.

Tomato Dressing
Chop tomatoes and mash with scallions until almost a paste. Add remaining ingredients except lettuce. Beat with wire whisk. Refrigerate.

When ready to serve, place lettuce in large salad bowl, pour dressing on top, and toss well. Serve immediately.

TOTAL GRAMS 28.0
GRAMS PER SERVING 2.3

Not Just Another Tossed Salad

12 servings

2 pounds large shrimp, peeled and deveined
½ cup garlic oil
½ pound fresh spinach, washed and dried
1 small head Boston lettuce, washed and dried
½ 7¼-ounce can large black olives, pitted, drained, and sliced
½ cup diced celery
5 scallions, diced
6 radishes, sliced
½ cup diced raw cauliflower florets
1 avocado, pitted, peeled, and diced
8 slices cooked bacon, crisp and crumbled
2 soft-boiled eggs (2 minutes), peeled
½ cup lemon juice
¼ cup peanut oil
¼ cup Parmesan cheese
seasoned salt to taste

Sauté shrimp in garlic oil until they turn pink. Refrigerate while you prepare salad.

Tear spinach and lettuce leaves into bite-size pieces. Toss all vegetables and bacon together in bowl.

Make dressing by beating eggs, lemon juice, oil, cheese, and salt together.

Top salad with shrimp. Pour dressing over salad and serve.

TOTAL GRAMS 65.0
GRAMS PER SERVING 5.4

Greek Salad

6 servings

1 large tomato, cubed
½ large green pepper, seeded and cubed
½ large cucumber, pared and cubed
½ 6-ounce can ripe pitted olives, drained
3 scallions, diced
2 tablespoons capers, drained
¼ pound feta cheese, crumbled
12 thin slices pepperoni
4 tablespoons olive oil
2 tablespoons wine vinegar
¼ teaspoon cracked pepper
½ teaspoon oregano

Combine tomato, pepper, cucumber, olives, scallions, capers, cheese, and pepperoni in salad bowl. Mix olive oil, vinegar, pepper, and oregano together in small bowl. Pour dressing over vegetables. Toss and serve.

TOTAL GRAMS 28.9
GRAMS PER SERVING 4.8

Honeydew and Seafood

6 servings

1 1-pound honeydew melon
1 6½-ounce can tuna fish, drained
1 4½-ounce can shrimp, drained
1 medium cucumber, peeled and cubed
½ pound raw mushrooms, sliced
½ cup mayonnaise
2 tablespoons tomato sauce
½ teaspoon seasoned salt

Cut melon in half. Scoop out center using a melon baller or cube. Leave ¼-inch-wide rim on rinds. Cut each rind half into thirds.

In bowl combine tuna fish, shrimp (save a few for garnish), cucumber, mushrooms, and melon balls.

Combine mayonnaise, tomato sauce, and salt. Pour dressing over seafood mixture. Mix well.

Fill melon shells. Garnish with some shrimp.

If you prefer low fat, eliminate dressing, and use juice of 1 lemon.

TOTAL GRAMS 47.0
GRAMS PER SERVING 7.8

Chicken Salad

2 servings

2 cups cooked chicken meat, peeled, boned, and diced
⅓ cup marinated artichoke hearts, drained
20 black olives, pitted
3 tablespoons onion, minced
1 tablespoon sweet butter, melted
2 tablespoons crème fraîche or sour cream
1 tablespoon mayonnaise
seasoned salt to taste

Toss first 5 ingredients together. Mix crème fraîche and mayonnaise

together. Add to chicken mixture. Mix well. Season with salt.
  Refrigerate.

TOTAL GRAMS 8.4
GRAMS PER SERVING 4.2

Poached Salmon Salad

2 servings

whole leaves of 1 endive
1 small tomato, peeled and quartered
1 small ripe avocado, pitted, peeled, and diced
¼ small onion, diced (Vidalia when possible)
6 pitted black olives
2 salmon fillets, poached and cut into 1-inch strips
1 recipe Lime Dill Dressing

Wash and dry endive leaves. Chop tomato, avocado, onion, and olives together in a wooden chopping bowl. Poach salmon and allow it to come to room temperature.

  Place endive leaves in a daisy formation in a round, shallow salad bowl. Make chopped tomato mixture the center of the daisy. Place strips of salmon in each of the endive leaves. Artistically dot with *Lime Dill Dressing,* page 91.

TOTAL GRAMS 19.8
GRAMS PER SERVING 9.9

Hot Beef Salad

6 servings

1 small head Boston lettuce
1 small Chinese cabbage
1 large cucumber, sliced thin
1 red onion, peeled and sliced thin
½ small daikon radish, sliced thin
2 small tomatoes, cut in eight pieces
6 mint leaves
6 coriander leaves (cilantro)
¼ cup walnut oil
1½ pound sirloin, sliced thin
½ teaspoon seasoned salt

Dressing:
5 garlic cloves, minced
¼ cup fresh lime juice
1 packet sugar substitute
1 tablespoon Tamari soy sauce
2 teaspoons crushed red pepper flakes
¼ cup sharp Cheddar cheese, diced for garnish

Wash and dry lettuce and cabbage. Tear into bite-sized pieces. Mix onions, radishes, tomatoes, and mint and coriander leaves together and pour over lettuce. Toss.

Heat oil in a nonstick skillet over medium heat. Add meat and seasoned salt. Cook quickly, stirring frequently, just until rare.

Artfully arrange cooked meat on salad. Mix dressing ingredients together and pour over salad. Top with Cheddar cubes.

TOTAL GRAMS 51.8
GRAMS PER SERVING 8.6

Leftover Lamb or Pork Salad

2 servings

1 pound cooked leftover lamb or pork
seasoned salt to taste
pepper to taste
3 tablespoons extra-virgin olive oil
2 tablespoons fresh rosemary, minced
1 tablespoon balsamic vinegar
1 teaspoon Dijon mustard
2 heads Bibb lettuce, cored, washed, and dried
¼ cup Parmesan cheese shavings

Thinly slice lamb or pork. Whisk together salt, pepper, oil, rosemary, vinegar, and mustard.

Place greens in a salad bowl with Parmesan shavings and toss them with the dressing. Arrange meat over greens.

TOTAL GRAMS 14.9
GRAMS PER SERVING 7.5

Salad Niçoise

12 servings

2 teaspoons Dijon mustard
2 tablespoons wine vinegar
1½ teaspoons salt
2 cloves garlic, minced
6 tablespoons peanut or vegetable oil
6 tablespoons olive oil
Freshly ground black pepper
1 teaspoon chopped fresh thyme (or ½ teaspoon dried)
2 pounds green beans
2 green peppers
4 celery stalks
1 pint cherry tomatoes
3 7-ounce cans tuna, drained
1 2-ounce can flat anchovies, drained
10 stuffed green olives
10 black olives
2 small or 1 large red onion
2 tablespoons chopped fresh basil (or 1 teaspoon dried)
⅓ cup finely chopped fresh parsley
¼ cup finely chopped scallions
6 hard-boiled eggs, quartered

Combine mustard, vinegar, salt, garlic, peanut and olive oil, pepper, and thyme in a bowl. Beat with a fork until well blended. Set aside.

Pick over beans and break into 1½-inch lengths. Place beans in a saucepan and cook, in salted water to cover, until crisp-tender. Run under cold water and drain in a colander. Set aside.

Remove cores, seeds, and white membranes from green peppers. Cut peppers in thin rounds. Set aside.

Trim celery stalks and cut crosswise into thin slices. Set aside.

Use a large salad bowl and make a more or less symmetrical pattern of the green beans, peppers, celery, and tomatoes. Flake the tuna fish and add to bowl. Arrange anchovies on top and scatter olives over all.

Peel onions and cut them into thin, almost transparent slices. Scatter onion rings over all. Sprinkle with basil, parsley, and scallions.

Serve with dressing. Garnish with eggs.

TOTAL GRAMS 116.0
GRAMS PER SERVING 9.7

Crunchy Seafood Salad

10 servings

1 6½-ounce can tuna fish
1 6-ounce can crabmeat
1 5-ounce can shrimp
1 large head lettuce
1 cup diced celery
½ cup diced green onions
½ medium ripe avocado, diced
½ cup chopped walnuts
½ cup roasted unsalted soybeans
½ cup sunflower seeds
2 hard-boiled eggs, diced
1 tomato cut in wedges

Drain the 3 cans of seafood, discard bony tissue from crab. Combine with shrimp. Place in a bowl and refrigerate.

Combine remaining ingredients except tomato in a large salad bowl, and toss well.

Add seafood and toss again.

Add salad dressing of your choice.

Toss again before serving, and decorate with tomato wedges.

TOTAL GRAMS 74.8
GRAMS PER SERVING 7.5

Tricolor Salad with Three Cheeses

8 servings

1 recipe Mustard Vinaigrette *(page 91)*
1 small head of radicchio
3 endive
1 head of romaine
3 ounces Parmesan cheese shavings
5 ounces Camembert, cut into 8 wedges
4 ounces herbed goat cheese, cut into 8 wedges
¼ cup pine nuts, toasted (or substitute Toasted Nuts*)*

Preheat oven to 450° F.

Prepare vinaigrette and place in refrigerator for ½ hour. Separate leaves of lettuces. Wash and dry greens (make sure they are very dry), and tear into bite-size pieces.

Place in large salad bowl. Toss in Parmesan cheese.

Place Camembert and goat cheeses on a nonstick cookie sheet to melt in oven for 1 minute.

Place cheese wedges on salad. Top with dressing and nuts and serve.

TOTAL GRAMS 34.7
GRAMS PER SERVING 4.3

Salad Dressings

Mustard Vinaigrette

20 tablespoons

1 teaspoon Dijon mustard
¼ teaspoon dry mustard
2 tablespoons fresh dill, minced
1 tablespoon balsamic vinegar
½ teaspoon seasoned salt
1 cup extra-virgin olive oil

Beat ingredients together in a small bowl until well blended. Refrigerate for ½ hour.

TOTAL GRAMS 4.5
GRAMS PER TABLESPOON 0.2

Lime Dill Dressing (vinegar-free)

18 tablespoons

1 cup extra-virgin olive oil
1 teaspoon Dijon mustard
¼ teaspoon dry mustard
juice of 1 lime
¼ teaspoon seasoned salt
1 clove garlic, minced
1 tablespoon dill, minced
pinch sugar substitute

Beat ingredients together in a small bowl. Refrigerate for ½ hour.

TOTAL GRAMS 3.0
GRAMS PER TABLESPOON 0.2

Tomato Mayonnaise (without vinegar)

20 tablespoons

1 organic egg
1 teaspoon lemon juice
½ teaspoon seasoned salt
¼ teaspoon dried mustard
¾ cup olive oil
1 small ripe tomato, peeled and seeded
2 tablespoons fresh basil, minced

Place first 4 ingredients in a food processor and blend. Add oil in a slow steady stream until it is fully blended. Chop tomato pulp and add to food processor with the basil. Blend for 30 seconds.

TOTAL GRAMS 5.9
GRAMS PER TABLESPOON 0.3

Basic Vinegar-Free Salad Dressing

16 tablespoons

1 teaspoon seasoned salt
¼ teaspoon black pepper
1 teaspoon dry mustard
dash of Tabasco sauce
¼ cup lemon juice
⅔ cup olive oil

Beat all ingredients together. Refrigerate.

TOTAL GRAMS 7.0
GRAMS PER TABLESPOON 0.5

Vinegar-Free Mayonnaise

20 tablespoons

1 organic egg
2 tablespoons lemon juice
1 teaspoon Dijon mustard
¼ teaspoon dry mustard
¼ teaspoon seasoned salt
1 cup olive oil

Place first 5 ingredients in a blender. Drizzle oil into blender very slowly in a steady stream until it is fully blended.

TOTAL GRAMS 3.9
GRAMS PER TABLESPOON 0.2

Vinegar-Free Mustard

2 tablespoons (1 serving)

2 tablespoons Vinegar-Free Mayonnaise
¼ teaspoon dry mustard

Blend well. For more of a mustard flavor, increase dry mustard.

TOTAL GRAMS 0.5

Our Favorite Roquefort Dressing

16 tablespoons

¼ cup tarragon vinegar
¼ teaspoon seasoned salt
3 turns of pepper mill
6 tablespoons olive oil
2 tablespoons heavy cream
½ teaspoon lemon juice
¼ cup crumbled Roquefort cheese

Beat all ingredients together except cheese. Stir in cheese.

TOTAL GRAMS 6.0
GRAMS PER TABLESPOON 0.4

Basic French Dressing

12 tablespoons

3 tablespoons tarragon vinegar
1 tablespoon lemon juice
½ teaspoon seasoned salt
3 turns of pepper mill
6 tablespoons olive oil
2 tablespoons vegetable oil
½ teaspoon Dijon mustard
¼ teaspoon dry mustard

Beat all ingredients together until well blended.

TOTAL GRAMS 4.7
GRAMS PER TABLESPOON 0.4

Vinaigrette Cream Dressing

32 tablespoons

½ cup tarragon vinegar
¾ teaspoon salt
¼ teaspoon cracked pepper
1½ cups olive oil (or ½ cup olive oil and 1 cup vegetable oil)
1 teaspoon chopped green olives
1 teaspoon chopped parsley
3 tablespoons sour cream
1 yolk from hard-boiled egg, finely chopped

Mix vinegar, salt, and pepper. Add oil, olives, parsley, sour cream, and chopped yolk.

Beat well with fork. Chill for several hours.

TOTAL GRAMS 9.3
GRAMS PER TABLESPOON 0.3

Dressing of the House

10 tablespoons

2 tablespoons olive oil
4 tablespoons vegetable oil
2 tablespoons tarragon vinegar
1 teaspoon seasoned salt
1 teaspoon Dijon mustard
¼ teaspoon garlic powder
1 tablespoon mayonnaise
¼ teaspoon sugar substitute

Put all ingredients in screw-top jar. Close jar and shake until everything is well blended. Refrigerate.

TOTAL GRAMS 3.8
GRAMS PER TABLESPOON 0.4

Thousand Island Dressing

20 tablespoons

6 scallions
1 kosher dill pickle
2 tomatoes
½ teaspoon garlic powder
1 teaspoon seasoned salt
2 tablespoons olive oil
2 tablespoons tarragon vinegar
2 tablespoons mayonnaise

Chop scallions, pickle, and tomatoes together in wooden chopping bowl. Add rest of ingredients and mix well. Refrigerate.

TOTAL GRAMS 18.8
GRAMS PER TABLESPOON   0.9

Creamy Celery-Seed Dressing

19 tablespoons

½ cup sour cream
½ cup mayonnaise
2 tablespoons tomato sauce
½ teaspoon Worcestershire sauce
½ teaspoon celery seed
½ teaspoon seasoned salt

Combine all ingredients in a screw-top jar. Shake well. Refrigerate.

TOTAL GRAMS 9.1
GRAMS PER TABLESPOON 0.5

Dill Vinaigrette Dressing

16 tablespoons

4 tablespoons tarragon vinegar
2 tablespoons olive oil
6 tablespoons safflower oil
2 tablespoons chopped olives
¼ teaspoon dry mustard
1 teaspoon Dijon mustard
1 teaspoon lemon juice
¼ teaspoon garlic powder
2 teaspoons dry dill (or 3 tablespoons chopped fresh dill)
½ packet sugar substitute
1 organic egg, beaten until frothy

Place all ingredients in a screw-top jar. Shake well. Refrigerate.

TOTAL GRAMS 9.0
GRAMS PER TABLESPOON 0.6

Curry Dressing

14 tablespoons

4 tablespoons tarragon vinegar
2 tablespoons olive oil
6 tablespoons safflower oil
1 teaspoon lemon juice
½ teaspoon curry
1 tablespoon sour cream
¼ teaspoon garlic powder
1 teaspoon sesame seeds
½ teaspoon seasoned salt
1 organic egg, beaten until frothy

Place all ingredients in a screw-top jar. Shake well. Refrigerate.

TOTAL GRAMS 7.4
GRAMS PER TABLESPOON 0.5

Italian Dressing

14 tablespoons

½ cup olive oil
¼ cup wine vinegar
1 clove garlic, minced
½ teaspoon seasoned salt
¼ teaspoon pepper

Combine all ingredients in a screw-top jar. Shake well. Refrigerate. Shake again before serving.

TOTAL GRAMS 5.1
GRAMS PER TABLESPOON 0.4

Parmesan Caesar Dressing

14 tablespoons

4 tablespoons tarragon vinegar
2 tablespoons olive oil
6 tablespoons safflower oil
1 teaspoon lemon juice
¼ teaspoon dry mustard
2 teaspoons Dijon mustard
1 teaspoon grated Parmesan cheese
¼ teaspoon garlic powder
1 teaspoon seasoned salt
½ packet sugar substitute
1 organic egg, beaten until frothy

Place all ingredients in a screw-top jar. Shake well. Refrigerate.

TOTAL GRAMS 7.4
GRAMS PER TABLESPOON 0.5

Meat

Oriental Beef Stir Fry

4 servings

½ pound spinach, steamed and drained
1½ pounds beef tenderloin
6 tablespoons hot sesame oil
4 tablespoons Tamari soy sauce
pepper to taste
½ pound shiitake mushrooms, sliced thin
1 onion, sliced thin
4 ounces bamboo shoots, cut into thin strips
3 stalks celery, cut into thin strips
2 tablespoons sake
½ cup Beef Stock (page 70)

Drain spinach well. Cut meat into thin strips and sauté in a large skillet using half of the hot sesame oil. Brown meat on both sides. Sprinkle with 2 tablespoons soy sauce and pepper. Remove meat from skillet. Put mushrooms, onion, bamboo shoots, and celery into skillet with remaining oil. Sauté for 3 minutes. Return beef to pan, add spinach and toss with remaining soy sauce, sake, and stock. Cook over low heat for 6–8 minutes or to desired doneness.

TOTAL GRAMS 37.2
GRAMS PER SERVING 9.3

Kayzie's Rabbit

6 servings

1 3–4 pound frying rabbit
½ cup olive oil plus olive oil for sautéing
juice of 1 large lemon
½ teaspoon rosemary
½ teaspoon fennel seeds
½ teaspoon seasoned salt
8 cloves garlic, minced
1 large onion, sliced thin
4 small carrots, sliced thin
2 bay leaves
¼ pound thick-sliced bacon
1 cup shiitake mushrooms, sliced
2 cups Chicken Stock *(page 68)*

Wash and dry rabbit.

Mix ½ cup olive oil, lemon juice, rosemary, fennel, salt, and garlic in a large bowl. Add onions and carrots.

Spread ½ of vegetable mixture on bottom of a roasting pan. Place rabbit pieces on top. Top with remaining vegetable mixture. Place bay leaves on top. Cover pan and place in refrigerator for 2 days. Sprinkle with olive oil daily.

To cook:
Remove rabbit from vegetable mixture, and save the vegetables.

Slice bacon into bite-size pieces and brown in a large skillet. Add ½ cup olive oil to skillet and brown rabbit pieces well on all sides. Remove and set aside.

Drain vegetable mixture. Place vegetables in hot skillet and lightly brown. Add rabbit back into skillet, cover with *Chicken Stock*, heat to a simmer. Cover and cook for 1½ hours, or until very tender.

TOTAL GRAMS 58.4
GRAMS PER SERVING 9.7

Mother's Pot Roast

6 servings

3½ pound rump roast
½ teaspoon garlic powder
1 teaspoon seasoned salt
2 medium onions, sliced
3 tomatoes, skinned and quartered
2 cloves of garlic

Rub garlic powder and seasoned salt into the meat. Place in refrigerator for ½ hour.

Place onions and garlic in a food processor. Push tomatoes through a strainer to rid them of seeds and place tomato pulp in food processor. Puree.

Place meat in a large pot. Cover with tomato sauce and simmer for 1½ hours. Turn meat and simmer about 1½ hours more or until fork-soft. Remove meat from pot to a wooden cutting board to cool. Place sauce in refrigerator to allow fat to rise to top. When meat is cool, slice. Remove fat that has formed on the sauce and place meat back in the sauce. Warm and serve.

TOTAL GRAMS 35.5
GRAMS PER SERVING 5.9

THE HAMBURGERS

Dr. Atkins' Fromage Burger

6 servings

2 pounds beef, ground
1 tablespoon chives, chopped
¾ teaspoon tarragon, crumbled
2 teaspoons seasoned salt
¼ cup fresh parsley, chopped
¼ cup scallions, minced
1 small tomato, diced
1 egg, beaten
6 ounces Cheddar cheese, coarsely grated
3 tablespoons butter, melted (optional)

Combine beef, chives, tarragon, salt, parsley, scallions, tomato, and egg. Mix well.

Shape into 12 equal balls. Flatten each ball to pancake shape. Divide cheese into 6 piles. Press cheese together. Place 1 pile of cheese in the center of 6 of the meat pancakes. Place second burger pancake on top. Press edges together to seal.

Dr. Atkins likes to cook these on an outdoor grill. If one is not available, broil in oven or sauté with butter in a nonstick skillet for five minutes on each side.

TOTAL GRAMS 12.3
GRAMS PER SERVING 2.1

Brit Burgers

2 servings

4 tablespoons butter
½ cup onions, chopped
1 pound beef, ground
½ teaspoon seasoned salt
½ teaspoon pepper

½ teaspoon sage

Melt 2 tablespoons butter in a skillet. Sauté onions until golden. Remove and set aside.

Combine beef, salt, pepper, and sage with onions and mix well. Shape into patties. In same skillet melt remaining 2 tablespoons butter. Sauté for 5 minutes on each side.

TOTAL GRAMS 7.3
GRAMS PER SERVING 3.6

Pizza Burgers

6 servings

2 pounds beef, ground
1 teaspoon seasoned salt
1 tablespoon parsley, chopped
⅛ teaspoon basil
⅛ teaspoon oregano
2 eggs, beaten
1 package fried pork rinds, crushed
¼ cup olive oil
6 slices mozzarella cheese
½ recipe Pasta Sauce *(pages 179–180)*
3 tablespoons grated Parmesan cheese

Preheat oven to 400° F.

Mix beef with salt, parsley, basil, and oregano

Shape into 6 patties ½-inch thick.

Dip patties into eggs, then coat with crushed pork rinds. Sauté patties in hot olive oil until well browned on both sides. Arrange in a shallow baking dish. They must not be touching. Top each patty with a slice of mozzarella cheese. Pour on *Pasta Sauce*. Sprinkle with Parmesan cheese. Bake for 15 minutes.

TOTAL GRAMS 66.2
GRAMS PER SERVING 11.0

Feta Burgers

2 servings

2 tablespoons butter
1 pound beef, ground
¼ cup crumbled feta cheese
¼ cup finely chopped black olives
½ teaspoon seasoned salt
½ teaspoon pepper

Melt butter in a heavy skillet.
    Mix remaining ingredients, and shape into patties.
    Sauté hamburgers for 5 minutes on each side.

TOTAL GRAMS 3.4
GRAMS PER SERVING 1.7

Curry Burgers

2 servings

2 tablespoons butter
1 pound beef, ground
1 tablespoon finely chopped walnuts
2 teaspoons curry powder
½ teaspoon seasoned salt

Melt butter in skillet.
    Mix remainder of ingredients and shape into patties.
    Sauté hamburgers for 5 minutes on each side.

TOTAL GRAMS 3.6
GRAMS PER SERVING 1.8

¡Ole! Burgers

2 servings

2 tablespoons butter
1 pound beef, ground
6 drops Tabasco sauce
½ teaspoon cumin
½ teaspoon chili powder
¼ teaspoon garlic powder

Melt butter in a skillet.
    Mix remainder of ingredients and shape into patties.
    Sauté hamburgers for 5 minutes on each side.

TOTAL GRAMS 1.7
GRAMS PER SERVING 0.9

U.S. Hamburgers

2 servings

6 strips lean bacon
1 ripe tomato, finely chopped
2 tablespoons butter
1 pound beef, ground
½ teaspoon seasoned salt
½ teaspoon pepper

Fry bacon until crisp. Remove from pan, and place on paper towels
to drain. Crumble bacon into a large bowl. Sauté tomato in bacon fat
until tender. Add it to the bacon. Pour off bacon fat and melt butter in
same skillet. Combine meat, salt, and pepper with bacon and tomato.
    Shape into patties.
    Sauté hamburgers for 5 minutes on each side.

TOTAL GRAMS 6.7
GRAMS PER SERVING 3.4

Steak Au Poivre

4 servings

4 shell steaks, pounded to ⅛-inch thickness
freshly ground black pepper
6 tablespoons butter
2 teaspoons rosemary
2 teaspoons sage
4 ounces cognac, warmed
6 ounces heavy cream
2 teaspoons Worcestershire sauce
2 tablespoons Dijon mustard

Cover surface of steaks on both sides with ground pepper.

Press pepper into steaks.

In a large skillet melt butter and add rosemary and sage.

Add steaks and brown quickly on both sides. Pour warm cognac over steaks and ignite. When fire goes out, remove steaks from skillet and keep warm.

Add cream, Worcestershire, and mustard to pan juices. Stir well and simmer for 3 minutes. Pour over steak and serve.

TOTAL GRAMS 14.2
GRAMS PER SERVING 3.6

Moussaka

6 servings

8 teaspoons sweet butter
3 egg yolks
1¼ cups water
¼ cup heavy cream
½ cup grated Parmesan cheese
1 medium eggplant
1 pound ground lamb or ½ pound ground chuck
6 tablespoons olive oil
1 large onion, chopped

1 large green pepper, chopped
2 cloves garlic, minced
1 8-ounce can tomato sauce
1½ teaspoons cumin
¼ teaspoon nutmeg
¼ teaspoon oregano
2 teaspoons salt

Preheat oven to 350° F.

To prepare cream sauce:
Place butter in top of double boiler over hot water. Add egg yolks one at a time. Beat constantly with rotary or hand electric beater. Add ¼ cup water, cream, and Parmesan cheese. Continue to beat until sauce thickens, about 10 minutes.

Pare and slice eggplant. Arrange eggplant on a large plate. Place plate in sink. Cover with another large plate, allowing plate to press eggplant. Let drain for ½ hour, then press each slice with a paper towel. Heat 2 tablespoons olive oil in a large skillet. Add onion and green pepper. Sauté until light golden brown. Add garlic and meat, and cook until browned.

Add tomato sauce, 1 cup water, cumin, nutmeg, oregano, and salt. Simmer for 15 minutes.

Heat remaining 4 tablespoons of olive oil, and sauté eggplant slices until lightly browned. Drain on paper towels. Place half the eggplant slices in a well-oiled baking dish. Spread with half the meat mixture. Place remaining eggplant slices on top and cover with the rest of the meat. Cover top with cream sauce.

Bake for 30 minutes.

TOTAL GRAMS 68.7
GRAMS PER SERVING 11.5

Calves Liver in Red Wine

4 servings

6 shallots or 1 small onion, finely chopped
1 cup dry red wine
juice of 1 lemon
4 tablespoons oil
½ teaspoon oregano
½ teaspoon seasoned salt
¼ teaspoon black pepper
1 pound calves liver, sliced
4 tablespoons butter

Combine shallots, wine, lemon juice, oil, oregano, salt, and pepper in a large bowl. Marinate liver for 1 hour, then turn it and marinate for another hour.

Remove liver from marinade.

Melt butter in a skillet, and sauté liver for 5 minutes on each side.

TOTAL GRAMS 20.9
GRAMS PER SERVING   5.2

Veal Rolatine

4 servings

4 veal cutlets, flattened with a mallet
½ teaspoon seasoned salt
4 slices prosciutto ham
6 slices Jarlsberg cheese
1 egg, beaten
¼ cup grated Parmesan cheese
4 tablespoons sweet butter
¼ cup dry white wine

Preheat oven to 350° F.

Wash and dry veal. Sprinkle with salt. Place 1 slice of ham and 1 slice of cheese on each cutlet. Roll up and tie with string. Dip rolls in egg and coat with Parmesan cheese. Place in refrigerator for ½ hour to set. Melt butter in a heavy skillet. Sauté veal rolls until they are brown on all sides. Remove rolls to a small baking dish. Add wine to pan juices and bring to a boil. Pour sauce over rolls. Top with 2 remaining slices of cheese. Bake for ½ hour. Remove string and serve.

Note: This may be used as an hors d'oeuvre by cutting rolls into pieces the size of half dollars.

TOTAL GRAMS 4.1
GRAMS PER SERVING 1.0

Gourmet Pork Chops

6 servings

12 pork chops
salt and pepper to taste
2 tablespoons garlic oil
2 tablespoons olive oil
1 onion, chopped
1 clove garlic, minced
1 pound mushrooms, sliced
1 cup hot Chicken Stock *(page 68)*
½ cup dry red wine
1 bay leaf
¼ cup sour cream (optional)

Preheat oven to 350° F.

Sprinkle pork chops with salt and pepper. In a heavy skillet brown chops in garlic oil over high heat. Remove and keep warm. Add olive oil to pan. Sauté onion, garlic, and mushrooms in olive oil until onion is golden. Pour in *Chicken Stock,* wine, and add bay leaf. Bring mixture to a boil and cook for about 3 minutes.

Arrange 6 pork chops in casserole. Top with half the sauce.

Put another layer of pork chops on top and pour over remaining mixture. Cover casserole tightly and bake for 1½ hours.

If desired, sour cream may be added to sauce mixture when served.

TOTAL GRAMS 36.9
GRAMS PER SERVING 6.2

Roast Veal

6 servings

1 4–5-pound veal roast (leg, loin, rump, shoulder, or breast)
1 clove garlic, minced
½ pound thick-sliced bacon
3 tablespoons olive oil
4 tablespoons chopped onion
2 celery stalks, diced
4 anchovies (optional)
½ cup white wine or Chicken Stock *(page 68)*

Preheat oven to 325° F.

Have the butcher bone and tie meat. Cut a few incisions in veal and insert minced garlic.

In roasting pan with cover, heat oil and brown veal. Add onion, celery, and wine (or stock) to pan. Arrange bacon on top. Place in oven. Cover and cook for 30 minutes to the pound, basting occasionally. Remove veal from pan, and let it set for 10 minutes for easier carving. Remove vegetables from pan juices, skim off excess fat, and pour pan juices over veal. Serve warm, or serve cold-sliced with *Vinaigrette Cream Dressing,* page 95.

TOTAL GRAMS 7.9
GRAMS PER SERVING 1.3

Veal Scaloppini at Its Best

6 servings

1½ pounds veal cut into scallops ¼-inch thick
salt and pepper to taste
6 tablespoons butter
¼ cup brandy
1 cup Chicken Stock *(page 68)*
¼ cup Chablis or other dry white wine
2 tablespoons dry sherry
1 pound porcini mushrooms, sliced
2 tomatoes, peeled and chopped
1 teaspoon garlic powder
½ cup grated Swiss cheese
¼ cup grated Parmesan cheese

Preheat broiler.

Pat salt and pepper into veal.

In a skillet melt butter, then add veal to brown.

Heat brandy. Pour over veal and ignite. Remove veal from skillet and keep warm. Pour *Chicken Stock*, Chablis, and sherry into skillet. Simmer until liquid reduces by half. Return veal to skillet. Simmer for 10 minutes. Keep warm until serving.

Sauté mushrooms in 2 tablespoons butter until brown. Add tomatoes and garlic powder. Simmer for 5 minutes. Place mushroom mixture in baking dish. Add veal and cover with wine sauce. Sprinkle with grated Swiss and Parmesan cheeses.

Broil until cheese is brown and bubbly. Serve immediately.

TOTAL GRAMS 38.9
GRAMS PER SERVING 6.5

My Grandmother's Veal Stew

4 servings

3 strips bacon, diced
3 tablespoons butter
1 tablespoon chopped onion
½ cup sliced mushrooms
2 pounds cubed veal
½ cup water or Chicken Stock *(page 68)*
1 cup sour cream
1 teaspoon salt
¼ teaspoon paprika

Preheat oven to 250° F.

Place bacon, butter, onion, and mushrooms in skillet. Sauté slowly until onion and bacon are lightly brown. Remove mixture with slotted spoon. Place in ovenproof serving dish. Leave bacon fat and butter in skillet, then add veal. Brown meat on all sides. Remove veal, leaving fat in skillet. Place meat in baking dish. Mix well with bacon mixture.

Add water (or stock), sour cream, salt, and paprika to fat in skillet. Heat just to boiling. Pour over meat mixture. Cover dish. Bake for 1 hour, or until veal is tender when pierced with fork.

TOTAL GRAMS 12.0
GRAMS PER SERVING 3.0

Garden Beef

8 servings

4 tablespoons vegetable oil
3 pounds stew beef (chuck, round), cubed
4 tablespoons onion, chopped
4 cups water
3 soup bones
2 teaspoons salt
½ cup rutabaga, cubed
½ medium green pepper, chopped
¼ small eggplant, chopped
½ cup zucchini, cubed
4 tablespoons tomato sauce
1 cup spinach

Heat oil in large heavy pot. Add meat and brown well on all sides. Push meat to one side of pot, and add onion. Cook 2 more minutes.

Add water, soup bones, and salt. Simmer for 2 hours.

Add rutabaga and simmer for 15 more minutes.

Add green pepper, eggplant, and zucchini. Simmer for 10 more minutes. Spoon in tomato sauce and spinach, and cook for 7 more minutes.

TOTAL GRAMS 20.8
GRAMS PER SERVING 2.6

Luscious Lamb

4 servings

8 lamb chops
garlic powder
2 tablespoons butter
2 tablespoons Worcestershire sauce
2 tablespoons lemon juice
2 tablespoons gin
1 teaspoon seasoned salt

Rub lamb chops with small amount of garlic powder and place in a dish. Melt butter in a small pan and add Worcestershire sauce, lemon juice, gin, and salt. Pour liquid over lamb chops. Allow to marinate in refrigerator for 30 minutes. Remove lamb from marinade. Broil or barbecue to desired doneness. Meanwhile, boil marinade in a small saucepan for 10 minutes. Top lamb with marinade before serving.

TOTAL GRAMS 9.9
GRAMS PER SERVING 2.5

Stuffed Leg of Lamb

8 servings

2 tablespoons butter
1 pound veal or beef, ground
3 tablespoons chopped onion
1 clove garlic, minced
½ cup white wine
1 8-ounce can tomato sauce
1 tablespoon dill
1 tablespoon chopped parsley
½ cup grated Parmesan cheese
salt and pepper to taste
1 leg of lamb, boned and flattened

Preheat oven to 300° F.

Melt 1 tablespoon butter in heavy skillet. Add ground meat, onion, and garlic. Brown lightly on all sides. Pour wine in pan slowly, and cook for 2 minutes. Add tomato sauce, dill, and parsley. Cook over medium heat for 10 minutes or until liquid has been absorbed. Remove from heat. Sprinkle with Parmesan cheese, salt, and pepper. Wipe lamb with damp cloth. Sprinkle with salt and pepper.

Spread ground meat mixture on lamb and roll up carefully. Use skewers to fasten it or tie with string.

Melt 1 tablespoon butter in medium-size roasting pan. Add lamb roll. Brown over medium heat.

Bake for 2 hours or until meat is tender. (If the pan gets dry, add 2 or 3 tablespoons water to pan.)

TOTAL GRAMS 25.3
GRAMS PER SERVING 3.2

Loin of Lamb with Horseradish Cream

6 servings

2 3-pound lamb loins, boned and trimmed of fat, bones reserved
3 bay leaves
3 ribs of celery, chopped
6 black peppercorns
4 cups water
1 clove garlic, quartered
1 onion, chopped
¼ cup walnut oil
salt and freshly ground pepper to taste
2 cups heavy cream
3 tablespoons white horseradish, drained
2 tablespoons snipped chives

Place lamb bones, bay leaf, celery, and peppercorns in 4 cups of water. Bring water to a boil, skimming broth, and simmer mixture until liquid is reduced to about 2½ cups. Strain stock through a fine sieve into a pan. Add garlic and onions. Bring liquid to a boil. Simmer until it is reduced to 1½ cups. Strain the stock.

In a large skillet, heat oil over medium heat until it is hot (do not allow it to smoke). Season lamb with salt and pepper and brown in oil. Turn lamb to brown well on all sides. Remove lamb from oil, cool for 10 minutes, and slice it into ½-inch-thick slices. Arrange it on a platter and keep it warm. Return stock to skillet, and stir in cream and horseradish. Gently simmer sauce until it thickens (do not boil). Adjust seasonings and spoon over lamb. Garnish with chives.

TOTAL GRAMS 29.2
GRAMS PER SERVING 4.9

Steak Pizzaiola

6 servings

⅛ cup garlic oil
¼ cup olive oil
2 tablespoons tarragon vinegar
1 teaspoon water
freshly cracked black pepper
3 pounds sirloin steak
8 Italian plum tomatoes, cut into strips (1 cup)
2 cloves garlic, crushed
1 tablespoon chopped parsley
1 teaspoon oregano
⅛ teaspoon seasoned salt
4 tablespoons pine nuts
½ packet sugar substitute

Combine garlic oil with ⅛ cup olive oil, vinegar, water, and pepper. Place steak in mixture and marinate in refrigerator for at least 2 hours, preferably overnight. Heat remaining olive oil, and add tomatoes, garlic, parsley, oregano, salt, and pine nuts. Cook over medium heat for 3 minutes. Remove from heat, add sugar substitute, and keep warm. Broil steak to desired doneness, slice, and pour mixture over it. Serve immediately.

TOTAL GRAMS 21.9
GRAMS PER SERVING 3.7

Cabbage Rolls Stuffed with Meat (Dolma)

6 servings

1 medium cabbage
1½ pounds lamb or beef, ground
4 tablespoons diced onion
4 tablespoons chopped parsley
2 eggs
1 teaspoon salt
pepper to taste
⅓ cup tomato sauce

Sauce:
1 cup chopped cabbage
½ cup water
⅔ can tomato sauce (6 ounces)
2 tablespoons lemon juice
2 packets sugar substitute

Clean cabbage and remove any damaged leaves. Pour boiling water over cabbage. Cover and let stand for ½ hour. Mix ground meat, onion, parsley, eggs, salt, pepper, and tomato sauce together.

Drain cabbage, core, and separate leaves.

To stuff:
Use 12 leaves. Put 3 full tablespoons of meat mixture in center of each leaf. Bring sides up over filling and roll leaf up. Set aside.

Sauce:
Chop remaining cabbage (the core and leaves not suitable for stuffing). Heat water in medium-size pot. Bring to boil. Add chopped cabbage, tomato sauce, salt, lemon juice, and sugar substitute. Reduce heat, cover, and simmer for 15 minutes.

Remove 1 cup sauce and set aside. Place cabbage rolls in pot with remaining sauce as close together as possible. Pour reserved sauce over cabbage rolls. Cover. Simmer for 1½ hours.

TOTAL GRAMS 61.6
GRAMS PER SERVING 10.2

Spicy Spareribs

4 servings

4 pounds pork spareribs (or beef ribs)
1 tablespoon paprika
2 teaspoons chili powder
¾ teaspoon salt
½ teaspoon dry mustard
¼ teaspoon garlic powder
⅛ teaspoon pepper

Preheat oven to 450° F.

Place single layer of ribs, meaty side down, in shallow roasting pan. Roast for ½ hour. Drain off fat. Combine rest of ingredients, sprinkle evenly over ribs.

Reduce oven to 350° F. Roast, meaty side up, for spareribs ½–1 hour longer. (Beef ribs will take about 1 hour longer.)

TOTAL GRAMS 7.2
GRAMS PER SERVING 1.8

Stuffed Steak

6 servings

garlic powder
3 pounds of any cut of steak (cut with pockets)
½ pound shiitake mushrooms
½ teaspoon thyme
3 sprigs parsley, chopped
5 slices smoked ham
2 tablespoons sweet butter
2 shallots or 1 small onion, finely chopped
1 clove garlic, chopped
2 tablespoons dry white wine

Rub garlic powder on steak and set aside.

Chop together mushrooms, thyme, parsley, and ham in large wooden chopping bowl.

Heat butter over low flame until melted. Brown shallots and garlic in butter. Add mushroom mixture and cook for 3 minutes, stirring occasionally. Add wine and cook 1 more minute. Remove from heat and spoon mushroom mixture into pockets in steak. Stuff firmly, and sew closed with a trussing needle and thread.

Broil steak to desired doneness.

Serve with hot *Parsley Butter Sauce,* page 183.

TOTAL GRAMS 17.5
GRAMS PER SERVING 2.9

Pork Loin with Mustard

6 servings

6 ½-inch slices of boneless pork loin
salt and freshly ground black pepper
2 tablespoons olive oil
2 tablespoons shallots, chopped
¼ cup dry white wine
2 teaspoons brandy
¾ cup Chicken Stock *(page 68)*
2 packets sugar substitute
1 tablespoon Dijon mustard

Season pork well with salt and pepper.

Heat oil in a large skillet over medium heat. Do not allow it to smoke. Brown pork in oil. Remove pork, lower heat, and add shallots. Cook them for about 3 minutes. Pour in wine and brandy and simmer until liquid has evaporated. Add stock and sugar substitute. Whisk mixture as it boils until liquid is reduced by half. Add pork and simmer for about 2 minutes until pork is warm and has absorbed some sauce. Remove pork to a serving plate. Whisk mustard into sauce, correct seasonings, and spoon remaining sauce over pork.

TOTAL GRAMS 7.2
GRAMS PER SERVING 1.2

Poultry

Chicken Cacciatore

8 servings

1 5-pound chicken, cut into 8 pieces
½ cup olive oil
4 tablespoons butter
⅓ cup chopped onion
½ pound shiitake mushrooms, sliced
3 cloves garlic
¾ cup dry white wine
2 bay leaves
1 teaspoon basil
½ teaspoon freshly ground black pepper
5 tablespoons tomato sauce
seasoned salt to taste
2 tablespoons brandy

In a large skillet, sauté chicken in olive oil until light golden brown, about 20 minutes.

Heat butter in a separate skillet until melted; add onion and mushrooms and sauté until golden. Add garlic. Cook for 4 more minutes. Spoon mushrooms, onions, and garlic over chicken. Pour on wine. Add bay leaves, basil, and pepper. Simmer for about 8 minutes, uncovered. Stir in tomato sauce. Salt to taste. Cook, uncovered, over low heat for 15 more minutes. Add brandy, and serve.

TOTAL GRAMS 31.1
GRAMS PER SERVING 3.8

Lemon-Basted Roast Chicken

4 servings

1 chicken, quartered
½ teaspoon oregano
¼ teaspoon garlic powder
¼ cup butter (½ stick)
salt and pepper to taste
juice of 2 lemons (6 to 8 tablespoons)

Preheat oven to 400° F.

Sprinkle chicken with oregano and garlic powder. Melt butter in roasting pan or casserole. Add chicken; turn to coat. Sprinkle with salt and pepper.

Roast chicken skin side up, uncovered, for 30 minutes or until golden brown. Turn pieces over and continue roasting until brown (about 30 more minutes). Reduce heat to 300° F. and cook until tender. Squeeze lemon juice over chicken.

Cover and let sit in turned-off oven for 15 minutes.

Remove to platter and serve.

TOTAL GRAMS 6.2
GRAMS PER SERVING 1.6

Coq Au Vin with Shiitake Mushrooms

8 servings

4 slices thick-sliced bacon
7 tablespoons butter
1 4-pound chicken, cut into 8 pieces
1 teaspoon seasoned salt
¼ cup cognac (or brandy)
1 cup dry red wine
1 cup Chicken Stock (page 68)
¼ teaspoon garlic powder
¾ teaspoon thyme
1 bay leaf
4 medium-size onions, sliced
½ pound shiitake mushrooms, sliced
chopped chives

Dice bacon and sauté in 4 tablespoons butter in large skillet until brown. Remove bacon from skillet and save.

Wash and thoroughly dry chicken. Brown in bacon fat and season with salt.

Put bacon back in pan, cover, and simmer for about 10 minutes.

Heat cognac in small pan. Ignite, and pour over chicken. Add wine, stock, garlic powder, and thyme. Add bay leaf to chicken, cover and simmer for 45 minutes. Remove chicken and keep warm.

Boil liquid in pan until it reduces by half.

In a separate pan, sauté onions and mushrooms in remaining 3 tablespoons butter until onions are golden.

Put chicken back into skillet. Cover with mushrooms and onions. Simmer for 5 minutes. Garnish with chives.

TOTAL GRAMS 39.8
GRAMS PER SERVING 5.0

Chicken à la Firenze

4 servings

4 boneless chicken breasts
2 eggs, beaten
½ package fried pork rinds, crushed
3 tablespoons butter
½ cup Sautérne
1 cup Chicken Stock *(page 68)*
1 clove garlic, crushed
dash of marjoram
dash of basil
⅓ cup cream
½ pound spinach, cooked*
¼ cup grated Parmesan cheese

Preheat oven to 350° F.

Dip chicken in eggs and dredge in crushed pork rinds until well coated. Sauté in butter until chicken begins to brown. Turn once. Lower heat. Add wine and cook until wine has almost evaporated. Remove from heat. Place chicken in casserole pan.

Mix together stock, garlic, marjoram, basil, and cream. Pour into skillet and heat with pan juices.

Place ½ spinach in bottom of casserole. Add chicken; top with remaining spinach. Pour sauce over top. Sprinkle with Parmesan cheese and bake for ½ hour.

TOTAL GRAMS 16.5
GRAMS PER SERVING 4.1

---

*To cook fresh spinach: Wash carefully several times to remove all sand. Place in pot with just enough water to cover it. Cook at low boil for about 10 minutes or until tender, but not limp. Press out water before serving. Two packages of frozen spinach may be substituted for fresh spinach. Cook to package directions. Whether fresh or frozen do not overcook.

Summer Day Chicken From Spain

4 servings

1 5-pound chicken, cut into pieces
¼ cup safflower oil
2 cloves garlic
juice of 1 lemon
1 teaspoon grated orange rind
2 bay leaves
½ cup vinegar
1 cup white wine
1 cup Chicken Stock (page 68)
½ teaspoon coarsely ground pepper
salt to taste

Wash and dry chicken. Heat oil in skillet. Lightly brown chicken over medium heat.

Combine remaining ingredients. Pour over chicken. Simmer, covered, for 1 hour. Add more stock, if necessary, to keep chicken covered.

Serve warm or chilled.

TOTAL GRAMS 18.6
GRAMS PER SERVING   4.7

Austrian Paprika Chicken

6 servings

2 tablespoons butter
2 tablespoons vegetable oil
2 chicken broilers, cut up, about 5 pounds
seasoned salt
4 small onions, quartered
1 clove garlic, minced
2 tablespoons paprika
1 cup Chicken Stock *(page 68)*
1 cup sour cream

Preheat oven to 350° F.

Heat butter and oil together. Brown chicken carefully in oil on all sides. Add salt. Remove chicken from pan.

Place onions and garlic in oil and sauté until onions are golden. Add paprika, stock, and sour cream. Stir constantly until mixture is smooth.

Place chicken in casserole and cover with mixture, making sure to scrape pan well of all drippings.

Bake, covered, for 1 hour.

Serve with *Tossed Salad with Tomato Dressing,* page 81.

TOTAL GRAMS 34.8
GRAMS PER SERVING 5.8

Chicken Croquettes

2 servings

1½ cups chicken, ground, about ¾ pound
2 egg whites
¼ teaspoon poultry seasoning
pinch of salt
canola oil for deep frying
2 tablespoons chopped onion
4 large mushrooms, chopped
1 tablespoon butter
Cream Sauce *(page 177)*

Preheat oven to 375° F.

Mix chicken, egg whites, poultry seasoning, and salt. Form into croquettes 1 inch wide and 3 inches long. Fry in canola oil until crisp.

Sauté mushrooms and onions in oil until lightly browned.

Prepare *Cream Sauce.*

Place mushrooms and onion in a casserole and arrange croquettes on top.

Pour sauce on top.

Bake for about 8–10 minutes until thoroughly heated.

To make a prettier dish, place sliced hard-boiled eggs between croquettes. Then add sauce. Sprinkle with paprika.

TOTAL GRAMS 7.4
GRAMS PER SERVING 3.7

Gourmet Game Hens

6 servings

¾ cup butter
¾ cup white port wine
3 tablespoons dried tarragon
6 garlic cloves
1½ teaspoons salt
¾ teaspoon pepper

garlic powder
6 frozen Rock Cornish hens, about 1¼ pounds each, thawed

Preheat oven to 400° F.

Melt butter in a saucepan. Add wine and 1 tablespoon dried tarragon. Heat thoroughly.

Place 1 garlic clove, 1 teaspoon tarragon, ¼ teaspoon salt, and ⅛ teaspoon pepper in each hen. Sprinkle outside liberally with garlic powder.

Pour wine sauce over hens and roast in large shallow pan, without rack, for about 1 hour or until well browned and drumstick twists easily. Baste frequently with sauce.

TOTAL GRAMS 16.8
GRAMS PER SERVING 2.8

Turkey à la King

4 servings

4 egg yolks
¼ teaspoon seasoned salt
½ teaspoon dry tarragon
1 cup heavy cream
1 cup Chicken Stock *(page 68)*
2 cups diced turkey meat
nutmeg

Preheat oven to 350° F.

Beat yolks until thick and lemon-colored. Add salt and tarragon. Beat in heavy cream. Stir in stock, then add turkey meat.

Pour into 4 small ovenproof bowls. Sprinkle with nutmeg. Set bowls in shallow pan half full with water, and bake for 30 minutes.

TOTAL GRAMS 9.4
GRAMS PER SERVING 2.4

Roast Turkey

Preheat oven to 400° F.

This is an easy, delicious way to cook a perfect, moist turkey. Have turkey at room temperature. Remove giblets from cavity. Run turkey under cold water to clean inside and out. Never soak a turkey in water. Dry turkey well. Rub turkey with garlic inside and out. Place sliced oranges and lemons in the cavity if you are not stuffing it or use the *Almond Stuffing* that follows. Insert poultry pins to draw open cavity together. Use string to lace between pins as you would lace a boot.

Tie legs together with string if not already tucked under a piece of string. Bend wing tips under body and tuck loose neck skin under turkey.

Place turkey, breast side up, in a stainless-steel roasting pan that has a cover. Cover turkey breast with slices of turkey bacon. Place cover on pan.

Bake at 400° F. for 20 minutes. Reduce to 350° F. Cook for 20 minutes per pound if turkey is over 10 pounds. If under 10 pounds, cook for 15 minutes per pound.

TOTAL GRAMS 0

Almond Stuffing

6 1/2-cup servings

½ *cup butter*
½ *cup finely chopped onion*
¼ *pound smoked ham, chopped fine*
¼ *cup chopped parsley*
½ *teaspoon thyme*
½ *teaspoon freshly ground pepper*
½ *cup fried pork rinds, crushed*
2 *eggs*
¼ *cup dry red wine*
⅔ *cup blanched almonds*

Melt butter in large skillet. Add onions. Cook until light brown. Add ham, parsley, and spices. Mix well. Combine mixture with pork rinds, eggs, wine, and almonds.

Use to stuff chicken, turkey, veal roast, or anything that needs a stuffing.

TOTAL GRAMS 24.5
GRAMS PER SERVING 4.1

Duck in Red Wine

4 servings

2 tablespoons butter or rendered chicken fat
1 5–6 pound duck, skin removed and cut into 8 pieces
2 cloves garlic, minced
2 cups dry red wine
8 shiitake mushrooms, thinly sliced
2 sprigs parsley, chopped
1 small bay leaf
¼ teaspoon thyme
1 teaspoon seasoned salt
8 small white pearl onions, peeled
2 carrots, peeled and quartered

Preheat oven to 350° F.

Melt butter in a large skillet. Brown pieces of duck in fat over medium heat.

Remove to a casserole.

Add garlic to fat and cook 1 minute. Add red wine, shiitake mushrooms, parsley, bay leaf, thyme, and salt. Bring to a boil, stirring constantly until sauce thickens. Place onions and carrots into casserole with duck. Top with sauce.

Cover and bake for 1¼ hours.

TOTAL GRAMS 60.4
GRAMS PER SERVING 15.1

Hal's Chicken

4 servings

1 chicken, cut into 8 pieces
Mustard Sauce *to cover (page 181)*
1 medium onion, sliced thin
1 medium tomato, sliced thin
2 tablespoons fresh dill, minced
seasoned salt to taste

Preheat oven to 350° F.

Wash and dry chicken. Place in a baking dish and cover with *Mustard Sauce.* Top with onion slices and then tomatoes. Sprinkle with dill and salt.

Cover and bake for 1 hour. Remove lid and bake 1 hour more.

TOTAL GRAMS 18.7
GRAMS PER SERVING 4.7

Joan's Chicken Mascarpone

4 servings

4 skinless, boneless chicken breasts
2 tablespoons butter
2 medium onions, sliced thin
½ teaspoon dried tarragon
3 tablespoons dry white wine
3 tablespoons mascarpone cheese

Preheat oven to 350° F.

Place chicken breasts in a glass baking dish. Sauté onions, garlic, and tarragon in the butter until onions become golden. Place on top of chicken. Swish wine in sauté pan and add mascarpone cheese. Allow cheese to melt (about 30 seconds), stir well to combine flavors and spoon over chicken and onions. Cover.

Bake for 1 hour.

TOTAL GRAMS 16.7
GRAMS PER SERVING 4.2

Tandoori Chicken

4 servings

1 5-pound chicken, cut in 8 pieces
4 cloves garlic
2-inch piece ginger, peeled
2 bay leaves
2 teaspoons chili powder
1 teaspoon sea salt
2 teaspoons turmeric
1 teaspoon coriander, ground
½ teaspoon cumin
½ teaspoon cinnamon, ground
½ teaspoon cloves, ground
½ cup olive oil
1½ cups sour cream
juice of 2 lemons

Place chicken in a covered glass baking dish large enough for pieces to lie side by side.

Place next 10 ingredients in a blender and grind to a paste.

Combine paste with sour cream and lemon juice.

Dip each piece of chicken into the mixture and coat it completely. Return chicken to baking dish.

Place in refrigerator to marinate overnight.

Bake chicken covered for 45 minutes, at 350° F.

TOTAL GRAMS 34.2
GRAMS PER SERVING 8.6

Goat Cheesy Chicken Rolls

4 servings

4 skinless, boneless chicken breasts, pounded thin
½ cup goat cheese, crumbled
½ cup fresh basil, minced
1 tablespoon sun-dried tomatoes, softened in olive oil and minced
¼ small onion, minced
½ teaspoon oregano
½ teaspoon seasoned salt
¼ cup dry white wine

Preheat oven to 350° F.

Oil a small glass baking dish.

In a small bowl combine all ingredients except chicken and wine and blend well. Spread mixture on chicken breasts and roll them. Fasten with a toothpick. Arrange in baking dish so rolled breasts do not touch each other. Pour wine over chicken rolls.

Bake for 45 minutes.

TOTAL GRAMS 15.6
GRAMS PER SERVING 3.9

Oriental Chicken with Broccoli Rabe

4 servings

3 teaspoons olive oil
2 teaspoons sesame oil
2 teaspoons ginger, minced
2 garlic cloves, minced
4 skinless, boneless chicken breasts, cubed
4 large shiitake mushrooms, sliced thin
2 scallions, minced
8 ounces broccoli rabe, coarsely chopped
1 tablespoon Tamari soy sauce
2 tablespoons dry sherry

Heat 2 teaspoons olive oil and 2 teaspoons sesame oil in a nonstick wok or skillet. Do not allow oil to smoke. Add ginger and garlic and stir for 30 seconds. Add chicken and mushrooms and stir 3 minutes more. Remove from skillet. Stir remaining olive oil into skillet. Add scallions and broccoli rabe. Stir-fry for 1 minute. Put back chicken and mushrooms and add soy sauce and sherry.

Remove chicken and vegetables with a slotted spoon. Place on a serving plate. Boil sauce until it reduces by half. Pour over chicken and serve immediately.

TOTAL GRAMS 32.5
GRAMS PER SERVING 8.1

Turkey Sausage Patties

8 patties

2 tablespoons garlic oil
1 small onion, chopped fine
1 clove garlic, minced
1 pound turkey, ground
3 tablespoons sour cream
10 pork rinds, crushed
½ teaspoon sage, minced
½ teaspoon seasoned salt
2 tablespoons walnut oil

Heat garlic oil in a nonstick skillet. Add onion and garlic and sauté until onions are golden.

Mix all other ingredients (except walnut oil) together in a bowl. Add onions and garlic and shape into eight balls. Flatten balls into patties. Heat walnut oil in skillet and sauté patties until brown on both sides.

TOTAL GRAMS 7.1
GRAMS PER SERVING 0.9

Ivan's Crisp Chicken

4 servings

1 5-pound chicken, cut in 8 pieces
4 tablespoons garlic oil
¼ cup white wine
1 medium-size red onion, sliced thin
seasoned salt to taste
¼ cup grated Jarlsberg cheese
¼ cup grated sharp Cheddar cheese

Preheat oven to 350° F.

Wash and dry chicken. Brush with garlic oil. Place in baking dish and sprinkle with wine. Cover with onions. Salt to taste and bake, covered, for ½ hour.

Uncover, sprinkle with cheeses and bake uncovered until chicken, onions, and cheeses are crisp, about 45 minutes.

TOTAL GRAMS 7.3
GRAMS PER SERVING 1.8

Fish and Shellfish

Sun Luck Scallops

4 servings

¼ cup Tamari soy sauce
⅛ cup sake
1 pound bay scallops
2 tablespoons sesame oil
6 shiitake mushrooms, sliced thin
½ cup sour cream

Preheat oven to 350° F.

Mix soy sauce and sake together. Place scallops in a glass baking dish. Pour soy sauce mixture over scallops and place in refrigerator for ½ hour. Heat sesame oil in a skillet. Sauté mushrooms for 2 minutes. Turn off heat and allow to cool in oil. Place scallops in oven and bake for 10 minutes. Spoon sour cream into a small dish. Spoon 1 tablespoon of sauce from scallops over mushrooms and artfully arrange them on top of sour cream. Enjoy eating by dipping a scallop in the mushroom sour cream mixture.

TOTAL GRAMS 33.4
GRAMS PER SERVING 8.4

Snappy Swordfish

6 servings

2½ pounds swordfish steak
juice of 1 lemon
3 teaspoons garlic paste (available in a tube)
2 tablespoons fresh dill (or 1 tablespoon dried, minced)
1 medium tomato, thinly sliced
½ pound shiitake mushrooms, sliced
3 tablespoons olive oil
½ cup shelled sunflower seeds
½ pound sugar snap peas, trimmed
¼ cup dry white wine
3 ounces herbed goat cheese, crumbled

Preheat oven to 350° F.

Wash and dry swordfish. Sprinkle both sides with lemon juice and place in a covered glass baking dish.

Spread garlic paste evenly on fish. Top with dill, tomato, and mushrooms. Sprinkle olive oil and sunflower seeds evenly across the top.

Spread snap peas over fish; pour wine over the peas.

Cover and place in oven for 20 minutes. Uncover, add goat cheese and cook for 10 minutes more, basting frequently.

TOTAL GRAMS 50.4
GRAMS PER SERVING 8.4

Poached Fish Fillets (Basic Recipe)

4 servings

4 fish fillets (sole, salmon, halibut, or flounder)
juice of 1 lemon
1 small onion
seasoned salt
1 tablespoon butter
3 large mushrooms, thinly sliced
¼ cup water
½ cup dry white wine

Preheat oven to 350° F.

Wash fillets in a mixture of water and lemon juice and dry. Place in a covered glass baking dish. Melt butter in a pan over medium heat. Add mushrooms, sprinkle with ½ teaspoon seasoned salt. Cook for 2 minutes. Stir in water and wine. Bring to a boil and pour over fish. Cover, place in oven, and poach for 15 minutes. For salmon, allow 5 minutes additional cooking time.

TOTAL GRAMS 10.4
GRAMS PER SERVING 2.6

Halibut Roll-Ups

4 servings

2 pounds halibut fillets
seasoned salt
3 slices bacon, diced
¼ pound shiitake mushrooms, sliced
¼ cup celery, diced
2 tablespoons onion, diced
1 clove garlic, minced
1 tablespoon parsley, minced
3 tablespoons sweet butter, melted
½ cup dry white wine
¼ cup Parmesan cheese
paprika to taste

Preheat oven to 350° F.

Sprinkle fillets with salt. Allow to stand for about 10 minutes. Place in a glass baking dish.

In skillet, sauté bacon, mushrooms, celery, and onion until vegetables are soft and bacon is crisp. Add garlic and cook 2 minutes more. Add parsley, and blend well.

Spread mixture over fillets, roll up, and fasten with toothpicks.

Place 1 tablespoon melted butter in bottom of baking dish. Add fish. Pour remaining butter over fish, and add wine.

Sprinkle with Parmesan cheese and paprika.

Bake for ½ hour.

TOTAL GRAMS 11.6
GRAMS PER SERVING 2.9

Fabulous Flounder

6 servings

3 pounds flounder fillets
lemon juice
salt and pepper
1 teaspoon dried tarragon
2 cups sour cream
1 tablespoon minced chives and parsley

Preheat oven to 350° F.

Oil a baking dish just large enough to hold fish fillets. Rub fillets with lemon juice, salt, and pepper, and place in dish.

Sprinkle with tarragon. Cover with sour cream and bake for 20 minutes, or until fish flakes easily.

Remove from oven, and sprinkle with chives and parsley. Serve immediately.

TOTAL GRAMS 22.5
GRAMS PER SERVING 3.8

Stuffed Flounder

6 servings

2 pounds flounder fillets
salt to taste
3 slices bacon, diced
¼ pound shiitake mushrooms, sliced
¼ cup diced celery
2 tablespoons diced onion
1 clove garlic, diced fine
1 tablespoon parsley, minced
3 tablespoons butter, melted
½ cup dry white wine
¼ cup grated Parmesan cheese
paprika

Preheat oven to 350° F.

Sprinkle fillets with salt. Allow to stand for about 10 minutes.

Sauté bacon, mushrooms, celery, and onion in a nonstick skillet until vegetables are soft and bacon crisp. Add garlic. Cook for 2 minutes more. Add parsley, and blend well.

Spread mixture over fillets, roll them up, and fasten with toothpicks. Place 1 tablespoon melted butter in bottom of baking dish. Add fish.

Pour remaining butter over fish, and add wine.

Sprinkle with Parmesan cheese and paprika.

Bake for ½ hour.

TOTAL GRAMS 11.7
GRAMS PER SERVING 2.0

Fennel Red Snapper

4 servings

4 fillets of red snapper, about 1½ pounds
½ stick butter, softened
1 teaspoon fennel seeds
½ teaspoon lemon juice
¼ teaspoon dried tarragon
1 clove garlic, minced
seasoned salt to taste
¼ cup olive oil
1 teaspoon grated lemon rind
½ bay leaf

Wash and dry fish. Combine butter, fennel seeds, lemon juice, tarragon, garlic, and salt. Spread butter mixture on fish fillets, roll them up, and fasten with toothpicks.

Combine oil, lemon rind, and bay leaf in baking dish. Add fish and marinate in refrigerator for 1 hour. Turn once. Drain fish and reserve marinade.

Preheat oven to 350° F.

Bake for 45 minutes. Serve with warmed marinade on side.

TOTAL GRAMS 1.5
GRAMS PER SERVING 0.4

Trout in Tomato Sauce

4 servings

4 trout fillets, about 1½ pounds
5 tablespoons tomato sauce
8 tablespoons cider vinegar
3 tablespoons olive oil
1 tablespoon minced onion
4 drops Tabasco sauce (optional)
½ packet sugar substitute

Cut fish into ½-inch pieces. Arrange attractively in shallow serving dish.

Combine remaining ingredients. Mix well. Pour over fish and cover. Place in refrigerator for 24 hours.

Preheat oven to 350° F.

Bake, uncovered for 45 minutes.

TOTAL GRAMS 13.4
GRAMS PER SERVING 3.4

Fresh Spring Salmon Mousse

10 servings

2 envelopes unflavored gelatin
1½ cups cold water
⅔ cup sour cream
1 cup mayonnaise
1½ pounds fresh salmon, cooked, skinned, and boned
½ teaspoon onion powder
1 tablespoon capers, drained
2 teaspoons dill
1 cup cucumbers, seeded, chopped, and peeled
1 teaspoon salt

Soften gelatin in cold water. Heat until completely dissolved. Cool.

Mix sour cream and mayonnaise together. Add gelatin, and chill until slightly thickened.

Flake salmon and add onion powder, capers, dill, cucumbers, and salt. Mix well with sour cream and mayonnaise.

Pour into 5-cup mold. Refrigerate until firm.

Unmold and serve.

TOTAL GRAMS 17.4
GRAMS PER SERVING 1.7

Tuna Loaf

4 servings

2 cups canned tuna, drained, or 1 pound fresh tuna, poached, skinned and boned
2 teaspoons diced onion
2 teaspoons capers
1 cup mayonnaise
½ cup water
½ cup heavy cream
½ teaspoon salt
¼ teaspoon paprika
½ teaspoon curry, or to taste

Preheat oven to 350° F.

Drain fish. In a small bowl flake fish. Add onion and capers to fish.

Combine mayonnaise, water, cream, salt, and paprika. Stir until smooth.

Add half the sauce to fish and mix. Place mixture in buttered loaf pan or baking dish. Bake for 30 minutes.

Add curry to remaining sauce. To serve, slice fish loaf and spoon sauce over slices.

TOTAL GRAMS 8.4
GRAMS PER SERVING 2.1

Oriental Shrimp

2 servings

2 tablespoons butter
2 tablespoons onion, chopped
3 slices boiled ham, cut into strips
1 clove garlic, minced
½ cup bean sprouts
¼ head cabbage, shredded
1 pound raw shrimp, shelled and deveined
4 servings Fish Stock *(page 71)*
paprika

Preheat oven to 350° F.

Melt butter in saucepan, add onion, and sauté until soft. Add ham and garlic, and sauté for 3 minutes. Add bean sprouts, and sauté for about 3 or 4 minutes until lightly browned.

Place shrimp in small casserole. Add uncooked cabbage to bean sprout mixture. Spread over shrimp.

Pour *Fish Stock* over all. Sprinkle with paprika. Cover dish with lid or aluminum foil and bake for 30 minutes.

TOTAL GRAMS 21.6
GRAMS PER SERVING 5.4

Shrimp Parmesan

4 servings

2 tablespoons olive oil
½ cup onion, minced
2 cloves garlic, minced
2 pounds raw shrimp, shelled and deveined
8 ounces tomato sauce
½ cup clam broth
1 teaspoon basil
¼ teaspoon oregano
2 teaspoons salt
pepper to taste
8 ounces shredded mozzarella cheese
¼ cup grated Parmesan cheese

Preheat broiler

Heat 1 tablespoon oil in skillet. Sauté onion until golden, add garlic, and sauté 1 minute.

Add shrimp and sauté for 3 minutes, remove from pan and place in a baking dish.

In skillet, heat remainder of oil, add tomato sauce, clam broth, oregano, and basil. Simmer for 15 minutes. Salt and pepper to taste.

Pour over shrimp and add shredded mozzarella cheese on top. Top with Parmesan and broil until bubbly.

TOTAL GRAMS 32.6
GRAMS PER SERVING 8.1

Shrimps and Scallops Marc

2 servings

½ pound medium shrimp, shelled and deveined
generous dash seasoned salt
generous dash garlic powder
1 egg, beaten
¼ cup grated Parmesan cheese

½ pound sea scallops
¼ cup heavy cream
2 tablespoons sweet butter
3 strips cooked bacon, diced
¼ cup dry white wine
¼ cup heavy cream
tarragon

Sprinkle shrimp with salt and garlic powder. Dip shrimp in egg and then coat with Parmesan cheese.

Sprinkle scallops with additional salt and garlic powder, dip into heavy cream, and then coat with Parmesan cheese.

Melt butter in pan. Add bacon, scallops, and shrimp. Brown on both sides; add wine and simmer for 10 minutes. Add ¼ cup cream and simmer gently for 10 minutes longer. Garnish with tarragon.

Total Grams 13.6
Grams per Serving 6.8

Broiled Tarragon Lobster Tails

2 servings

4 frozen lobster tails, thawed
½ stick butter
1 tablespoon fresh chopped ginger (or ½ tablespoon dried)
1 teaspoon dried tarragon
½ teaspoon dry mustard
seasoned salt

Preheat broiler.

Remove soft part of lobster tail with scissors. Hit hard shell slightly with mallet or cleaver to make it lie flat. Melt butter. Add ginger, tarragon, mustard, and salt. Spoon generously over tails and allow to stand 20 minutes.

Broil about 4 inches from heat for 10–15 minutes with meaty side up. Baste often.

TOTAL GRAMS 2.8
GRAMS PER SERVING 1.4

Crabmeat Almond Pie

8 servings

¼ cup chopped toasted almonds (see Toasted Nuts *recipe, page 67)*
2 eggs plus 2 egg yolks
2 teaspoons Dijon mustard
2 teaspoons seasoned salt
2 tablespoons chives, minced
2 cups grated fontina cheese
4 ounces frozen or canned, drained crabmeat
1½ cups heavy cream

Preheat oven to 300° F.

Place toasted almonds on the bottom of 9-inch pie plate.

Put eggs and yolks in bowl and beat well. Add mustard, salt, chives, cheese, and crabmeat.

Scald heavy cream by bringing it right to the boiling point (do not boil).

Add heavy cream to mixture and pour into pie plate.

Bake for 1 hour.

TOTAL GRAMS 40.7
GRAMS PER SERVING 5.1

Curried Crabmeat

4 servings

¾ *cup onion, chopped*
¼ *cup olive oil*
2 tablespoons curry powder
1 pound lump crabmeat, flaked and picked over for bones
2 tablespoons fresh parsley, minced
¼ *teaspoon crushed red pepper*
2 tablespoons lemon juice
½ *teaspoon seasoned salt*
½ *teaspoon black pepper*
¼ *teaspoon oregano*
½ *cup grated Parmesan cheese*
2 tablespoons butter
1 lemon, cut into wedges
Preheat broiler.

Sauté onion in oil until soft. Add curry powder and cook, stirring constantly, for 1 minute.

Stir in crabmeat, parsley, and red pepper, and sauté for 2 minutes. Add lemon juice, salt, pepper, and oregano. Sauté for 1 minute more.

Divide crabmeat mixture among 4 buttered scallop shells or small baking cups, sprinkle each serving with Parmesan cheese, and dot tops with butter. Put shells under broiler for 2–3 minutes, or until cheese is golden. Serve with wedges of lemon.

TOTAL GRAMS 26.6
GRAMS PER SERVING   6.7

Houston's Ceviche

4 servings

1 pound fresh whitefish cut into bite-size pieces
½ pound medium shrimp, shelled and deveined
½ pound bay scallops
juice of 6 limes
juice of 4 lemons
3 tablespoons garlic, minced
6 slices ginger root, peeled
1 medium onion, sliced thin
1 teaspoon cilantro, minced

Wash and dry fish and shellfish. Mix all remaining ingredients together. Place in a glass baking dish just large enough to fit fish, shrimp, and scallops. Mix fish, shellfish, and citrus mixture and refrigerate for 2 days until fish and shellfish "cook." The fish and shellfish will be opaque and appear to have been cooked.

Serve cold.

TOTAL GRAMS 49.6
GRAMS PER SERVING 12.4

Pasta

Manicotti

12 crepes

1 recipe Pasta Sauce *(pages 179–180)*
1 recipe Pasta *(page 155)*
Stuffing for Pasta:
1 pound ricotta cheese
6 ounces mozzarella cheese
2 teaspoons parsley
5 tablespoons grated Parmesan cheese
2 eggs

Preheat oven to 300° F.

Prepare 7 cups *Pasta Sauce* and 12 *Pasta Crepes*; set aside.

In a bowl mix ricotta cheese, mozzarella cheese, parsley, 2 tablespoons Parmesan cheese, and eggs.

Cover the bottom of large baking pan with thin layer of *Pasta Sauce*.

Place about 3 full tablespoons of ricotta mixture in center of crepe. Roll crepe around stuffing. Place crepe in baking pan, seam side down. Repeat with each crepe, placing them side by side in baking pan. Pour remaining sauce over crepes.

Sprinkle remaining 3 tablespoons Parmesan cheese on top. Bake for 20 minutes.

TOTAL GRAMS 97.0
GRAMS PER MANICOTTI 7.6

Gnocchi

8 servings

1 pound ricotta cheese, pressed of liquid
½ pound cream cheese or Boursin cheese
3 eggs, beaten
2 tablespoons soy flour
dash of salt, cayenne pepper, and nutmeg
½ pound sweet butter, melted
½ cup grated Parmesan cheese

Push ricotta cheese and cream cheese through a fine strainer. (The easiest and fastest way is with your hands.)

Beat eggs into mixture with electric or rotary beater. Blend in soy flour and seasonings. Refrigerate for about 1 hour. Bring large pot of water to rolling boil. Lower heat to simmer. Drop cheese mixture into water by teaspoonfuls. (They will drop and then rise to the top.)

Allow gnocchi to poach (simmer on top of water) for about 20 minutes. Remove gnocchi carefully with a slotted spoon and allow to drain on paper towel.

Melt ¼ pound butter in large baking dish. Place drained gnocchi in dish. Cover with remaining melted butter and grated Parmesan cheese.

Gnocchi may be served immediately, kept warm in a low oven or refrigerated and reheated.

The substitution of Boursin for cream cheese will give you a much spicier gnocchi. Adding ¼ package of frozen spinach that has been thawed and squeezed dry makes a delicious Spinach Gnocchi.

TOTAL GRAMS 27.2
GRAMS PER SERVING 3.4

Enchiladas

6 servings

1 recipe Pasta *(page 155)*
1½ pounds pork, ground
3 cloves garlic, minced
3 teaspoons chili powder
3 tablespoons cider vinegar
1 tablespoon oil
3 tablespoons chopped onion
1 8-ounce can tomato sauce
1 cup water
½ teaspoon cumin
1 teaspoon chili powder
6 drops Tabasco sauce, or to taste
1 teaspoon salt, or to taste
1½ cups shredded Cheddar cheese

Prepare *Pasta* recipe. Place *Pasta* on wax paper, and set aside.

Preheat oven to 350° F.

In bowl combine ground pork, garlic, 2 teaspoons chili powder, and vinegar.

Heat oil in skillet, and sauté onion over medium heat for 3 or 4 minutes until soft.

Add pork mixture to onion, and brown. Cook thoroughly. Pour off all fat. Set aside.

Sauce:

In saucepan combine tomato sauce, water, cumin, chili powder, Tabasco sauce, and salt. Simmer for ½ hour.

Pour ½ cup sauce in 13×9-inch baking pan. Fill crepes with 2 tablespoons pork and 1 tablespoon cheese. Fold over and place crepes seam side down in baking pan. Repeat until you use all crepes. Pour remaining sauce over all. Bake for 15 minutes. Cover with remaining cheese. Bake for 5 minutes more or until cheese is hot and bubbly.

TOTAL GRAMS 44.4
GRAMS PER SERVING 7.4

Pasta

12 crepes

⅓ cup soy flour
½ cup water
3 eggs
1 tablespoon oil

Put all ingredients in blender. Blend until smooth. Use a crepe pan or a 5- or 6-inch skillet. Cover bottom of pan lightly with small amount of oil. When pan is hot enough to sizzle a drop of water, pour about 3 tablespoons of crepe mixture into pan. Tilt pan to distribute mixture evenly. Crepes should be thin. Lightly brown on both sides (about 1 minute on each side). Place on wax paper until all crepes are finished.

The crepes are very delicate, so handle carefully. If you have trouble the first time, try again. Oil pan again if necessary.

They can be made a day ahead and stored in refrigerator separated by sheets of wax paper.

TOTAL GRAMS 10.8
GRAMS PER SERVING 0.9

Cannelloni

4 servings

3 chicken livers
1 boned chicken breast
4 tablespoons butter
5 thin slices prosciutto ham
¼ teaspoon marjoram
¾ cup grated Parmesan cheese
1 recipe Cream Sauce *(page 177)*
1 recipe Pasta *(page 155)*

Sauté chicken livers and chicken breast in butter over medium heat until brown on both sides. Grind livers, chicken breast, and prosciutto in food grinder with medium blade. Mix in marjoram and ½ cup grated Parmesan cheese. Add 10 tablespoons *Cream Sauce*. Place 2 tablespoons chicken mixture in center of each crepe. Roll up crepes.

Butter baking dish, and place crepes seam side down. Cover with remaining sauce and Parmesan cheese. Bake for 1½ hours.

TOTAL GRAMS 13.0
GRAMS PER SERVING 3.3

Bread

4 Grain and Seed Bread

12 slices

1 tablespoon unbleached flour
1 tablespoon whole wheat flour
1 tablespoon sesame seeds
1 tablespoon cornmeal
½ teaspoon baking powder
2 eggs, separated
1 packet sugar substitute
⅛ teaspoon seasoned salt
2 tablespoons ricotta cheese, whole milk
2 tablespoons butter
⅛ teaspoon cream of tartar
1 tablespoon pumpkin seeds

Preheat oven to 350° F.

Mix flours, seeds, cornmeal, and baking powder together. Beat in egg yolks. Sprinkle with sugar substitute and seasoned salt. Mix cheese with butter. Add dry ingredients to cheese mixture and blend well.

Beat egg whites with cream of tartar until stiff. Fold into cheese mixture.

Spoon into a small, oiled loaf pan. Sprinkle with pumpkin seeds and bake for 50 minutes. Cool on a wire rack.

TOTAL GRAMS 24.6
GRAMS PER SERVING 2.1

Rye Bread

12 slices

2 tablespoons unbleached flour
1 tablespoon whole wheat flour
1 tablespoon rye flour
1 tablespoon caraway seeds
½ teaspoon baking powder
1 packet sugar substitute
2 eggs, separated
⅛ teaspoon seasoned salt
2 tablespoons ricotta cheese
2 tablespoons butter, melted
⅛ tablespoon cream of tartar

Preheat oven to 350° F.

Mix flours and caraway seeds together. Beat in egg yolks and sprinkle with seasoned salt and sugar substitute. Mix cheese with butter, add dry ingredients, and blend well. Beat egg whites with cream of tartar until stiff. Spoon into a small oiled loaf pan and bake for 50 minutes. Remove from oven and cool on rack.

TOTAL GRAMS 23.7
GRAMS PER SERVING 2.0

Zucchini Bread

12 slices

2 tablespoons unbleached flour
1 tablespoon whole wheat flour
1 cup zucchini, grated and pressed to remove liquid
½ teaspoon baking powder
¼ teaspoon seasoned salt
1 packet sugar substitute
2 eggs, separated
2 tablespoons ricotta cheese
2 tablespoons grated Parmesan cheese
⅛ teaspoon cream of tartar
10 walnuts

Preheat oven to 350° F.

Mix flours, salt, sugar substitute, baking powder, and zucchini. Beat in one egg yolk at a time. Mix in ricotta and Parmesan cheeses. Beat egg whites with cream of tartar until stiff. Spoon into small loaf pan and place walnut halves on top.

Bake for 50 minutes. Remove from oven and cool on a rack.

TOTAL GRAMS 34.7
GRAMS PER SERVING 2.9

Vegetables

Eggplant Parmigiana

8 servings

1 large eggplant, cut into ½-inch slices
4 tablespoons olive oil
1 large onion, chopped
2 cloves garlic, minced
1 pound chuck, ground
1 8-ounce can tomato sauce
1 cup water
1 teaspoon oregano
½ cup grated Parmesan cheese
1 8-ounce package mozzarella cheese, sliced

Preheat oven to 350° F.

Soak eggplant in salted water for 1 hour. Dry with paper towels.

Heat 2 tablespoons olive oil in a skillet and lightly brown chopped onion. Add garlic and sauté one more minute. Add ground chuck, stir and cook. When meat turns brown, add tomato sauce and water. Simmer for 15 minutes. Place remaining olive oil in a separate large skillet over medium heat, and sauté a few eggplant slices at a time until golden brown; add a little more oil if needed.

Oil a baking dish and arrange half of the eggplant slices on the bottom. Cover with half of the tomato mixture. Sprinkle with half of the Parmesan cheese and half of the mozzarella. Repeat these layers.

Bake for 25 to 30 minutes until golden brown.

TOTAL GRAMS 62.6
GRAMS PER SERVING 7.8

Broccoli in Cheese Sauce

6 servings

1 pound broccoli
1 recipe Cheese Sauce *(page 183)*

Prepare broccoli by removing hard stem and reserving florets. Place in a steamer and steam for 10 to 15 minutes, depending on how soft you like your vegetables. Serve with *Cheese Sauce* (3 tablespoons per serving).

TOTAL GRAMS 35.7
GRAMS PER SERVING 5.9

Baked Spinach

4 servings

¾ cup cooked spinach
3 tablespoons olive oil
3 tablespoons butter
3 tablespoons onion, minced
1 clove garlic, minced
2 slices prosciutto, diced
5 eggs
3 tablespoons heavy cream
pinch of black pepper
3 tablespoons grated Parmesan cheese

Preheat oven to 350° F.
    Heat olive oil and butter in skillet.
    Add onion, garlic, and prosciutto to skillet. Cook slowly until onion is light brown. Add onion mixture to spinach, and place in a baking dish.
    Beat eggs with cream, and add pepper. Pour over spinach. Sprinkle with Parmesan cheese.
    Bake for 30 minutes, or until set.

TOTAL GRAMS 13.9
GRAMS PER SERVING 3.5

Stuffed Zippy Zucchini

4 servings

2 medium-size zucchini
3 ounces ricotta cheese
1 teaspoon minced parsley
1 onion, chopped
1 egg white, beaten stiff
1 8-ounce can tomato sauce

Preheat oven to 300° F.

Cut zucchini into halves lengthwise and scoop out pulp, leaving a ½-inch shell.

Combine ricotta, parsley, and onion. Mix well. Fold in egg white.

Stuff mixture into halved zucchini. Place in baking dish and pour tomato sauce over top.

Bake for 10 minutes. Lower heat to 250° F. and cook for 30 more minutes. Baste often.

TOTAL GRAMS 42.7
GRAMS PER SERVING 10.7

Zucchini Stuffed with Cream Sauce

6 servings

6 medium-size zucchini
3 tablespoons mayonnaise
2 tablespoons grated Parmesan cheese
½ cup sliced mushrooms
4 slices lean prosciutto, diced
1 egg yolk
1 teaspoon salt
½ teaspoon pepper
½ teaspoon oregano
3 tablespoons olive oil

Preheat oven to 375° F.

Cut zucchini into halves lengthwise. Scoop out pulp and reserve.

Mix together pulp from zucchini, mayonnaise, Parmesan cheese, mushrooms, prosciutto, egg yolk, salt, pepper, and oregano.

Place zucchini halves in greased baking dish and fill each zucchini half with mixture. Sprinkle with olive oil. Bake for 30 minutes.

TOTAL GRAMS 50.6
GRAMS PER SERVING 8.4

String Beans Almandine

4 servings

1 pound fresh or frozen string beans
½ pound shiitake mushrooms, sliced
4 tablespoons butter
½ teaspoon seasoned salt
¼ cup slivered almonds

Prepare string beans for cooking. Simmer in small amount of water for 10 minutes. In a skillet sauté mushrooms in butter until brown. Add salt and almonds.

Add string beans to skillet. Toss well. Simmer for 4 minutes. Correct seasoning to taste.

TOTAL GRAMS 43.2
GRAMS PER SERVING 10.8

Mock Potato Dumplings

12 dumplings

½ head cauliflower (1 cup mashed)
2 eggs, beaten
½ cup grated Parmesan cheese
1 teaspoon parsley
1 teaspoon nutmeg
4 tablespoons soy flour
1 tablespoon salt
4 tablespoons butter

Boil cauliflower until soft, for about 25 minutes. Mash with fork or potato masher.

Add eggs, Parmesan cheese, parsley, nutmeg, and soy flour. Shape into walnut-size balls.

Bring large pot of water to rolling boil. Add salt. Drop cauliflower balls into water. When they rise, remove with slotted spoon.

Heat butter in skillet. Fry balls until brown on all sides. Drain on paper towel.

TOTAL GRAMS 18.1
GRAMS PER SERVING 1.5

Chinese Snow Pea Pods

6 servings

2 tablespoons vegetable oil
1 onion, chopped fine
1 clove garlic, chopped fine
½ teaspoon seasoned salt
¼ cup sliced water chestnuts
½ pound snow pea pods
1 tablespoon Tamari soy sauce
¼ cup Chicken Stock *(page 68)*

Heat oil in heavy skillet. Add onion, garlic, salt, and water chestnuts. Sauté until onion is golden. Add pea pods, soy sauce, and *Chicken Stock.* Cover and cook for 5 minutes. Uncover and cook for 5 more minutes.

TOTAL GRAMS 28.4
GRAMS PER SERVING 4.7

Eggplant Little Shoes

8 servings

4 medium eggplants
2 tablespoons butter
4 tablespoons onion
1 clove garlic
1 pound beef or lamb, ground
1 8-ounce can tomato sauce
1 teaspoon cumin
1 teaspoon parsley
1 teaspoon seasoned salt
pepper to taste
1 egg
1 tablespoon water
1 tablespoon lemon juice
¼ cup grated Parmesan cheese

Preheat oven to 350° F.

Wash eggplants. Do not peel. Parboil whole eggplants in salted boiling water for 5 minutes. Remove. Cut in half lengthwise. Spoon out center pulp carefully and chop, leaving about ¼-inch around rim.

Melt butter in saucepan. Add onion and garlic. Sauté for 3 minutes. Add meat and eggplant pulp. Stir. Brown lightly. Add tomato sauce, cumin, parsley, salt, and pepper. Cook over low heat until all liquid is absorbed.

Place eggplants in lightly oiled roasting pan or large casserole dish. Stuff with chopped meat mixture. Beat egg, water, and lemon juice together. Pour over eggplants. Sprinkle with Parmesan cheese. Bake for 20 minutes until lightly browned.

TOTAL GRAMS 57.2
GRAMS PER SERVING 7.2

Cheese-Stuffed Eggplant

8 servings

4 medium-size eggplants
2 medium-size onions, chopped
3 tablespoons butter
3 cups crumbled feta cheese
½ cup grated Parmesan cheese
¼ cup ricotta cheese
1 egg
2 tablespoons chopped parsley
seasoned salt

Preheat oven to 350° F.

Slice eggplants in half. Scoop out pulp, chop it, and set aside. Reserve shells. Sauté onions in butter until golden. Add eggplant pulp and continue to sauté for about 5 more minutes. Transfer mixture to bowl and let cool. Add cheeses to mixture; beat in egg and parsley. Stuff mixture in eggplant shells. Sprinkle with salt. Bake for 40 minutes.

TOTAL GRAMS 62.3
GRAMS PER SERVING 7.8

The Most Delicious Cucumbers

4 servings

4 cucumbers, peeled and seeded
½ tablespoon seasoned salt
½ tablespoon tarragon vinegar
¼ cup butter, melted
1 tablespoon minced dill
1 tablespoon minced chives
1 tablespoon minced onion
¼ cup heavy cream
2 tablespoons minced parsley
grated Parmesan cheese

Preheat oven to 375° F.

Slice cucumbers to bite-size pieces. Add salt and vinegar. Allow to stand at room temperature for at least 2 hours. Drain and dry thoroughly with paper towels.

Put cucumbers in casserole with butter, dill, chives, and onion. Bake for 25 minutes.

Remove from oven; add heavy cream. Stir over medium heat on top of stove for about 5 minutes (do not allow to boil). Cream will thicken. Sprinkle with parsley and small amount of Parmesan cheese. Serve hot.

TOTAL GRAMS 23.2
GRAMS PER SERVING 5.8

Crazy Cabbage

8 servings

1 cabbage, trimmed
1 onion, chopped
¼ pound bacon
2 garlic cloves
2 tablespoons olive oil
¼ cup chopped parsley
1 egg
1 tablespoon grated Parmesan cheese
1 cup Chicken Stock *(page 68)*
seasoned salt

Preheat oven to 375° F.

Boil cabbage in salted water for 15 minutes. Remove and run under cold water. Core cabbage, leaving outer leaves intact. Chop core and inner leaves. Sauté cabbage, onion, bacon, and garlic together in olive oil.

Mix parsley with egg and Parmesan cheese. Beat well.

Mix egg mixture into sautéed cabbage.

Oil a deep casserole. Place large outer cabbage leaves in casserole. Fill middle with sautéed mixture. Pour *Chicken Stock* over mixture. Add seasoned salt to taste. Cover and bake for 1 hour. Remove cover and bake for 30 more minutes. Serve.

TOTAL GRAMS 37.4
GRAMS PER SERVING 4.7

Ratatouille

12 ½-cup servings

4½ tablespoons olive oil
3 medium-size zucchini, unpeeled, quartered, cut into 1-inch lengths
½ medium-size eggplant, unpeeled, cut into 1½-inch cubes
salt and pepper to taste
2 medium-size onions, chopped
5 cloves garlic, finely minced
2 green peppers, seeded and chopped
1 8-ounce can tomato sauce
½ teaspoon thyme
1 teaspoon basil
¼ cup finely chopped parsley
lemon wedges

Preheat oven to 350° F.

Heat 2½ tablespoons olive oil in large skillet, add zucchini, eggplant, salt, and pepper. Cook, stirring occasionally, for about 10 minutes.

Heat remaining 2 tablespoons olive oil in another skillet. Add onions, garlic, and peppers, and cook until lightly browned. Add tomato sauce and simmer, stirring occasionally, for about 10 minutes.

Add zucchini and eggplant mixture, then thyme, basil, and parsley. Pour in casserole, cover, and bake for about 20 minutes, or until vegetables are tender.

Can be served warm, or cold with lemon wedges.

TOTAL GRAMS 73.7
GRAMS PER SERVING 6.1

Basic Fried Green Tomatoes

Not always available, I treat green tomatoes like jewels when I have them. The following recipes are easy to prepare and enjoy.

1 green tomato, washed and sliced
1 tablespoon garlic oil
1 tablespoon sweet butter

Heat garlic oil and butter together in small nonstick skillet. Place tomato slices in skillet and fry over medium heat on both sides until brown.

TOTAL GRAMS 6.3

Variation 1: Sprinkle with sugar substitute while cooking.
Variation 2: Sprinkle with seasoned salt while cooking.
Variation 3: Dip tomatoes in egg and then in grated Parmesan cheese before frying.

TOTAL GRAMS 7.3

Variation 4: Spoon ½ teaspoon of white wine on each slice as it cooks.

TOTAL GRAMS 6.5

Variation 5: When finished frying, place a slice of Gruyère cheese and crumbled bacon on top of each slice and broil until cheese begins to bubble.

TOTAL GRAMS 6.4

Variation 6: Top with warm goat cheese and serve on lettuce, garnished with ½ avocado for a delicious lunch salad.

TOTAL GRAMS 13.6

Porcini Mushrooms

4 servings

4 large porcini mushrooms
2 tablespoons butter
2 tablespoons garlic oil
2 tablespoons white wine
4 tablespoons mascarpone cheese
2 tablespoons Tamari soy sauce

Wash, dry, and cut off stems of mushrooms, leaving caps intact.

Heat butter and garlic oil in a large skillet. Add mushrooms and cook for 3 minutes over medium heat. Turn once. Add wine to the pan. Turn mushrooms again. Place 1 tablespoon of mascarpone cheese in center of each mushroom. Sprinkle with soy sauce. Cook 1 minute longer and serve hot.

TOTAL GRAMS 12.6
GRAMS PER SERVING   3.2

Spicy Cauliflower Bake

6 servings

2 tablespoons butter
½ onion, minced
4 cloves garlic, minced
2 cups cauliflower, chopped
2 eggs, beaten
1 cup Parmesan cheese
5 slices bacon, cooked crisp and crumbled

Preheat oven to 350° F.

Heat butter in a skillet. Add onions and garlic and cook until onions turn golden. Add cauliflower and continue to cook 1 minute more. Remove to a bowl. Add eggs, Parmesan cheese, and crumbled bacon.

Spoon into a buttered baking dish. Bake for 1 hour, or until brown.

TOTAL GRAMS 21.5
GRAMS PER SERVING 3.6

Crispy White Radish

2 servings

1 medium daikon white radish
garlic oil
seasoned salt

Using the large holes on a four-sided grater, shred radish. Fill a 9-inch skillet ¼ full with garlic oil. Heat oil until very hot. Fry radish until golden brown. Remove from oil with slotted spoon and drain on brown paper. Sprinkle with seasoned salt.

Better than French fries!

TOTAL GRAMS 3.6
GRAMS PER SERVING 1.8

Cheesy Brussels Sprouts

4 servings

20 Brussels sprouts, washed and trimmed
garlic oil
2 tablespoons grated Parmesan cheese

Slice Brussels sprouts in half. Heat enough garlic oil to ¼ fill a skillet. Fry Brussels sprouts until golden on both sides.

Remove with a slotted spoon and allow to drain on brown paper. Place in a bowl and toss with Parmesan cheese.

TOTAL GRAMS 34.4
GRAMS PER SERVING 8.6

Rutabaga Home Fries

6 servings

½ large rutabaga, peeled and quartered
2 tablespoons of sweet butter
2 medium-size onions, sliced thin
5 shiitake mushrooms, sliced thin

Boil rutabaga in water until fork-soft. Drain and return to pan. Heat 2 minutes more to dry. Slice to size of half dollars.

Melt butter in a nonstick skillet. Add onions and sauté until transparent. Add mushrooms and continue sautéing until soft. Add rutabagas and sauté until brown and crisp.

TOTAL GRAMS 51.1
GRAMS PER SERVING 8.5

Irene's Turnips

4 servings

4 medium-size turnips, trimmed
seasoned salt to taste
2 tablespoons sweet butter
3 slices no-nitrate bacon

Boil turnips in salted water until fork-soft. Drain well and, using a potato masher, mash turnips with butter until smooth. Cook bacon in a nonstick skillet. Remove bacon and leave fat in pan. Spoon turnips into pan and sauté in bacon fat until turnips absorb fat. Remove to a bowl, crumble bacon on top and serve.

TOTAL GRAMS 38.6
GRAMS PER SERVING 9.7

Chic Asparagus

4 servings

1 pound asparagus
3 tablespoons extra-virgin olive oil
2 tablespoons white wine
2 ounces goat cheese
2 sun-dried tomatoes in olive oil, minced

Wash and trim asparagus, and place in a glass baking dish. Mix olive oil and wine together and sprinkle over asparagus. Dot with goat cheese and sun-dried tomatoes. Microwave on low speed for 5 minutes or until crisp-tender.

TOTAL GRAMS 21.4
GRAMS PER SERVING 5.4

Green Bean Chokes

4 servings

1 pound green beans
1 6-ounce jar marinated artichoke hearts, undrained
2 ounces Parmesan cheese shavings

Wash green beans and cut off ends. Place in a glass baking dish. Top with marinade from artichokes. Quarter artichoke hearts and spread over string beans. Add Parmesan shavings. Place in a microwave oven and cook at low speed for 5 minutes.

TOTAL GRAMS 43.2
GRAMS PER SERVING 10.8

Sauces

Cream Sauce

24 tablespoons

¼ pound sweet butter
3 egg yolks
¼ cup water
¼ cup heavy cream
dash of nutmeg

Place butter in top of double boiler over hot (not boiling) water. Add egg yolks one at a time. Beat constantly with rotary or hand electric beater. Add water and heavy cream. Continue to beat until sauce thickens, about 7 to 10 minutes. Add nutmeg as a garnish.

TOTAL GRAMS 4.1
GRAMS PER TABLESPOON 0.2

Frozen Horseradish Cream

19 tablespoons

1 cup heavy cream
2 tablespoons white horseradish
1 teaspoon seasoned salt
2 teaspoons Dijon mustard

Whip heavy cream until stiff.

Mix together horseradish, salt, and mustard. Carefully fold mixture into whipped cream. Freeze until firm.

TOTAL GRAMS 10.5
GRAMS PER TABLESPOON 0.6

Hollandaise Sauce

24 tablespoons

2 tablespoons tarragon vinegar
½ teaspoon seasoned salt
1 tablespoon cold water
4 egg yolks
2 sticks butter, at room temperature
1 teaspoon lemon juice
1 tablespoon heavy cream

Combine vinegar and salt in saucepan and cook rapidly to reduce by half. Remove from heat and add water. Place yolks in saucepan and beat with wire whisk until creamy. Place pan over double boiler and add butter a little at a time, beating with whisk as butter is melting. When sauce is thick, add lemon juice and heavy cream. Beat again. Keep warm until ready to serve.

TOTAL GRAMS 3.0
GRAMS PER TABLESPOON 0.1

Tartare Sauce

15 tablespoons

¾ cup mayonnaise
1 tablespoon tarragon vinegar
1 teaspoon finely chopped onion
1 teaspoon capers, drained
1 teaspoon finely chopped pickles
1 teaspoon finely chopped olives
1 teaspoon finely chopped parsley

Combine all ingredients. Mix well.
    Store in covered jar in refrigerator. Will keep for several weeks.

TOTAL GRAMS 4.6
GRAMS PER TABLESPOON 0.3

Cocktail Sauce

16 tablespoons

1 8-ounce can tomato sauce
1 tablespoon horseradish
1 teaspoon Worcestershire sauce
1 teaspoon lemon juice

Mix all ingredients. Chill thoroughly.

TOTAL GRAMS 19.2
GRAMS PER TABLESPOON 1.2

Pasta Sauce

24 ¹/₂-cup servings

2 pork chops
5 tablespoons olive oil
6 8-ounce cans tomato sauce
3 8-ounce cans water
3 large cloves garlic, minced
1 teaspoon salt
1 pound sweet or hot Italian sausages
1 pound chuck, ground
1 teaspoon oregano
1 teaspoon thyme
2 packets sugar substitute

Place pork chops and 2 tablespoons olive oil in a large heavy pot. Brown chops well. Add tomato sauce, water, garlic, and salt.

Bring to slow boil. Allow to simmer.

Meanwhile, place sausages in heavy skillet without any oil. Prick sausages with fork. Cook until well browned on all sides. Slice into one-half-inch pieces. Drain well and discard drippings. Add to pork chop mixture.

Brown ground chuck in skillet with 3 tablespoons olive oil. As chuck is browning, slowly break up into small pieces. When meat is lightly browned, add to pork chop mixture.

Simmer for 3 hours, stirring occasionally.

Remove pork chops from sauce; bone, chop meat, and return to sauce.

Add oregano and thyme the last ½ hour. When mixture is finished cooking, add sugar substitute.

TOTAL GRAMS 120.6
GRAMS PER SERVING   5.0

Green Sauce for Pasta

26 tablespoons

5 cloves garlic, minced
2 tablespoons dried basil
¼ teaspoon thyme
¼ cup grated Parmesan cheese
4 tablespoons chopped walnuts
6 tablespoons olive oil
6 tablespoons butter
2 tablespoons chopped parsley

Place garlic, basil, thyme, Parmesan cheese, walnuts, and 2 teaspoons oil in blender. Blend until smooth. Add remaining oil, 2 tablespoons at a time, and blend. Serve on pasta topped with 1 tablespoon butter per serving.

TOTAL GRAMS 10.9
GRAMS PER SERVING   0.4

Mustard Sauce

20 tablespoons

4 tablespoons Dijon mustard
1 cup sour cream
2 tablespoons chopped chives

Mix ingredients well. Refrigerate.

TOTAL GRAMS 13.0
GRAMS PER TABLESPOON 0.7

Hot Barbecue Sauce

20 tablespoons

2 tablespoons butter
1 medium onion, chopped
1 clove garlic, minced
¼ cup tomato sauce
2 tablespoons wine vinegar
Tabasco sauce to taste
3 packets sugar substitute
1 teaspoon salt
1 teaspoon dry mustard
¼ cup water

Melt butter in saucepan. Sauté onion and garlic until golden. Add remaining ingredients and bring to boil. Store in covered jar and refrigerate.

TOTAL GRAMS 16.7
GRAMS PER TABLESPOON 0.8

Lemon Barbecue Sauce

12 tablespoons

1 small clove garlic
½ teaspoon salt
½ cup oil
¼ cup lemon juice
2 tablespoons chopped onion
½ teaspoon thyme
1 packet sugar substitute

Mash garlic clove in bowl. Add salt. Mix in oil and add remaining ingredients. Chill to blend flavors.

Excellent on grilled fish.

TOTAL GRAMS 8.8
GRAMS PER TABLESPOON 0.7

Cranberry Sauce

8 ½-cup servings

2½ cups fresh cranberries
1½ cups water
1 package diet lemon or orange gelatin
8 packets sugar substitute
2 tablespoons cranberry or orange liqueur
1 tablespoon No-Cal raspberry syrup
pinch salt

Cook cranberries in water over low heat until they pop open. Drain and press through sieve, and add boiling water to make 1½ cups liquid.

Dissolve gelatin, sugar substitute, liqueur, and syrup in hot liquid. Add cranberry pulp if desired.

Chill until firm. Slice to serve.

TOTAL GRAMS 48.1
GRAMS PER SERVING 6.0

Cheese Sauce

18 tablespoons

³/₄ cup heavy cream
¹/₃ cup water
³/₄ pound (1¹/₂ cups) Cheddar cheese, diced
1 teaspoon mustard
1 teaspoon salt
¹/₂ teaspoon paprika

In top of double boiler combine all ingredients. Simmer slowly over hot water, stirring constantly until smooth.

Total Grams 11.9
Grams per Tablespoon 0.7

Parsley Butter Sauce

4 2-tablespoon servings

4 sprigs parsley, chopped (tops only)
1 small clove garlic, chopped fine
¹/₄ pound sweet butter, melted
¹/₄ teaspoon Worcestershire sauce

In a skillet add parsley and garlic to melted butter. Cook for 1 minute over medium heat. Add Worcestershire sauce.
    Serve immediately.
    (If you must reheat this sauce, use very low heat.)

Total Grams 2.3
Grams per Serving 0.6

Joan's Ricotta Sauces

10 tablespoons

For Pork:
½ cup ricotta cheese
2 tablespoons olive oil
1 packet sugar substitute
1 teaspoon orange rind
¼ teaspoon nutmeg
⅛ teaspoon ground cloves
⅛ teaspoon cinnamon

Mix all ingredients together. Refrigerate for ½ hour.

TOTAL GRAMS 6.0
GRAMS PER TABLESPOON 0.6

For Chicken:
½ cup ricotta cheese
½ teaspoon curry powder
¼ teaspoon turmeric
¼ teaspoon cumin
2 tablespoons sour cream

Mix ingredients together and refrigerate for ½ hour.

TOTAL GRAMS 6.0
GRAMS PER TABLESPOON 0.6

For Fish:
½ cup ricotta cheese
2 tablespoons heavy cream
1 teaspoon tarragon
1 teaspoon grated lemon peel
1 packet sugar substitute

Mix all ingredients together and refrigerate for ½ hour.

TOTAL GRAMS 6.7
GRAMS PER TABLESPOON 0.7

Tomato Paste

8 tablespoons

10 tomatoes, chopped
½ teaspoon salt

Place tomatoes in a saucepan. Sprinkle with salt. Simmer for ½ hour uncovered. Strain, mashing pulp through strainer. Cool. Store in refrigerator.

TOTAL GRAMS 53.0
GRAMS PER TABLESPOON 6.6

Vinegar- and Sugar-Free Ketchup

40 tablespoons

2 cups Tomato Paste
½ cup lemon juice
½ cup water
½ teaspoon salt
1 teaspoon oregano
⅛ teaspoon cumin
⅛ teaspoon nutmeg
⅛ teaspoon pepper
½ teaspoon dry mustard
dash garlic powder

Place all ingredients in a blender or food processor and blend well. Refrigerate.

TOTAL GRAMS 23.6
GRAMS PER TABLESPOON 0.6

Desserts

Mac-Nut Candy

10 candies

2 tablespoons No-Cal chocolate syrup
2 packets sugar substitute
6 tablespoons unsweetened coconut
10 large macadamia nuts

Mix syrup and sweetener. Spoon over coconut and mix well. Allow flavors to blend for 2 minutes. Roll nuts in coconut mixture until well covered. Place on wax paper in freezer for 10 minutes before serving.

To store: Wrap well in wax paper and place in freezer bag.

TOTAL GRAMS 26.4
GRAMS PER SERVING 2.7

Almond Balls

12 balls

¼ teaspoon almond extract
2 packets sugar substitute
1 tablespoon coconut
3 tablespoons almond butter*
1 tablespoon mascarpone cheese

Mix almond extract and 1 packet sugar substitute. Spoon over coconut and mix well. Mix almond butter, cheese, and 1 packet sugar substitute until fully blended.

Roll into ¼-inch balls, roll in coconut, and place in freezer for 10 minutes.

To store: Wrap well in waxed paper and store in freezer bag.

TOTAL GRAMS 14.5
GRAMS PER SERVING 1.2

---

*Available at health food stores.

Almond Ball Cookies

12 cookies

1 Almond Ball *recipe (page 186)*
2 tablespoons coconut

Preheat oven to 325° F.
　Follow *Almond Ball* recipe, add coconut mixture and additional coconut.
　Drop by teaspoonsful onto greased cookie sheet.
　Bake for 10 minutes or until golden brown. Be careful not to burn bottoms.

TOTAL GRAMS 21.5
GRAMS PER SERVING 1.8

Pistachio Popcorn Balls

6 balls

1¼ cups fresh popped corn
3 tablespoons roasted pistachio nut butter*
1 dozen cold pistachio nuts

Mix all ingredients and form into tablespoon-size balls. Serve.

TOTAL GRAMS 21.1
GRAMS PER SERVING 3.5

Basic Frosting

13 tablespoons

¼ cup sugar-free vanilla pudding
2 cups heavy cream
¼ cup mascarpone cheese

---

*Available at health food stores.

¼ cup ricotta cheese
1 teaspoon vanilla extract
3 packets sugar substitute

Prepare pudding using heavy cream as liquid.

Place mascarpone, pudding, ricotta, and extract in bowl and whisk together.

Chocolate or butterscotch frosting may be made by substituting appropriate pudding flavor.

Use frosting on one of our sponge cakes.

TOTAL GRAMS 27.7
GRAMS PER SERVING 2.1

Creme Caramel

2 ½-cup servings

1 Basic Frosting *recipe (page 187)*
1 tablespoon No-Cal Pancake Syrup

Preheat oven to 350° F.

Place *Basic Frosting* in 2 small ramekins or custard cups. Bake for ½ hour or until set. Remove from oven and spoon pancake syrup on top. Serve immediately.

TOTAL GRAMS 17.2
GRAMS PER SERVING 8.6

Cannoli Custard Frosting

13 tablespoons, fills 1 cake

Follow *Basic Frosting* recipe directions and place mixture in freezer until frosting is the consistency of soft custard. May be used as cake frosting, between two cake layers, or enjoyed as a custard.

TOTAL GRAMS 14.9
GRAMS PER SERVING 1.1

Ice Cream

Ice cream is a very important part of this diet. It has long been enjoyed as the special, delicious climax of afternoon picnics, informal lunches, and formal dinners. Dr. Atkins has been known to eat it watching football on a Sunday afternoon.

Because we all love it so much, I have perfected seven (one for each day of the week) no-fail ice cream recipes. Two of the recipes (*Vanilla* and *Coffee*) you may have from the beginning of the diet. *Coconut Macadamia, Butter Pecan,* and *Maple Walnut* may be added to the Ongoing Weight Loss. Premaintenance welcomes *Raspberry Rapture* and *Chocolate*. Maintenance offers *Chunky Chocolate Fudge Ice Cream* plus two frozen yogurts and two sorbets.

Preparing these creamy delights is easy. All you need are these recipes and an ice cream maker. This may sound expensive but it need not be. Hand-churned ice cream makers sell for as low as $25. Using them is easy. The preparation time is a little longer because the custard must be refrigerated for two hours before you can churn it. The electric machines start at about $70 and go up. Two that are under $90 are The Big Chill® and Gelato Modo 11®. Both make delicious ice cream from these recipes. The custard is churned in a container you prefreeze in your freezer. The entire process takes about ½ hour once the prepared custard is cooled at room temperature. You will rejoice at the way these ice cream makers make dessert (ice cream) while you eat dinner.

Basic Ice Cream Custard

6 ½-cup servings

2 cups heavy cream
4 egg yolks
½ vanilla bean, slit open and scraped
8 packets sugar substitute

Heat cream in a heavy sauce pan over a low heat. Whisk in one egg yolk at a time. Add vanilla bean scrapings and whisk until custard begins to thicken. Remove from heat and cool. Beat one packet of sugar substitute at a time into cooled custard. At this point the custard is ready to add recipe ingredients that make it ice cream (see recipes that follow). Do not overlook the value of refrigerating the custard as it is and using it as a delicious, rich dessert. Or you could whisk in a tablespoon of brandy or brandy flavoring and serve it over berries. An elegant dessert, indeed.

TOTAL GRAMS 20.8
GRAMS PER SERVING 3.5

Chocolate Ice Cream

8 ½-cup servings

1 recipe Basic Ice Cream Custard *(page 193)*
½ cup unsweetened cocoa
2 packets sugar substitute
2 tablespoons No-Cal chocolate syrup
2 tablespoons Sugar-Free Jell-O Chocolate Instant Pudding powder

Prepare *Basic* recipe. Whisk in cocoa. Beat until smooth. Remove from stove and whisk in sugar substitute, chocolate syrup, and pudding powder. Cool to room temperature. Place custard in ice cream maker. Churn according to manufacturer's directions.

TOTAL GRAMS 58.8
GRAMS PER SERVING 7.4

Chunky Chocolate Fudge Ice Cream

9 ½-cup servings

1 recipe Chocolate Ice Cream *(page 190)*
½ recipe Chocolate Fudge *(page 209)*

Prepare *Chocolate Ice Cream* and *Chocolate Fudge* recipes. Cut fudge into ¼-inch squares. Add to ice cream maker just before ice cream is ready.

TOTAL GRAMS 72.5
GRAMS PER SERVING 8.0

Raspberry Rapture Ice Cream

8 ½-cup servings

1 recipe Basic Ice Cream Custard *(page 190)*
2 tablespoons No-Cal raspberry syrup
1 tablespoon Framboise (red raspberry liqueur)
1 cup whole raspberries
2 packets sugar substitute

Prepare *Basic Ice Cream Custard.* Allow to cool.

Mix syrup and Framboise together. Place raspberries in a small bowl. Sprinkle with sugar substitute. Add syrup and Framboise. Chill to allow flavors to blend (about 5 minutes).

Whisk raspberry mixture into cooling custard. Cool to room temperature. Place in ice cream maker and churn.

TOTAL GRAMS 39.4
GRAMS PER SERVING 4.9

Vanilla Ice Cream

6 ½-cup servings

1 recipe Basic Ice Cream Custard *(page 190)*
1 tablespoon vanilla extract
2 tablespoons Sugar-Free Jell-O Vanilla Instant Pudding powder

Prepare *Basic Ice Cream Custard.* While cooling, whisk in vanilla extract and pudding powder. Cool to room temperature.

Place in ice cream maker and churn according to manufacturer's directions.

TOTAL GRAMS 32.2
GRAMS PER SERVING 5.4

Butter Pecan Ice Cream

8 ½-cup servings

1 recipe Basic Ice Cream Custard *(page 190)*
2 tablespoons sweet butter
1 cup pecan halves
2 packets sugar substitute
1 tablespoon Sugar-Free Jell-O Butterscotch Instant Pudding powder

Prepare *Basic Ice Cream Custard.* Allow to cool.

Melt butter in a small skillet. Add nuts to pan. Sauté for one minute. Sprinkle with sugar substitute. Remove from heat and mix well, coating nuts completely. Whisk butterscotch pudding powder into cooling custard. Blend until smooth. Whisk nuts in. Cool to room temperature. Place in ice cream maker and churn according to manufacturer's directions.

TOTAL GRAMS 61.2
GRAMS PER SERVING 7.7

Coconut Macadamia Ice Cream

8 ½-cup servings

1 recipe Basic Ice Cream Custard *(page 190)*
¼ cup unsweetened coconut
½ teaspoon rum extract
½ cup whole unsalted macadamia nuts
1 tablespoon Sugar-Free Jell-O Vanilla Instant Pudding powder
2 packets sugar substitute

Prepare *Basic Ice Cream Custard.* Allow to cool.

Place coconut in a small bowl and sprinkle rum extract on it. Stir to combine flavors. Whisk coconut, macadamia nuts, pudding powder, and sugar substitute into cooling custard. Cool to room temperature. Place in ice cream maker and churn according to manufacturer's directions.

TOTAL GRAMS 40.8
GRAMS PER SERVING 5.1

Maple Walnut Ice Cream

8 ½-cup servings

1 recipe Basic Ice Cream Custard *(page 190)*
1 tablespoon maple extract
2 tablespoons sweet butter
2 packets sugar substitute
1 cup walnut halves

Prepare *Basic Ice Cream Custard.* Whisk in maple extract. Melt butter in a skillet. Add nuts and sauté for 1 minute. Sprinkle with sugar substitute and mix well. Add nuts to custard and cool to room temperature. Place in ice cream maker and churn according to manufacturer's directions.

TOTAL GRAMS 34.6
GRAMS PER SERVING 4.3

Decaf-Coffee Ice Cream

8 ½-cup servings

1 recipe Basic Ice Cream Custard *(page 190)*
1 cup very strong decaffeinated coffee
2 tablespoons sugar-free French vanilla creme coffee*

Prepare *Basic Ice Cream Custard* recipe. Brew coffee by using 2 cups water and 4 tablespoons decaf. When brewed, simmer over a low flame until it reduces by half. Remove from heat. Whisk in vanilla creme coffee and allow to cool. Whisk coffee mixture into *Basic Ice Cream Custard.* Cool to room temperature. Place in ice cream maker and churn according to manufacturer's directions.

TOTAL GRAMS 28.0
GRAMS PER SERVING   3.5

Peach Melba Frozen Yogurt

8 ½-cup servings

2 cups Dannon Lite vanilla yogurt
2 egg yolks
8 packets sugar substitute
3 Stewed Peaches, *diced (page 211)*
1 tablespoon No-Cal raspberry syrup

Whisk yogurt, egg yolks, and sugar substitute together over a low heat. Stir until mixture begins to thicken. Remove from heat. Add peaches and raspberry syrup. Mix well. Cool to room temperature. Place in ice cream maker and churn according to manufacturer's directions.

TOTAL GRAMS 65.7
GRAMS PER SERVING   8.2

---

*Available in coffee department of supermarket.

Chocolate Yogurt

4 ½-cup servings

2 cups Dannon Lite vanilla yogurt
2 egg yolks
4 packets sugar substitute
2 tablespoons No-Cal chocolate syrup

Heat yogurt on low heat. Whisk in egg yolks, sugar substitute, and No-Cal syrup. Stir until mixture begins to thicken. Remove from heat and cool to room temperature. Place in ice cream maker and churn according to manufacturer's directions.

TOTAL GRAMS 65.7
GRAMS PER SERVING 16.4

Raspberry Sorbet

8 ½-cup servings

1 cup heavy cream
2 egg yolks
1 teaspoon lemon extract
8 packets sugar substitute
1 cup raspberries
½ cup No-Cal raspberry syrup
½ cup Framboise (red raspberry liqueur)

Heat cream on low heat. Whisk in egg yolks one at a time. Add lemon extract and 4 packets of sugar substitute. Whisk until mixture begins to thicken. Remove from heat.

Wash and dry raspberries. Place in a bowl. Sprinkle with 4 packets of sugar substitute. Add raspberry syrup and Framboise. Mix well.

Whisk raspberry mixture into cream mixture. Cool to room temperature.

Place mixture in ice cream maker and churn according to manufacturer's directions.

TOTAL GRAMS 37.4
GRAMS PER SERVING 4.7

Grapefruit Sorbet

8 ½-cup servings

1 cup heavy cream
2 egg yolks
8 packets sugar substitute
1 cup fresh grapefruit juice
1 package sugar-free lemon Jell-O
½ cup Cointreau (orange liqueur)

Heat heavy cream on low heat. Whisk in one egg yolk at a time. Remove from heat. Whisk in sugar substitute.

Heat grapefruit juice to boiling. Pour over Jell-O and mix until Jell-O completely dissolves. Whisk in Cointreau. Mix grapefruit mixture with heavy cream. Blend very well. Place in ice cream maker and churn according to manufacturer's directions.

TOTAL GRAMS 52.7
GRAMS PER SERVING 6.6

Italian Rum Cake

12 servings

1 recipe Lemon Sponge Cake *(page 199)*
1 recipe Cannoli Custard Frosting *(page 188)*
1 tablespoon rum or rum extract
1 recipe Chocolate Basic Frosting *(page 187–188)*

Bake two layers of *Sponge Cake* and cool. Mix rum with *Custard.* Spread custard on top of one cake layer. Add second layer. Cover with *Frosting.*

TOTAL GRAMS 85.7
GRAMS PER SERVING 7.1

Confetti Mold

8 servings

1 package diet strawberry gelatin
1 package diet lime gelatin
1 package diet orange gelatin
3 packages diet lemon gelatin
1 cup heavy cream
1 teaspoon vanilla extract

Prepare first 3 diet gelatins separately, using 1½ cups water each. Refrigerate each in separate shallow pans until thoroughly firm. Dice each into tiny cubes.

Mix all 3 packages of lemon diet gelatin with 2¾ cups water. Allow to thicken. When mixture is very thick, but not firm, add heavy cream. Thicken again. Fold in all flavors of gelatin cubes and vanilla extract. Chill until thoroughly firm, in a decorative mold.

TOTAL GRAMS 23.0
GRAMS PER SERVING 2.9

Chocolate Peanut Butter Cookies

24 cookies

¾ *cup soy flour*
2 *teaspoons cocoa*
1½ *teaspoons baking powder*
4 *packets sugar substitute*
pinch salt
⅓ *cup peanut butter*
1 *egg, beaten*
1 *teaspoon melted butter*
½ *cup heavy cream*
1 *teaspoon vanilla extract*
½ *teaspoon chocolate extract*

Preheat oven to 375° F.

Sift dry ingredients into bowl.

Combine peanut butter with remaining ingredients and add to flour mixture. Stir until blended.

Drop by teaspoon onto greased cookie sheet. Bake for 10–12 minutes until brown.

TOTAL GRAMS 47.9
GRAMS PER COOKIE 2.0

Lemon Sponge Cake

8 servings

½ cup heavy cream
1 cup soy flour
1½ teaspoons baking powder
dash salt
3 eggs
8 packets sugar substitute
2 teaspoons vanilla extract
1 teaspoon lemon extract

Preheat oven to 300° F.

Scald cream and remove from heat.

Sift flour, baking powder, and salt together.

Beat eggs and sugar substitute thoroughly until thick and lemon colored. Blend in flour mixture just until smooth. Add warm cream and extracts to mixture. Pour batter immediately into a 9-inch greased tube pan. Bake for 45 minutes, or until done.

TOTAL GRAMS 56.0
GRAMS PER SERVING 7.0

Spice Cake

8 servings

½ cup heavy cream
1 cup soy flour
1½ teaspoons baking powder
pinch salt
½ teaspoon cinnamon
⅛ teaspoon ground cloves
¼ teaspoon nutmeg
3 eggs
8 packets sugar substitute
1 teaspoon brandy extract
2 teaspoons vanilla extract

Preheat oven to 325° F.

Scald cream and remove from heat. Sift flour, baking powder, salt, and spices together.

Beat eggs with sugar substitute until very thick. Blend in flour mixture until smooth. Add warm cream and extracts to mixture. Pour batter immediately into 8-inch greased layer pan. Bake for 40 minutes, or until done.

TOTAL GRAMS 53.7
GRAMS PER SERVING 6.7

Chocolate Sponge Layer Cake

8 servings

½ cup soy flour
½ teaspoon baking powder
pinch salt
1 tablespoon unsweetened cocoa
2 eggs
8 packets sugar substitute
1 teaspoon vanilla extract
1 teaspoon chocolate extract

Preheat oven to 325° F.

Sift flour, baking powder, salt, and cocoa together.

Beat eggs with sugar substitute until very thick.

Stir in extracts. Fold in flour mixture. Bake in 8-inch greased layer pan for 30 minutes or until done. Makes 1 layer.

TOTAL GRAMS 30.9
GRAMS PER SERVING 3.9

Marzipan

24 1-inch forms

1 7-ounce package unsweetened grated coconut
1 package diet gelatin (any fruit flavor)
1 cup ground almonds
½ cup heavy cream
4 packets sugar substitute
½ teaspoon vanilla extract
½ teaspoon almond extract

Combine all ingredients. Shape into any designs you like—fruits, vegetables, and so forth. (Food coloring may be added to simulate true details.)

Chill until forms hold their shape.

TOTAL GRAMS 95.3
GRAMS PER SERVING 4.0

Almond Pie Crust

1 pie crust

1 cup soy flour
½ cup ground almonds
2 packets sugar substitute
pinch cinnamon
⅓ cup butter, chilled

Preheat oven to 400° F.

Stir first 4 ingredients together. Cut in butter. Work well into dry ingredients.

Cover with wax paper and refrigerate for 1 hour.

Place in pie pan patting crumb mixture over sides and bottom with back of spoon. Use fork tines to decorate edges of pie crust and to prick holes in bottom and sides of crust. Place empty disposable pie plate over pie (to keep crust from puffing). Bake for 30 minutes until solid and brown around edges. Remove second pan, cover edges with foil, and allow center to brown thoroughly (about 5 minutes). Cool.

Substitute for *Pie Shell* when on Maintenance.

TOTAL GRAMS 42.1

Lemon Chiffon Pie

8 servings

3 egg yolks, beaten
1½ cups water
2 packets sugar substitute
1 package diet lemon gelatin
2 tablespoons lemon juice
1 teaspoon lemon extract
½ teaspoon grated lemon rind
3 egg whites
⅛ teaspoon salt
1 recipe Pie Shell, *baked (page 211)*

Combine egg yolks, 1 cup water, and sugar substitute in a saucepan. Simmer, stirring constantly, until mixture begins to boil. Remove from heat, and stir in gelatin. Add remainder of water, lemon juice, lemon extract, and rind. Chill until somewhat thickened.

Beat egg whites and salt until mixture stands in stiff peaks. Stir gelatin mixture slightly, and fold in egg whites. Pour into prepared *Pie Shell*. Chill until firm.

TOTAL GRAMS 27.4
GRAMS PER SERVING 3.4

Coconut Cream Pie

10 servings

½ cup coconut
⅛ cup Cointreau
1 tablespoon butter
2½ cups heavy cream
1 envelope unflavored gelatin
¼ cup cold water
6 packets sugar substitute
4 egg whites at room temperature
2 teaspoons vanilla
1 recipe Pie Shell, *baked (optional) (page 211)*

Place coconut in flameproof bowl. Heat Cointreau and ignite. Pour over coconut. (Flames will be high.)

Heat butter in skillet. Add coconut and lightly toast it. Remove 2 tablespoons toasted coconut and set aside. Add 1 cup heavy cream to skillet. Simmer 4 minutes.

Sprinkle gelatin over cold water. Mix well to dissolve. Add to cream mixture. Simmer and stir until it begins to thicken. Remove from heat. Add 3 packets sugar substitute. Cool.

Beat egg whites until stiff with 1 packet of sugar substitute.

Fold egg whites into cool cream mixture.

Pour mixture into pie plate sprayed with oil substitute, or into prepared and baked *Pie Shell*.

Refrigerate until firm.

Beat 1½ cups heavy cream with vanilla and 2 packets sugar substitute. Pile on top of firm cream mixture. Refrigerate for at least 2 hours before serving. Sprinkle with reserved coconut.

TOTAL GRAMS 37.3
GRAMS PER SERVING 3.7

Chocolate Mint Pie

8 servings

½ cup chopped pecans or walnuts
1 recipe Pie Shell *(page 211)*
2 ounces unsweetened chocolate
2 tablespoons hot water
2 tablespoons peppermint extract
1 teaspoon vanilla
1 tablespoon crème de cacao
9 packets sugar substitute
2 cups heavy cream

Preheat oven to 275° F.

Sprinkle chopped nuts over *Pie Shell* and bake for 1 hour until lightly browned and crisp to touch. Cool, preferably leaving in oven until cool.

Melt chocolate in double boiler, stir in water, and cook until smooth. Remove from heat, and add peppermint extract, vanilla, crème de cacao, and sugar substitute.

Whip heavy cream with 1 packet of sugar substitute. Fold 1 cup whipped cream into chocolate mixture.

Spoon into pie shell and chill for 2–3 hours.

Just before serving, spread remaining 1 cup whipped cream over top.

TOTAL GRAMS 63.4
GRAMS PER SERVING 7.9

Cheesecake

12 servings

16 ounces cream cheese at room temperature
3 eggs
1 cup crème fraîche or sour cream
½ vanilla bean, scraped
12 packets sugar substitute

Preheat oven to 350° F.

Place all ingredients in a blender and blend for 15 minutes. Pour mixture into a 9-inch springform pan. Place in a pan of hot water in oven. If water evaporates during baking, add more hot water as needed. Bake for 1 hour, turn off oven and leave cake in oven 1 hour more.

TOTAL GRAMS 33.0
GRAMS PER SERVING 2.8

Coffee Cream Layer Cake

10 servings

5 egg whites, at room temperature
6 packets sugar substitute
2 cups heavy cream
1½ teaspoons instant decaffeinated coffee
½ tablespoon gelatin
1 tablespoon cold water
3 tablespoons butter, at room temperature
4 egg yolks at room temperature
2 teaspoons mocha extract
½ cup chopped walnuts

Preheat oven to 275° F.

Butter 3 round layer cake pans.

Beat egg whites until they form soft peaks. Add 1 packet sugar substitute and beat until stiff. Divide whites among 3 pans. Bake for 45 minutes.

Combine 1 cup heavy cream and instant decaf coffee in top of double boiler. Stir with wire whisk until powder dissolves. Dissolve gelatin in cold water. Add gelatin to coffee mixture and heat just to boiling. Stir constantly with whisk. Remove from heat. Beat in 4 egg yolks, 1 yolk at a time. Add butter and beat well until dissolved. Add extract and remaining sugar substitute. Put in freezer to cool.

Whip remaining cup heavy cream until stiff.

When coffee mixture is cool, fold into whipped cream and refrigerate until layers are cooked and cooled. Pile cream between layers of meringue as you would frost a layer cake. Top with cream, making sure to cover sides.

Sprinkle nuts on top and sides. Refrigerate until serving time.

TOTAL GRAMS 30.2
GRAMS PER SERVING 3.0

Lemon-Lime Mousse

8 servings

½ cup butter
9 egg yolks
juice of 2 lemons
juice of 2 limes
6 packets sugar substitute
2 teaspoons grated lemon rind
4 egg whites
1½ cups heavy cream
1 teaspoon vanilla extract

Melt butter in saucepan over low heat.

Beat in egg yolks, one at a time, with wire whisk. Remove from heat. Add juice from lemons and limes, 4 packets sugar substitute, and lemon rind. Beat well. Cool.

Beat egg whites with 1 packet sugar substitute and vanilla extract. Fold into chilled mixture. Refrigerate for at least 2 hours.

TOTAL GRAMS 31.1
GRAMS PER SERVING 3.9

Pumpkin Chiffon

8 servings

1 envelope unflavored gelatin
½ teaspoon salt
½ teaspoon nutmeg
½ teaspoon cinnamon
¼ teaspoon ginger
½ cup cold water
2 egg yolks, slightly beaten
1 cup heavy cream
1¼ cups canned pumpkin
8 packets sugar substitute
2 egg whites

Combine gelatin, salt, and spices. Add ¼ cup water. Stir. Mix egg yolks with heavy cream, ¼ cup water, and pumpkin in top of double boiler. Add gelatin mixture. Cook over boiling water for 10 minutes, stirring constantly. Refrigerate until thick as unbeaten egg whites. Stir occasionally. Add sugar substitute (taste for sweetness).

Beat egg whites until stiff. Fold chilled pumpkin mixture into egg whites. Be careful not to break down volume of egg whites. Turn into 1½-quart soufflé dish. Refrigerate.

TOTAL GRAMS 39.9
GRAMS PER SERVING 5.0

The "Pop" Pop

6 popsicles

1½ cups sugar-free fruit-flavored soft drink
6 teaspoons cream
sprinkle of sugar substitute (optional)

Mix all ingredients together.

Fill plastic molds for popsicles (1 mold holds 6 popsicles) with mixture. Insert stick if desired. (It is best to do this when popsicles are partially frozen.)

Freeze.

TOTAL GRAMS 4.5
GRAMS PER SERVING 0.8

Peanut Butter Cookies

40 cookies

½ cup chunk-style, sugar-free peanut butter
¾ cup heavy cream
½ cup chopped pecans
2 teaspoons vanilla
4 packets sugar substitute
2 tablespoons soy flour
1 teaspoon baking powder

Preheat oven to 375° F.
    Spray a cookie sheet with oil substitute.
    Mix all ingredients in bowl. Blend well.
    Drop on cookie sheet by teaspoonfuls. Bake for about 10 minutes.

TOTAL GRAMS 47.6
GRAMS PER SERVING 1.2

Chocolate Fudge

15 squares

1 package Sugar-Free Jell-O Chocolate Instant Pudding
4 packets sugar substitute
½ cup heavy cream
1 tablespoon crème de cacao
3 heaping tablespoons chunk-style, sugar-free peanut butter

Mix all ingredients together except peanut butter. Place over low heat and add peanut butter. Heat until peanut butter melts. Stir until well blended.
    Spray a small baking pan with oil substitute. Spoon mixture into pan. Refrigerate until firm. Slice into at least 15 squares.

TOTAL GRAMS 56.9
GRAMS PER SQUARE 3.8

Brownies

30 squares

½ cup butter, at room temperature
2 eggs
1 1-ounce square unsweetened chocolate
2 teaspoons chocolate extract
2 tablespoons water
2 tablespoons soy flour
½ cup coarsely chopped walnuts
8 packets sugar substitute
3 tablespoons crème de cacao

Preheat oven to 350° F.

Cream butter with electric hand mixer. Add eggs one at a time, beating well.

Melt chocolate with extract and water in top of double boiler. (If it gets too thick, add a little more water.)

Add melted chocolate, soy flour, chopped walnuts, and sugar substitute to butter. Mix well. Taste for sweetness. Add more sugar substitute if needed.

Grease a 1½-quart flat baking dish.

Pour in chocolate mixture. Bake 15 minutes. Do not overcook. Remove from oven. Sprinkle crème de cacao over top. Cool. Cut into at least 30 squares.

TOTAL GRAMS 49.0
GRAMS PER SQUARE 1.6

Pie Shell

1 pie shell

4 egg whites
1 teaspoon cream of tartar
pinch of salt
4 teaspoons crème de cacao

Preheat oven to 250° F.

Place egg whites, cream of tartar, and salt in bowl. Beat together until frothy. Gradually add crème de cacao. Continue beating until whites are stiff, glossy, and stand in stiff peaks.

Grease a pie plate. Pour meringue into pie plate and form crust with back of spoon.

Bake for 1 hour.

How to Beat Egg Whites for Meringues:

Eggs will beat better at room temperature, but separate better when cold. The trick is to separate them when cold, then let stand until they reach room temperature.

The best way to beat egg whites is with an electric hand beater; however, a rotary beater will also do the job.

TOTAL GRAMS 7.4

Stewed Peaches

10 peach halves

5 ripe summer peaches, pitted and peeled, cut in halves
3 tablespoons No-Cal raspberry syrup

Place peaches and syrup in a small pan. Simmer covered for 20 minutes.

Serve hot or refrigerate.

TOTAL GRAMS 49.0
GRAMS PER PEACH HALF 4.9

Snappy Raspberries and Lemons

4 ½-cup servings

1 package sugar-free raspberry Jell-O
1 cup boiling water
1 cup cold diet Snapple raspberry iced tea

Dissolve Jell-O in hot water. Cool. Add iced tea. Refrigerate until jelled.
   For lemon, use lemon Jell-O and diet Snapple lemon iced tea.

TOTAL GRAMS 1.4
GRAMS PER SERVING 0.4

Raspberry or Lemon Jell-O Cream

8 ½-cup servings

1 package sugar-free raspberry Jell-O
1 cup diet Snapple raspberry iced tea, heated to boiling
1 cup sour cream

Dissolve Jell-O in hot Snapple. Cool to room temperature.
   Whisk in sour cream, beating until blended. Refrigerate until jelled.
   For lemon cream, use diet lemon Jell-O and diet Snapple lemon iced tea.

TOTAL GRAMS 10.2
GRAMS PER SERVING   1.3

Tomato Lemon Jell-O

4 ½-cup servings

½ cup boiling water
1 package sugar-free lemon Jell-O
1½ cups Piquant V-8 Juice, chilled

Bring water to a boil. Dissolve Jell-O in water. Cool.
   Add V-8 and chill until firm.

TOTAL GRAMS 15.2
GRAMS PER SERVING   3.8

Strawberry-Banana Cream

4 ½-cup servings

1 cup water
1 teaspoon banana extract
1 package sugar-free strawberry-banana Jell-O
2 tablespoons No-Cal strawberry syrup
½ cup diet strawberry soda
6 tablespoons heavy cream

Heat water to a boil. Add banana extract. Pour over Jell-O and completely dissolve it. Cool. Add syrup, soda, and cream. Whisk until well blended. Refrigerate until firm.

TOTAL GRAMS 2.4
GRAMS PER SERVING 0.6

Beverages

Hot Chocolate

1 serving

⅓ cup cream
⅔ cup water
1 teaspoon unsweetened cocoa
1 packet sugar substitute
½ teaspoon vanilla

Place all ingredients in saucepan. Heat to boiling point, but do not boil. Stir constantly.
   Serve in mug.

TOTAL GRAMS 5.4

Cappuccino

1 serving

1 recipe Hot Chocolate *(page 214)*
½ teaspoon instant coffee
½ teaspoon brandy extract
1 cinnamon stick

Make *Hot Chocolate.* Add coffee and brandy extract.
   Serve in mug with cinnamon stick.

TOTAL GRAMS 8.1

Spicy Cocktail

2 servings

2 cups Beef Stock *(page 70)*
4 teaspoons tomato sauce
½ teaspoon onion juice or grated onion
½ teaspoon Worcestershire sauce
2 drops Tabasco sauce

Combine all ingredients. Mix well. Serve hot or cold.

TOTAL GRAMS 4.1
GRAMS PER SERVING 2.1

Orange Cooler

4 servings

1 package sugar-free orange Jell-O
2 egg whites, beaten stiffly
2 teaspoons lemon rind, grated
1 teaspoon orange extract
2 packets sugar substitute
4 strawberries
4 ice cubes
4 lemon slices

Prepare gelatin according to package directions and cool.

Beat in stiff egg whites with wire whisk. Add lemon rind, orange extract, and sugar substitute.

Place in blender. Add strawberries and ice cubes. Blend at medium speed for 30 seconds.

Pour into glasses and garnish with lemon slices.

TOTAL GRAMS 10.2
GRAMS PER SERVING 2.5

Black and White Ice Cream Soda

1 serving

⅔ *glass diet chocolate soda*
1 tablespoon No-Cal chocolate syrup
2 tablespoons heavy cream
2 scoops Vanilla Ice Cream *(page 192)*

Mix No-Cal syrup and heavy cream into soda. Add *Ice Cream*.

TOTAL GRAMS 6.0

Blender-Thick Raspberry Shake

2 servings

2 scoops Vanilla Ice Cream *(page 192)*
3 tablespoons heavy cream
2 tablespoons No-Cal raspberry syrup
1 8-ounce bottle diet ginger ale

Place all ingredients in blender. Blend for 1 minute at medium speed.

TOTAL GRAMS 7.9
GRAMS PER SERVING 4.0

Chocolate Shake

1 serving

1 envelope unflavored gelatin
1 cup diet chocolate soda
1 tablespoon unsweetened cocoa
4 ice cubes
⅓ cup heavy cream
1 packet sugar substitute
dash of salt

Place gelatin, ¼ cup soda, and cocoa in saucepan. Stir well. Heat slowly to boiling point. Be sure gelatin dissolves completely. Cool.

Place ice cubes in blender. Add cooled gelatin mixture, heavy cream, ¾ cup soda, sugar substitute, and salt. Blend at high speed for 30 seconds.

Serve in tall glass. It will become thicker as it sets. Stir vigorously.

TOTAL GRAMS 5.8

Shape-Up Shake

1 serving

1 envelope sugar-free lime Jell-O
1 cup diet lime soda
4 ice cubes
⅓ cup heavy cream
1 packet sugar substitute

Place gelatin and ¼ cup soda in saucepan. Heat to boiling point, stirring constantly. Be sure gelatin dissolves.

Cool.

Place ice cubes in blender, add gelatin mixture, heavy cream, ¾ cup soda, and sugar substitute.

Blend at high speed for 30 seconds.
Serve in tall glass. It will become thicker as it sets. Stir vigorously.

TOTAL GRAMS 3.7

Mocha Drink

1 serving

1 cup brewed decaffeinated coffee
1 cup diet chocolate soda
1 tablespoon No-Cal chocolate syrup
4 ice cubes
¼ teaspoon cinnamon
2 tablespoons heavy cream
1 organic egg
1 packet sugar substitute (optional)

Place all ingredients in a blender and blend until smooth.

TOTAL GRAMS 3.9

Spiced Iced Decaf Coffee

4 servings

2 tablespoons decaffeinated instant coffee
5 whole allspice
5 whole cloves
dash cinnamon
3 cups boiling water
8 ice cubes
4 teaspoons heavy cream

Combine all ingredients except cream in a 1-quart container. Cover and refrigerate 1 hour or more.

Strain. Pour over ice cubes into 4 tall glasses.

Add 1 teaspoon cream to each glass.

TOTAL GRAMS 3.8
GRAMS PER SERVING 1.0

Sweet Lemonade with Lecithin

4 servings

1 cup water
¼ cup lemon juice
2 packets sugar substitute
2 egg whites
1 teaspoon vanilla
½ teaspoon orange extract
dash salt
8 ice cubes
2 teaspoons lecithin

Place all ingredients except ice cubes and lecithin in a blender. Blend until thick.

Add 1 ice cube at a time and blend until frothy.

Remove from blender and stir in lecithin. Pour into 4 glasses. Stir again and serve immediately.

TOTAL GRAMS 21.7
GRAMS PER SERVING   5.4

Hot Mint Chocolate Nog

1 servings

1 cup Pelican Punch herbal tea*
2 teaspoons No-Cal chocolate syrup
1 teaspoon chocolate extract
1 packet sugar substitute
1 organic egg
2 tablespoons heavy cream

Place all ingredients in blender. Blend well.

TOTAL GRAMS 4.4

*Available in specialty and health food stores.

Appendices

Special Menus for Entertaining

FORMAL DINNER

Serves 12

HORS D'OEUVRES

Fran's Special Pâté
Deviled-Salmon Eggs
Caribbean Crabmeat

APPETIZER

Honeydew and Seafood

SOUP

Cold Avocado Soup

SALAD

Tricolor Salad with Three Cheeses

ENTRÉE

Stuffed Steak
or
Stuffed Flounder

VEGETABLES

Spicy Cauliflower Bake
Cheesy Brussels Sprouts

TO CLEAR THE PALATE

Small scoop of Grapefruit Sorbet

DESSERT

Spice Cake with Coconut Macadamia Ice Cream

BEVERAGES

Cappuccino
tea
decaffeinated coffee with cream and sugar substitute

BARBECUE

Serves 12

WHEN FOLKS ARRIVE

Guacamole with cucumber slices
Sour Cream Clam Dip with pork rinds
cheese tray

ON THE COALS

Dr. Atkins' Fromage Burgers
Luscious Lamb
Broiled Tarragon Lobster Tails (cook on coals instead of broiling)
chicken marinated in Hot Barbecue Sauce

THE SALADS

Cole Slaw
Mock Potato Salad

SWEETS

Confetti Mold
Decaf-Coffee Ice Cream
Almond Ball Cookies
Chocolate Sponge Layer Cake

DRINKS

Spicy Cocktail
Sweet Lemonade with Lecithin
Orange Cooler

BUFFET DINNER

Serves 20

APPETIZING TABLE

Fresh Spring Salmon Mousse
Spicy Spare ribs
Heavenly Wings
Salad Niçoise with Fresh Tuna
assorted olives

ENTRÉE TABLE

Kayzie's Rabbit
Moussaka
Shrimp and Scallops Marc
Coq Au Vin with Shiitake Mushrooms

DESSERT TABLE

Lemon-Lime Mousse
Chocolate Mint Pie
Cheesecake
Raspberry Rapture Ice Cream

CANDY TRAY

Almond Balls
Chocolate Fudge
Pistachio Popcorn Balls

BEVERAGES

Cappuccino
tea
decaffeinated coffee with cream and sugar substitute

DESSERT BUFFET ATKINS STYLE

Serves 12

2 CAKES

    Italian Rum Cake
    Coffee Cream Layer Cake

2 PIES

    Coconut Cream Pie
    Lemon Chiffon Pie

3 KINDS OF COOKIES

    Chocolate Peanut Butter Cookies
    Pistachio Popcorn Balls
    Brownies

2 FLAVORS OF ICE CREAM

    Butter Pecan Ice Cream
    Chocolate Ice Cream

BEVERAGES

    Spiced Iced Tea
    Cappuccino
    Hot Chocolate

Nutritional Supplementation

Twenty years ago I was almost a voice crying in the wilderness when I said you'd live a longer and healthier life if you ate a healthy diet *and* consumed vitamin and mineral supplements than you would if you ate a healthy diet alone. I have stubbornly persisted because the experiences of my forty thousand patients have affirmed and reaffirmed the correctness of that view. Now the virtues of supplements are becoming commonplace, supported by an increasing number of highly orthodox medical scientists and loudly proclaimed from the covers of major newsmagazines. In the end my viewpoint may become the conventional one, which would be a change of pace.

For all of you who are doing the Atkins diet I must insist on the importance of your supplements. During the two-week Induction phase of the diet, you will need supplements to maintain a proper nutritional balance. After that, you should go right on taking them because they're good for you.

Following is my Dieter's Formula. Find a multivitamin that gives you something close to this formula, and then take three capsules a day. People who weigh 200 pounds or more are to use the second, larger doses, provided in parentheses, of certain vitamins.

Dieter's Formula

Vitamin A	200 IU
Beta-Carotene	500 IU
Vitamin D-2	15 IU
Thiamine (HC1)(B$_1$)	5 mg
Riboflavin (B$_2$)	4 mg
Vitamin C (Calcium Ascorbate)	120 mg (150 mg)
Niacin (B$_3$)	2 mg
Niacinamide	5 mg
Pantethine (80%)	25 mg (30 mg)
Calcium Pantothenate (B$_5$)	25 mg
Pyridoxal-5-Phosphate	2 mg
Pyridoxine (HCl)(B$_6$)	20 mg
Folic Acid	100 mcg
Biotin	75 mcg
Cyanocobalamin (B$_{12}$)	30 mcg
Vitamin E (D alpha tocopherol)	2 IU
Copper (Sulfate)	200 mcg
Magnesium (Oxide)	8 mg
Chlorine (Bitartrate)	100 mg
Inositol	80 mg
PABA	100 mg
Manganese (Chelate)	4 mg
Zinc (Chelate)	10 mg
Citrus Bioflavonoids	150 mg
Chromium (Picolinate)	50 mcg
Molybdenum (Sodium)	10 mcg
Vanadyl Sulfate	15 mcg
Selenium	40 mcg
Octacosanol	150 mcg
N-Acetyl-1-cysteine	20 mg
L-Glutathione (reduced)	5 mg

The recommended formula comes in a base of lactobacillus, bulgaris and bifidus acidophilus, B-Complex, and growth factors.

In addition to this formula, the next most important nutritional group for long-range supplementation are the essential fatty acids. You won't find these in a multivitamin formula because they exist physically as oils and don't mix with a dry powder capsule. There are two types of essential fatty acids that most of us need. One type is the omega-3 series that provides you with alpha linolenic acid (ALA). The other type is the omega-6 series called gamma linolenic acid (GLA).

To supplement with these important nutrients, take an essential oils formula containing approximately the following:

Flaxseed oil	400 mg
Borage oil	400 mg
Super EPA	400 mg

Carbohydrate Gram Counter

Foods	*Grams of Carbohydrate*
BEANS (COOKED)	
Black-eyed peas (1 cup)	35.5
Lima (½ cup), Fordhook/baby	16.0/21.2
Navy (1 cup), dried, boiled	47.9
Peanuts (2 oz.), oil rstd./dry rstd.	9.8/12.0
Red kidney (½ cup)	20.2
Soybeans (½ cup), green, boiled	10.0
Split peas (1 cup), boiled	41.4
Tofu (3½ oz.), raw, firm	5.4
CONDIMENTS	
Anchovies (1 oz.)	0.0
Cocoa (1 Tbsp. unsweetened)	2.8
Horseradish (1 tsp.)	0.5
Mayonnaise (1 Tbsp.)	0.4
Mustard:	
Dijon (1 tsp.)	0.3
regular (1 tsp.)	0.3
Pickles (1 medium dill)	1.4
Soy sauce (1 Tbsp.)	2.0
Syrup:	
No-Cal chocolate	0.0
No-Cal strawberry	0.0
Vinegar:	
balsamic (1 Tbsp.)	3.0
cider (1 Tbsp.)	0.9
tarragon (1 Tbsp.)	0.9
wine (1 Tbsp.)	0.9
Worcestershire sauce (1 Tbsp.)	2.7

Foods	**Grams of Carbohydrate**
FATS/OILS	
Canola	0.0–trace
Olive	0.0–trace
Peanut	0.0–trace
Safflower	0.0–trace
Walnut	0.0–trace
FRUIT	
Apple, medium (2¾")	21.1
Applesauce, unsweetened (½ cup)	13.8
Apricots (3 fresh)	11.8
Avocado:	
California	12.0
Florida	27.1
Banana (1 medium)	26.7
Blackberries (1 cup)	18.4
Blueberries (1 cup)	20.5
Cantaloupe (1 cup, pieces)	13.4
Cherries (½ cup raw, sweet)	11.2
Cranberries (1 cup)	11.0
Grapefruit (½, pink)	9.5
Grapefruit juice (4 oz.)	11.2
Grapes (1 cup)	15.8
Honeydew (¼ cup)	7.7
Kiwi (1 medium)	11.3
Lemon (1 medium)	5.4
Lemon juice (1 Tbsp., fresh)	1.3
Lemon peel (1 tsp.)	0.3
Lime juice (1 oz.)	2.8
Mango (½ medium)	17.1
Olives:	
black (10 olives)	3.0
green, pitted	0.5

Foods	**Grams of Carbohydrate**

FRUIT (continued)

Orange (1 medium)	16.3
Orange rind (1 tsp.)	0.5
Papaya (⅓ medium)	9.9
Peach (2½")	9.7
Pear (3½")	25.1
Pineapple (1 cup)	19.2
Plum (1 medium)	8.6
Prunes, cooked (½ cup)	29.8
Raspberries (1 cup)	14.2
Rhubarb (4 oz.)	3.5
Stewed peaches (1 cup)	20.0
Strawberries (1 cup)	10.5

GELATIN

Gelatin	0.0
Sugar-Free Jell-O (all flavors)	0.0

GRAINS

Bagel (1) (approx. 2 oz.)	30.9
Bread:	
pumpernickel (1 slice)	15.4
whole-wheat (1 slice)	11.4
Corn muffin (homemade/mix)	17.0/20.0
Cornmeal (1 cup, cooked)	25.7
Farina (1 cup reg, ckd)	27.8
Noodles (1 cup enriched)	37.3
Oatmeal (1 cup old fash)	27.8
Pancake (1 buckwheat ¼ oz. dry mix)	21.3
Popcorn (popped, 1 cup)	4.6
Rice:	
cooked (1 cup white, enriched)	49.6
puffed (1 cup whole)	19
Soy flour (1 cup)	27.1
Waffle from mix, (7")	27.2

Foods	**Grams of Carbohydrate**

HERBS

Allspice (1 tsp.)	1.4
Basil (1 tsp. ground)	0.9
Caraway (1 tsp. seeds)	1.1
Celery (1 tsp.)	0.8
Cinnamon (1 tsp.)	1.8
Coriander leaf (1 tsp. dried)	0.3
Dill seed (1 tsp.)	1.2
Garlic clove (1)	1.0
Ginger root:	
fresh (1 oz.)	3.6
ground (1 tsp.)	1.3
Saffron (1 tsp.)	0.5
Tarragon (1 tsp.)	0.8
Thyme (1 tsp.)	0.4
Vanilla, double strength (1 tsp.)	3.0

MILK PRODUCTS

Butter (½ cup)	0.0
Cheese:	
American (1 oz.)	0.5
Boursin (1 oz.)	0.1
Camembert (1 oz.)	0.1
Cheddar (1 oz.)	0.4
cottage, creamed (1 cup)	5.6
cottage, uncreamed (1 cup)	2.7
cream (1 oz.)	0.8
feta (1 oz.)	1.2
fontina (1 oz.)	0.4
goat (1 oz.)	1.0
Jarlsberg (1 oz.)	1.0
mascarpone (1 oz.)	0.5
mozzarella (1 oz.)	0.6
muenster (1 oz.)	0.3
Parmesan (1 oz.)	0.4
provolone (1 oz.)	0.6
ricotta (1 oz., whole/part skim)	1.0/1.6

Foods	**Grams of Carbohydrate**

MILK PRODUCTS (continued)

Roquefort (1 oz.)	0.6
Swiss (1 oz.)	1.0
Cream:	
heavy (1 oz.)	2.0
light (1 oz.)	0.8
sour (1 oz.)	1.0
whipped (1 oz.)	0.8
Half-and-half (1 oz.)	1.2
Milk (whole, 1 cup)	11.4
Yogurt, plain:	
lite (1 cup)	15.0
skim (1 cup)	17.4
whole (1 cup)	10.6

NUTS AND SEEDS

Almond paste (1 oz.)	12.4
Almonds:	
1 oz. dried	5.8
12–15 nuts	2.9
Brazil (4 nuts)	1.8
Cashews (1 oz.)	9.3
Coconut (1 piece 2"x2"x$\frac{1}{2}$")	6.9
Grated coconut, unsweetened (1 oz. dried)	6.7
Hazelnuts (1 oz.)	5.0
Macadamia nuts (6 nuts)	3.9
Mixed (8–12 nuts, oil rstd.)	6.1
Peanut butter:	
regular (1 oz.) (ave. of several brands)	4.0–7.0
sugar-free (1 oz.) (ave. of several brands)	3.0
Peanuts (1 oz. dry rstd.)	6.0
Pecans (10 halves)	3.5
Pine nuts (Pignoli, 1 oz.)	4.0
Pistachio (30 nuts, dried)	4.5
Pumpkin seeds (1 oz./142 seeds, dried/rstd.)	5.1/3.8
Sesame seeds (1 oz.)	7.0
Soynuts (1 oz.)	10.1

Foods	Grams of Carbohydrate
NUTS AND SEEDS *(continued)*	
Sunflower seeds (1 oz., dried)	5.3
Walnuts (8–10 halves)	6.7
Water chestnuts (1 oz.)	7.4
PROTEIN (LEAN, WITHOUT SKIN OR BREADING)	
Eggs	0.6
Egg yolk	0.0–trace
Egg white	0.0–trace
Fish	0.0–trace
Meat	0.0–trace
Poultry	0.0–trace
SOUPS	
Chicken Consommé (1 cup)	1.8
Chicken Gumbo (1 cup)	9.2
Clam Stock (1 oz)	0.6
Cream of Chicken (1 cup)	9.3
Cream of Mushroom (1 cup)	9.3
Turkey Rice (1 cup)	7.2
VEGETABLES	
Asparagus (6 spears)	4.0
Bamboo shoots (1 cup)	4.2
Bean sprouts (1 cup)	6.2
Beans:	
green (½ cup, boiled)	4.9
yellow or wax (½ cup, boiled)	3.7
Broccoli (½ cup steamed)	4.3
Brussels sprouts (4, or ½ cup)	6.8
Cabbage (½ cup, raw, shredded)	1.9
Carrot (7")	7.3
Cauliflower (1 cup cooked)	5.8
Celery (1 stalk, 7½" long)	1.5
Chinese Cabbage (1 cup)	3.0
Cole slaw (4 oz. homemade)	15.0

Foods	**Grams of Carbohydrate**

VEGETABLES (continued)

Food	Grams
Collards (1 cup, boiled, chopped)	5.0
Corn (1 ear, 5", yellow)	28.7
Cucumber (6 slices, $\frac{1}{8}$")	1.5
Dandelion ($\frac{1}{2}$ cup, boiled, chopped)	3.3
Eggplant (diced, 1 cup)	6.4
Endive ($\frac{1}{2}$ cup)	.8
Kale ($\frac{1}{2}$ cup)	3.7
Kohlrabi ($\frac{2}{3}$ cup, slices, cooked)	5.5
Lettuce:	
Boston (2 leaves)	.4
iceberg (1 leaf)	.4
Romaine (2 leaves)	.7
Mushrooms:	
regular (10 small or 4 large, $\frac{1}{2}$ cup pieces)	1.6
porcini (1 cup)	4.0
shiitake (4 ckd, 2.2 oz)	10.3
Mustard greens ($\frac{1}{2}$ cup, boiled, chopped)	1.5
Okra ($\frac{1}{2}$ cup slices)	5.8
Onion ($\frac{1}{2}$ cup chopped)	5.9
Parsley (1 Tbsp., fresh)	0.3
Parsnips ($\frac{1}{2}$ cup slices, boiled)	1.9/15.2
Peas (cooked, 1 cup)	25.0
Peppers:	
green (2 rings)	1.4
red (dried, 1 oz.)	5.0
Potato, baked ($4\frac{3}{4}$" x $2\frac{1}{3}$")	21.0
Potato salad ($\frac{1}{2}$ cup)	14.0
Pumpkin:	
fresh ($\frac{1}{2}$ cup mashed, boiled)	6.0
canned ($\frac{1}{2}$ cup)	9.9
Radish (4 medium)	0.5
Rutabagas (1 cup)	13.2
Scallions (1 Tbsp.)	0.4
Spinach ($\frac{1}{2}$ cup cooked)	3.4

Foods	**Grams of Carbohydrate**
VEGETABLES (continued)	
Squash:	
summer (½ cup slices, cooked)	3.5
winter (½ cup cubes, baked)	8.9
String beans (1 cup)	5.9
Sweet potato (5" x 2", baked)	30.0
Tomato:	
cooked (½ cup)	6.8
juice (½ cup)	5.1
paste (1 oz.)	5.7
raw (2½", approx. 4 oz.)	5.3
sauce (1 oz.)	2.2
sun-dried (average)	2.0–5.0
V-8 Juice (5.5-oz. can)	7.0
Turnips:	
cooked (1 cup)	7.6
greens (1 cup, chopped, cooked)	6.2
SAMPLES OF CARBOHYDRATE-RICH "FATTENING" ITEMS	
Apple pie (1 slice, homemade)	61.0
Apple turnover	31.1
Banana split	91.0
Blueberry Muffin (1 average)	17.0
Brownie (1 average homemade, with icing)	12.7
Burrito, bean	51.9
Cheeseburger (¼ pounder)	33.0
Corn bread stuffing (¼ cup)	69.0
Devil Dog	30.0
Donut (1 glazed)	22.0
Egg roll (1)	30.0
French toast (2 slices)	34.0
Hot dog with bun (1)	24.0
Ice cream soda (1 cup)	49.0
Jam (1 Tbsp. grape)	15.0
Macaroni and cheese (1 cup)	40.0

Foods	**Grams of Carbohydrate**
"FATTENING" ITEMS (continued)	
Onion rings (fast food order)	33.5
Pancake (1 buttermilk, plain)	15.0
Pecan pie (1 piece, homemade)	41.0
Pizza (1 slice)	39.1
Pop-Tart (frosted, blueberry)	34.0
Popsicle	17.0
Roast beef sandwich	38.8
Shake (medium) average range	46–65
Sherbet (½ cup lemon)	45.0
Taco, beef	14.0
Tapioca, cream (½ cup)	22.0
Vanilla shake (1 average)	50.8
Waffles (1 homemade, plain)	45.0
Whaler	64.0

Index

Dr. ATKINS' NEW

Carbohydrate Gram Counter

Contents

Introduction

Are You What You Eat?

You've counted calories; you've counted fat—but nothing has worked. And now I tell you to count carbohydrate grams—you may ask, "why?"

I bet that most of you reading this already know the answer. My best-selling book, *Dr. Atkins' New Diet Revolution*, describes the diet's four phases, and the medical and clinical research behind them. Thousands of people are trying the diet for the first time or coming back to the only diet that worked for them. They don't worry about fat grams or calories because they have discovered the real culprit in weight gain: the **carbohydrate**.

Carbohydrates Versus Calories and Fat

As Americans have followed calorie-counting and low-fat diets faithfully, they have become fatter. And not by just a few pounds. Twenty million more people are obese today than a decade ago. Every man and woman is ten pounds, on average, heavier. And for children, the situation is even worse. Their obesity rates have doubled during the last ten years. Obviously, counting calories and fat grams has not worked.

But these statistics are not surprising to me. Along with our weight, our carbohydrate consumption has gone way up, too—by 50 grams a day! In my experience, treating thousands of patients, I have found that as many as 90 percent of those who are overweight have a metabolic disorder, not an eating disorder. Once their metabolism changes, their bodies adjust automatically to a new method of burning fat. And there is a scientific tool to alter this metabolic pattern: following the low-carbohydrate, high-protein diet.

Being overweight—especially to a significant degree—often represents the identifiable metabolic disorder called *hyperinsulinism*. When carbohydrates are consumed, insulin floods the bloodstream, but the body is incapable of utilizing it efficiently. You are left with excess insulin, otherwise known as the fat-producing hormone. This reaction can be bypassed by decreasing the carbohydrate intake.

On the Atkins diet, carbohydrates are restricted to a point at which your own fat is burned as the primary source of energy. With the absence of carbohydrates to fuel the body, a signal is sent out to release fat mobilizers. This burning of stored fat is a **natural** mechanism of our bodies. And, if you need to lose weight, restricting carbohydrates is the easiest, most hunger-free form of dieting.

Add Up the Carbs, Subtract the Weight

Most of us are unfamiliar with the carbohydrate content of most foods. We need to re-train our way of thinking about foods and become aware that carbohydrates can be found in unlikely places. Because understanding the carbohydrate content of foods is a difficult task, I have created this *Carbohydrate Gram Counter* as a tool for low-carbohydrate dieting. It will be of immediate help in two important ways.

First, success on the Atkins diet is dependent on accurately counting the total carbohydrate grams consumed each day. You should plan meals and snacks, monitoring the carbohydrate grams you consume. To do this with ease, even when dining out, you'll need a handy and thorough reference guide.

Secondly, the Federal government has established food labeling laws making it easier to find out carbohydrate grams of a food. But it can still be difficult to ascertain the actual carbohydrate gram count of everything you eat. The count listed on packages is for "serving sizes," which may be only a minute part of the whole product and can, therefore, be misleading. Also, you may find a label stating "less than one gram" of carbohydrates—but remember, it may contain as high as 0.99 of a gram. When added up, these counts can lead you astray, especially in the Induction Phase of the diet when carbohydrates are most restricted.

Remember that we have included foods in this book that are **not** recommended on the Atkins diet. We have even included some of the worst carbohydrate culprits, so you can compare your previous diet to a low-carbohydrate diet.

To ensure that you always have an accurate account of the carbohydrates you consume, you need a precise *Carbohydrate Gram Counter*. It is for you that I have created this user-friendly tool as an assistant to your dieting success.

—ROBERT C. ATKINS, M.D.
New York

HOW TO USE THIS BOOK

Take this book with you to your grocery store, or use it to make out your shopping list in advance. Plan your daily or weekly menu by adding up all the carbohydrate grams in the foods you plan to eat.

Pick foods with low carbohydrate counts.

High-carbohydrate foods often are made with refined sugars or starches, which should be avoided. Try to pick natural foods.

Find low-carbohydrate foods you love for your everyday eating, and also find the treats you can allow yourself on a Premaintenance or Lifetime Maintenance Diet.

Fat and protein grams are listed for reference, but on your low-carb diet, it's the carbohydrate grams that are most important to count.

Consult your doctor when undertaking serious dieting. The advice in this book is not intended to be a substitute for the advice of your personal physician.

For delicious, easy-to-use recipes, plus a summary of Dr. Atkins' diet plan, see *Dr. Atkins' New Diet Cookbook*. For the entire Atkins diet plan, refer to *Dr. Atkins' New Diet Revolution*.

RESTRICTING CARBOHYDRATES ON THE ATKINS DIET

On the 14-day Induction diet, no more than 20 grams a day are allowed.

While on the Ongoing Weight Loss diet, increase your daily carbohydrate consumption by 5 grams every week until you stop losing weight. You have reached your Critical Carbohydrate Level for Losing (the maximum number of carb grams you can eat and still lose weight). Eat below this level of carb grams until you have come to within five or ten pounds of your ideal weight.

When starting the Pre-Maintenance diet, you can add another 10 grams a day, or give yourself a 20 gram carbohydrate treat two or three times a week. But be careful—you should continue to lose weight at a very slow rate.

Your Critical Carbohydrate Level for Maintenance (the maximum number of carb grams you can eat without gaining weight) on the Maintenance diet will be tailored to your own metabolism. Most people's will be between 40 and 90 grams a day, but people with high metabolic resistance may find their maintenance level as low as 25 grams. To maintain your ideal weight, keep eating at this level of carb grams.

Dr. ATKINS' NEW

Carbohydrate Gram Counter

ABBREVIATIONS AND SYMBOLS

C = cup
dia. = diameter
fl. oz. = fluid ounce
gr = gram
lb. = pound
lg. = large
med. = medium
oz. = ounce
pkt. = packet
sm. = small
sq. = square
t = teaspoon
T = tablespoon
w/ = with
w/o = without
" = inch
< = less than

Dashes [—] denote lack of reliable data for a constituent believed to be present in a measurable amount.

Nutritive values in parentheses denote estimated values usually from another form of the food or from a similar food.

BEANS AND LEGUMES (Cooked)

Food (Serving)	Carbo/gr	Protein/gr	Fat/gr
Bean dip, Master Choice:			
black bean (2T)	**6.0**	(2.0)	1.0
pinto (2T)	**5.0**	1.0	1.0
Beans and franks,			
canned (1C)	**32.1**	19.4	18.1
Beans and rice: *See* Rice			
and Beans *in* Pasta			
and Rice			
Beans w/pork and tomato sauce,			
canned (1C)	**48.5**	15.6	6.6
Beans w/tomato sauce,			
canned (1C)	**58.7**	16.1	1.3
Chickpeas or garbanzos (1C)	**122.0**	41.0	9.6
Chili, canned:			
con carne w/beans (1C)	**31.1**	19.1	15.6
turkey w/beans (1C)	**25.0**	19.0	3.0
vegetarian w/beans (1C)	**38.0**	12.0	(12.0)
Cowpeas or black-eyed peas (1C)	**29.9**	13.4	1.3
Falafel (½C)	**42.0**	15.0	4.0
Great Northern (1C)	**38.2**	14.0	1.1
Hummus tahini (2T)	**5.0**	2.0	3.0
Lentil pilaf, Near East			
dry mix (2 oz.)	**37.0**	10.0	4.0
Lentils (1C)	**38.6**	15.6	trace
Lima (1C)	**33.7**	12.9	0.9
Pea or Navy (1C)	**40.3**	14.8	1.1
Peas, split (1C)	**41.6**	16.0	0.6
Pinto (1C)	**38.0**	14.0	0.8

Food (Serving)	Carbo/gr	Protein/gr	Fat/gr
Red kidney (1C)	**39.6**	14.4	0.9
Refried beans,			
Old El Paso (½C)	**17.0**	6.0	2.0
Soybeans (1C)	**19.4**	19.8	10.3
Tofu or soybean curd (2" cube)	**2.9**	9.4	5.0

BEVERAGES

Food (Serving)	Carbo/gr	Protein/gr	Fat/gr
Beer, nonalcoholic:			
Cutter (12 fl. oz.)	**17.1**	0.8	0
O'Doul (12 fl. oz.)	**15.0**	0.7	0
Sharp (12 fl. oz.)	**12.1**	0.4	0
Beer: *See* Liquor *in this section*			
Chocolate Milk: *See* Milk and Milk Products			
Coffee:			
ground and instant, regular and			
decaffeinated	**trace**	trace	trace
flavored instant, General Foods			
Café Francais (4t)	**7.0**	<1.0	3.5
Cappuccino (4t)	**10.0**	<1.0	1.5
French Vanilla (4t)	**10.0**	<1.0	2.5
Hazelnut Belgian (4t)	**12.0**	<1.0	2.0
Suisse Mocha (4t)	**9.0**	<1.0	2.0
Gatorade, most flavors (1C)	**14.0**	0	0
Hot chocolate, Swiss Miss:			
Cocoa and Cream (1 pkt.)	**25.0**	2.0	5.0
diet (1 pkt.)	**4.0**	2.0	0
fat free (1 pkt.)	**9.0**	3.0	0
lite (1 pkt.)	**17.0**	1.0	0.5
Marshmallow Lovers (1 pkt.)	**27.0**	2.0	3.0
Juices, fruit and vegetable:			
apple (1C)	**29.5**	0.2	trace
apricot nectar (1C)	**36.6**	0.8	0.3
banana nectar (1C)	**34.0**	0	0
Clamato (1C)	**24.0**	1.0	0
Cranapple (1C)	**41.0**	0	0

Food (Serving)	Carbo/gr	Protein/gr	Fat/gr
Juices, fruit and vegetable (*continued*):			
Cranberry cocktail (1C)	**41.7**	0.3	0.3
Cran-Cherry (1C)	**39.0**	0	0
Five Alive (1C)	**30.0**	0	0
Fruit Punch, Hawaiian (1C)	**30.0**	0	0
grape (1C)	**42.0**	0.5	trace
grapegruit			
fresh, pink, red or white (1C)	**23.0**	1.0	trace
canned, white, unsweetened (1C)	**24.0**	1.0	trace
sweetened (1C)	**32.0**	1.0	trace
carton (1C)	**23.0**	<1.0	0
frozen concentrate,			
unsweetened (1C)	**24.0**	1.0	trace
guava nectar (1C)	**39.0**	0	0
mango (1C)	**37.0**	0	0
mango guava (1C)	**33.0**	0	0
orange			
fresh (1C)	**26.0**	2.0	trace
carton (1C)	**27.0**	<1.0	0
frozen concentrate (1C)	**29.0**	2.0	trace
peach nectar (1C)	**36.0**	<1.0	0
pear nectar (1C)	**38.0**	0	0
pineapple (1C)	**33.8**	1.0	0.3
prune (1C)	**48.6**	1.0	0.3
tangerine (1C)	**29.9**	1.2	0.5
tomato (1C)	**10.4**	2.2	0.2
V-8 (1C)	**10.0**	1.0	0
Lemonade:			
bottled, Snapple (8 fl. oz.)	**27.0**	0	0
canned concentrate (1C)	**28.0**	trace	trace
powdered,			
Country Time (18 gr)	**17.0**	0	0
Limeade,			
canned concentrate (1C)	**27.0**	trace	trace
Liquor:			
beer			
regular (12 fl. oz.)	**13.7**	1.1	0
light (12 fl. oz.)	**6.0**	1.0	0

Food (Serving)	*Carbo/gr*	*Protein/gr*	*Fat/gr*
hard liquor (whisky, Scotch, vodka, Bourbon, gin, etc.),			
any proof (1 fl. oz.)	**trace**	trace	trace
wine, dessert (3½ fl. oz.)	**7.9**	0.1	0
table (3½ fl. oz.)	**4.3**	0.1	0
Milk, *see* Milk and Milk Products			
Nantucket Nectars:			
cranberry (8 fl. oz.)	**36.0**	0	0
guava (8 fl. oz.)	**31.0**	0	0
orange mango (8 fl. oz.)	**31.0**	0	0
pink grapefruit (8 fl. oz.)	**26.0**	0	0
Ovaltine (4T)	**18.0**	1.0	0
Rice Dream:			
original (1C)	**25.0**	1.0	2.0
chocolate (1C)	**36.0**	1.0	3.0
vanilla (1C)	**28.0**	1.0	2.0
Rice and Soy Milk,			
EdenBlend (1C)	**16.0**	7.0	3.0
Snapple,			
most fruit flavors (1C)	**28.5**	0	0
Sodas:			
club soda (12 fl. oz.)	**0**	0	0
Coke (12 fl. oz.)	**39.0**	0	0
cranberry, Cape Cod (12 fl. oz.)	**44.0**	0	0
cream soda			
A & W (12 fl. oz.)	**42.0**	0	0
Doctor Brown's (12 fl. oz.)	**44.0**	0	0
Mug (12 fl. oz.)	**48.0**	0	0
diet, all varieties (12 fl. oz.)	**0**	0	0
Doctor Brown's			
Black Cherry (12 fl. oz.)	**45.0**	0	0
Cel-Ray (12 fl. oz.)	**34.0**	0	0
Dr. Pepper (12 fl. oz.)	**40.0**	0	0
ginger ale			
Seagram's (12 fl. oz.)	**36.0**	0	0
Schweppes (12 fl. oz.)	**33.0**	0	0
grape			
Minute Maid (12 fl. oz.)	**48.0**	0	0

Food (Serving)	Carbo/gr	Protein/gr	Fat/gr
Sodas (*continued*):			
Welch's (12 fl. oz.)	**51.0**	0	0
Mountain Dew (12 fl. oz.)	**46.0**	0	0
orange			
Minute Maid (12 fl. oz.)	**47.0**	0	0
Slice (12 fl. oz.)	**51.0**	0	0
Pepsi (12 fl. oz.)	**41.0**	0	0
RC Cola (12 fl. oz.)	**43.0**	0	0
root beer			
A & W (12 fl. oz.)	**44.0**	0	0
Doctor Brown's (12 fl. oz.)	**42.0**	0	0
Mug (12 fl. oz.)	**43.0**	0	0
seltzer, flavored and plain (12 fl. oz.)	**0**	0	0
7-Up (12 fl. oz.)	**39.0**	0	0
Sprite (12 fl. oz.)	**38.0**	0	0
Soy milk, Eden:			
original (1C)	**13.0**	10.0	4.0
vanilla and carob (1C)	**23.0**	6.0	3.0
Sport Shake:			
chocolate (11 oz.)	**63.0**	13.0	13.0
strawberry and vanilla (11 fl. oz.)	**55.0**	13.0	14.0
Sunny Delight:			
California Style (1C)	**33.0**	0	0
Florida Citrus (1C)	**30.0**	0	0
passion fruit (1C)	**35.0**	0	0
Tea, both herbal and traditional blends	**trace**	trace	trace
Tea, iced:			
canned or bottled			
Lipton (12 fl. oz.)	**33.0**	0	0
Nestea (12 fl. oz.)	**33.0**	0	0
Snapple (8 fl. oz.)	**25.0**	0	0
fruit flavored teas (8 fl. oz.)	**26.9**	0	0
powdered mix			
Crystal Light (1 gr)	**0**	0	0
Lipton (5T)	**22.0**	0	0
Nestea (2T)	**19.0**	0	0
Water, bottled			
(Perrier, Evian, etc.) (8 fl. oz.)	**0**	0	0
Yoo-Hoo (1C)	**29.0**	2.0	1.0

BREADS, CRACKERS AND PASTRIES

Food (Serving)	Carbo/gr	Protein/gr	Fat/gr
Apple cinnamon rolls w/icing, Pillsbury (1)	**23.0**	2.0	6.0
Bagel, 3" dia.:			
egg (1)	**28.0**	6.0	2.0
water (1)	**30.0**	6.0	1.0
Lender's, plain (1)	**30.0**	6.0	1.0
Biscuit:			
homemade, 2" dia. (1)	**14.6**	2.0	2.6
bake and serve, Pillsbury			
buttermilk (3)	**29.0**	4.0	2.0
country (3)	**29.0**	4.0	2.0
Grands (1)	**24.0**	4.0	10.0
Hungry Jack (1)	**14.0**	2.0	4.5
Bread:			
cracked-wheat (1 slice)	**13.0**	2.2	0.6
French (1 slice)	**12.6**	2.4	1.0
Italian (1 slice)	**11.3**	1.8	0.2
oatmeal (1 slice)	**17.5**	4.0	2.0
raisin (1 slice)	**13.4**	1.7	0.7
rye (1 slice)	**13.0**	2.3	0.3
pumpernickel (1 slice)	**17.0**	2.9	0.4
white (1 slice)	**14.1**	2.4	0.9
whole wheat (1 slice)	**11.0**	2.4	0.7
Bread stick:			
plain (1)	**7.0**	1.0	1.0
sesame (1)	**7.0**	1.0	2.5

Food (Serving)	Carbo/gr	Protein/gr	Fat/gr
Cinnamon roll w/icing,			
Sara Lee (1)	**53.0**	5.0	15.0
Coffee cake, crumb:			
Drake (1)	**23.0**	2.0	6.0
Sara Lee (⅛)	**32.0**	3.0	9.0
Cornbread (2½" sq.)	**27.5**	3.8	5.8
Crackers:			
Buttercrisp (9)	**19.0**	2.0	7.0
Club (6)	**13.5**	1.5	4.5
crispbreads, Scandinavian			
Finn Crisp, dark (3)	**12.0**	2.0	0
Kavli,			
thick (2)	**15.0**	2.0	0.5
thin (3)	**13.0**	1.0	0
Ryvita,			
dark rye (2)	**11.0**	2.0	0
flavorful fiber (2)	**10.0**	2.0	0
Wasa,			
fiber rye (1)	**4.0**	1.0	1.0
light rye (1)	**5.0**	<1.0	0
toasted wheat (1)	**9.0**	1.0	1.0
flat breads			
low fat			
garlic (1)	**7.0**	1.0	1.0
poppy (1)	**7.0**	1.0	1.0
sesame (1)	**8.0**	2.0	1.5
fat free			
garden vegetable (1)	**8.0**	1.0	0
plain (1)	**8.0**	1.0	1.0
pumpernickel (1)	**8.0**	1.0	0
graham			
regular and honey (8)	**22.0**	2.0	3.0
cinnamon (8)	**26.0**	2.0	3.0
Harvest Crisp (13)	**23.0**	3.0	3.5
matzoh (1)	**22.0**	3.0	0.5
melba toast (3)	**11.0**	2.0	0
Oat Thins (18)	**20.0**	3.0	6.0

Food (Serving)	Carbo/gr	Protein/gr	Fat/gr
rice or corn cake			
puffed, plain,			
Quaker (1)	**7.0**	1.0	0
mini cakes, Hain's			
apple cinnamon (6)	**13.0**	1.0	0
caramel (5)	**14.0**	1.0	0
white cheddar (6)	**10.0**	1.0	3.0
Rice Snaps, brown (4)	**13.0**	1.0	0
Ritz (5)	**10.0**	1.0	4.0
Saltines, regular or multigrain (5)	**10.0**	1.0	1.5
SnackWell's			
Golden (6)	**11.0**	1.0	1.0
Wheat (5)	**12.0**	2.0	0
Sociables (7)	**9.0**	1.0	4.0
soda, Export (3)	**10.0**	1.0	2.0
Town House (5)	**9.0**	1.0	4.5
Triscuits (7)	**21.0**	3.0	5.0
Uneeda Biscuit (2)	**11.0**	1.0	1.0
water (2 lg./4 med.)	**12.0**	2.0	1.0
Waverly (5)	**10.0**	1.0	3.5
Wheat Thins (17)	**21.0**	2.0	4.0
Wheat, Stoned, mini (19)	**21.0**	3.0	3.0
Wheatables (26)	**18.0**	3.0	7.0
Wheatsworth (5)	**10.0**	2.0	3.5
Zwieback (1)	**6.0**	1.0	1.0
Croissants, Sara Lee:			
original (1)	**20.0**	4.0	8.0
petite (2)	**26.0**	6.0	11.0
Danish:			
plain ring (⅛)	**19.4**	3.1	10.0
individual (5 oz.)	**64.8**	10.5	33.4
Donut:			
cake type, 3⅝" dia. (1)	**29.8**	2.7	10.8
yeast leavened, glazed, 3¾" dia. (1)	**22.0**	3.0	11.0
English muffin, Thomas':			
original (1)	**25.0**	4.0	1.0
oat bran (1)	**26.0**	4.0	1.0

Food (Serving)	Carbo/gr	Protein/gr	Fat/gr
English muffin, Thomas' (*continued*):			
raisin (1)	**31.0**	4.0	1.0
sourdough (1)	**25.0**	4.0	1.0
French toast, frozen,			
Aunt Jemima			
original (2)	**38.0**	9.0	6.0
cinnamon (2)	**37.0**	9.0	6.0
Muffin:			
blueberry w/crumb topping:			
Duncan Hines mix (1)	**32.0**	2.0	6.0
Sara Lee (1)	**27.0**	3.0	11.0
corn			
homemade (1)	**20.0**	2.8	4.2
Sara Lee (1)	**30.0**	3.0	14.0
Thomas's Toaster Cake (1)	**19.0**	2.0	4.0
Pancakes:			
dry mix w/eggs and milk			
buckwheat, 6" dia. (1)	**17.4**	5.0	6.6
regular, 6" dia. (1)	**23.7**	5.3	5.3
frozen			
Aunt Jemima			
original (3)	**40.0**	6.0	3.0
low fat (3)	**33.0**	4.0	1.5
Downyflake (3)	**45.0**	5.0	7.0
Hungry Jack, buttermilk (3)	**46.0**	5.0	4.0
Pita, Sahara:			
original (1)	**31.0**	6.0	1.0
mini (1)	**15.0**	3.0	0
Rolls:			
bakery			
cloverleaf (1)	**14.8**	2.3	1.6
frankfurter/hamburger bun (1)	**21.2**	3.3	2.2
round or kaiser (1)	**29.8**	4.9	1.6
bake and serve, Pillsbury			
crescent (2)	**22.0**	4.0	11.0
Dinner (1)	**18.0**	4.0	2.0
Stuffing, Stove Top dry mix:			
corn (28 gr)	**21.0**	3.0	8.0

Food (Serving)	Carbo/gr	Protein/gr	Fat/gr
chicken (½C)	**19.0**	3.0	8.0
long grain and wld rice (30 gr)	**22.0**	4.0	9.0
Toaster pastries:			
Pop Tarts, Kellogg's (1)	**36.0-39.0**	2.0	5.0-7.0
Toaster Pastries, Snack Well's (1)	**37.0**	2.0	1.0
Toastettes, Nabisco (1)	**35.0**	2.0	5.0
Turnovers, Pepperidge Farm:			
apple (1)	**48.0**	4.0	14.0
blueberry (1)	**45.0**	4.0	16.0
Waffles:			
dry mix w/egg and milk			
regular, 9" sq. (1)	**72.4**	17.6	21.2
frozen:			
Aunt Jemima			
original (2)	**29.0**	5.0	7.0
low fat (2)	**33.0**	5.0	1.0
blueberry (2)	**28.0**	5.0	6.0
buttermilk (2)	**29.0**	6.0	7.0
Downyflake original (2)	**29.0**	4.0	4.0
Eggo			
blueberry (2)	**33.0**	5.0	8.0
buttermilk (2)	**30.0**	5.0	8.0
homestyle (2)	**30.0**	5.0	8.0
Nutri-Grain (2)	**30.0**	5.0	6.0
Special K (2)	**29.0**	6.0	0

CEREALS AND GRAINS

Food (Serving)	Carbo/gr	Protein/gr	Fat/gr
Cereals:			
cold w/o milk or sugar			
All-Bran (½C)	**22.0**	4.0	1.0
Alpen (⅔C)	**41.0**	6.0	3.0
amaranth flakes (¾C)	**24.0**	3.0	0
Apple Jacks (1C)	**27.0**	2.0	0
Bran Buds (⅓C)	**24.0**	3.0	0.5
Cheerios (1C)	**23.0**	3.0	2.0
Cocoa Puffs (1C)	**27.0**	1.0	1.0
Complete Bran Flakes (¾C)	**24.0**	3.0	0.5
Corn or Rice Chex (1C)	**26.0**	2.0	0
corn flakes (1C)	**24.0**	6.0	1.5
Corn Pops (1C)	**28.0**	1.0	0
Cracklin' Oat Bran (¾C)	**40.0**	4.0	8.0
Crispix (1C)	**25.0**	2.0	0
Crispy Brown Rice (1C)	**25.0**	2.0	0
Crunchy Corn Bran (¾C)	**23.0**	2.0	1.0
Fiber One (½C)	**24.0**	2.0	1.0
Frosted Flakes (¾C)	**28.0**	1.0	0
Frosted Mini-Wheats (1C)	**41.0**	5.0	1.0
Fruit Loops (1C)	**28.0**	2.0	1.0
granola			
apple-cinnamon (½C)	**34.0**	5.0	3.0
wheat-free, corn-free (½C)	**40.0**	7.0	6.0
Grape-Nuts (½C)	**47.0**	6.0	1.0
Grape-Nut Flakes (¾C)	**24.0**	3.0	1.0
Honey Bunches of Oats (¾C)	**25.0**	2.0	1.5
Honey Comb (1⅓C)	**26.0**	2.0	0.5

Food (Serving)	Carbo/gr	Protein/gr	Fat/gr
kashi, puffed, plain (1C)	**13.0**	3.0	<1.0
honey puffed (1C)	**25.0**	3.0	1.0
Kix			
plain (1⅓C)	**26.0**	2.0	0.5
Berry-Berry (¾C)	**26.0**	1.0	1.0
Life (¾C)	**25.0**	3.0	1.5
Lucky Charms (1C)	**25.0**	2.0	1.0
millet, puffed (1C)	**19.0**	3.0	0.5
Müeslix, Kellogg's (⅖C)	**42.0**	4.0	3.0
Nut and Honey Crunch (1¼C)	**45.0**	4.0	4.0
Nutri-Grain			
almond raisin (1¼C)	**38.0**	4.0	3.0
golden wheat (¾C)	**24.0**	3.0	1.0
Oatios			
original (1C)	**21.0**	4.0	1.0
Apple-n-Cinnamon (1C)	**18.0**	3.0	1.5
Honey-n-Almond (1C)	**22.0**	3.0	1.0
Oatmeal Squares (1C)	**43.0**	7.0	2.5
Product 19 (1C)	**25.0**	2.0	0
puffed rice or wheat (1C)	**11.5**	1.5	0
Raisin Bran (1C)	**47.0**	6.0	1.5
Raisin Nut Bran (1C)	**41.0**	5.0	4.5
Rice Krispies (1¼C)	**29.0**	2.0	0
Shredded Wheat:			
original (2 biscuits)	**38.0**	5.0	0.5
Spoon Size (1C)	**41.0**	5.0	0.5
'N Bran, Spoon Size	**47.0**	7.0	1.0
Smacks, sugared			
puffed wheat (¾C)	**26.0**	2.0	0.5
Special K (1C)	**22.0**	6.0	0
spelt flakes (1C)	**22.0**	5.0	1.0
Toasted Oatmeal Flakes			
Original (1¼C)	**44.0**	5.0	2.0
Honey Nut (1C)	**39.0**	5.0	2.5
Total			
Raisin Bran (1C)	**43.0**	4.0	1.0
Whole Grain (¾C)	**24.0**	3.0	1.0
Trix (1C)	**26.0**	1.0	1.5

Food (Serving)	Carbo/gr	Protein/gr	Fat/gr
Cereals, cold (*continued*):			
Wheaties (1C)	**24.0**	3.0	1.0
cooked, w/o milk or sugar			
Brown Rice Cream (¼C*)	**36.0**	5.0	1.0
cream of buckwheat (⅛C*)	**21.0**	1.0	0
cream of wheat			
regular (1C)	**25.0**	3.0	0.5
instant (1 pkt.)	**21.0**	3.0	0.5
Farina, H.O. Quick (1C)	**26.0**	3.0	0
grits			
old fashioned (¼C*)	**32.0**	3.0	0.5
quick (¼C*)	**29.0**	3.0	0.5
instant (½C*)	**33.0**	4.0	0.2
Maltex (⅓C*)	**37.0**	5.0	0.5
Maypo, Maple Oatmeal,			
instant (½C)	**36.0**	6.0	2.0
oatmeal			
old fashioned (½C*)	**27.0**	5.0	3.0
quick (½C*)	**27.0**	5.0	3.0
instant (1 pkt.)	**19.0**	4.0	2.0
quinoa flakes,			
instant (⅓C*)	**23.0**	3.0	1.0
rice cereal (⅓C*)	**43.0**	4.0	2.0
Wheatena (⅓C*)	**32.0**	5.0	1.0
Granola or cereal bars:			
Cereal, SnackWell's (1 bar)	**29.0**	1.0	0
Chewy Granola,			
Quaker (1 bar)	**21.0**	2.0	3.5
Kudos (1 bar)	**18.0-19.0**	2.0	4.5-5.0
Nutri-Grain, Kellogg's (1 bar)	**27.0**	2.0	3.0
Grains:			
barley			
quick cooking (⅓C)	**37.0**	5.0	1.0
cornmeal, cooked (1C)	**25.7**	2.6	0.5
couscous mix (⅓C)	**45.0**	6.0	1.0

*(An * after serving size indicates dry, uncooked measure, not cooked serving size.)*

Food (Serving)	Carbo/gr	Protein/gr	Fat/gr
flour			
barley (¼C)	**19.0**	3.0	0.5
buckwheat (1C)	**78.0**	6.0	1.0
quinoa (¼C)	**28.0**	5.0	2.0
soy (1C)	**21.3**	25.7	14.2
spelt (¼C)	**24.0**	4.0	0.5
wheat, all purpose baking (¼C)	**22.0**	3.0	0
whole wheat (¼C)	**25.0**	5.0	0.5
Oat Bran (1 oz.)	**15.0**	4.0	2.0
Polenta mix (⅜C)	**46.0**	8.0	5.0
Rice, *see* Pasta and Rice			
Tabouli mix (¼C)	**26.0**	4.0	0.5
Wheat Bran Flakes (½ oz.)	**10.0**	2.0	1.0
Wheat Germ (1T)	**3.0**	1.8	0.7

CONDIMENTS, SEASONINGS AND SAUCES

Food (Serving)	Carbo/gr	Protein/gr	Fat/gr
Anchovies (5 pieces)	**0.1**	3.8	2.1
A.1. steak sauce (1T)	**3.0**	0	0
Apple Butter (1T)	**8.2**	0.1	0.1
Bacon chips:			
Bacon Flavor, Bac-Os (1T)	**2.0**	3.0	1.0
Bacon Bits, Hormel (1T)	**0**	3.0	1.5
Barbecue sauce (1C)	**20.0**	3.8	17.3
Béarnaise sauce, Knorr, prepared (2T)	**3.7**	<1.5	7.0
Catsup (1T)	**3.8**	0.3	0.1
Chili sauce (1T)	**4.0**	0	0
Cocoa powder (1T)	**2.8**	0.9	1.0
Cranberry sauce, canned			
jellied (¼C)	**27.0**	0	0
whole berry (¼C)	**28.0**	0	0
Creamers, non-dairy:			
Coffee-Mate (1T)	**1.0**	0	0.5
Cremora (1T)	**1.0**	0	1.0
Ginger root, fresh (1 oz.)	**3.0**	0.4	0.3
Gravies from cans, jars, or dry mix			
beef or brown (¼C)	**3.5**	1.0	1.5
chicken (¼C)	**3.5**	.75	1.0
mushroom (¼C)	**3.0**	1.0	1.0
turkey (¼C)	**4.0**	1.0	1.0
Hazelnut spread, Nutella (2T)	**19.0**	2.0	9.0
Herbs and spices: 1 teaspoon of most herbs and spices provides trace			

Food (Serving)	Carbo/gr	Protein/gr	Fat/gr
amounts per serving. (eg. garlic, basil, oregano, turmeric, etc.)			
Hollandaise sauce, Knorr, prepared (2T)	**3.7**	<1.5	7.0
Horseradish (1t)	**0.5**	0.1	trace
Jams, jellies, marmalades and preserves:			
Polaner			
All Fruit, most flavors (1T)	**10.0**	0	0
preserves, most flavors (1T)	**13.5**	0	0
reduced sugar, most flavors (1T)	**5.5**	0	0
Smucker's			
jam and marmalade,			
most flavors (1T)	**13.0**	0	0
low sugar, most flavors (1T)	**6.0**	0	0
Trappist Preserves, most flavors (1T)	**13.0**	0	0
Welch's grape jelly (1T)	**13.0**	0	0
Wilkin and Sons Ltd,			
most flavors (1T)	**13.0**	0	0
Malted milk powder, Carnation (3T)	**15.0**	3.0	2.0
Mayonnaise: *See* Fats, Oils and Salad Dressings			
Miracle Whip: *See* Fats, Oils and Salad Dressings			
Mustard:			
Dijon (1t)	**<1.0**	<1.0	0
yellow or brown (1t)	**0.3**	0.2	0.2
Olives:			
green, large (10)	**0.5**	0.5	4.9
ripe, large (10)	**1.2**	0.5	6.5
oil cured (10)	**2.3**	0.6	9.5
Peppers, B & G:			
hot cherry peppers (1)	**2.0**	0	0
jalapenos, hot whole (1)	**1.0**	0	0
peperoncini (3)	**2.0**	0	0
roasted red peppers (1 oz.)	**1.0**	0	0
sweet peppers (1)	**2.0**	0	0
Pickles:			
B & G			
bread and butter chips (6)	**7.0**	0	0

Food (Serving)	Carbo/gr	Protein/gr	Fat/gr
Pickles, B & G (*continued*):			
sweet mixed (6½)	**8.0**	0	0
sweet or India relish (1T)	**4.0**	0	0
Vlasic			
hamburger dill chips (10)	**1.0**	0	0
Kosher dill spears (1)	**1.0**	0	0
sweet gherkins (3)	**10.0**	0	0
Salsa (2T)	**2.5**	0	0
Sandwich spread w/pickle (1T)	**2.4**	0.1	5.4
Seafood cocktail sauce (¼C)	**14.0**	1.0	0
Sesame tahini (2T)	**8.0**	5.0	15.0
Soy sauce (1T)	**1.7**	1.0	0.2
Spaghetti sauce:			
Healthy Choice			
traditional (½C)	**10.0**	2.0	0.5
extra chunky, Italian style (½C)	**8.0**	2.0	0
garlic and herb (½C)	**10.0**	2.0	0.5
Prego			
traditional (½C)	**23.0**	2.0	4.5
extra chunky, garden combo (½C)	**16.0**	2.0	1.0
marinara (½C)	**12.0**	2.0	6.0
meat (½C)	**21.0**	3.0	6.0
mushroom (½C)	**23.0**	2.0	5.0
tomato and basil (½C)	**19.0**	2.0	3.0
Ragú			
traditional (½C)	**10.0**	2.0	3.0
hearty w/onion, garlic (½C)	**18.0**	2.0	4.0
light, chunky garden (½C)	**11.0**	2.0	0
tomato and basil (½C)	**11.0**	2.0	0
marinara (½C)	**9.0**	2.0	4.5
meat (½C)	**9.0**	2.0	3.5
mushroom (½C)	**10.0**	2.0	3.0
Syrup:			
chocolate			
Bosco (2T)	**27.0**	0	0
Hershey (2T)	**24.0**	1.0	0
Nestlé's Quick (2T)	**25.0**	0	0.5
No-Cal Chocolate (2T)	**0**	0	0

Food (Serving)	Carbo/gr	Protein/gr	Fat/gr
Yoo-Hoo (2T)	**25.0**	0	0.5
strawberry			
Hershey (2T)	**26.0**	0	0
Nestlé's Quik (2T)	**27.0**	0	0
No-Cal Strawberry (2T)	**0.1**	0.1	0
Tabasco sauce (1t)	**0.1**	0.1	0
Tamari sauce (1T)	**1.0**	2.0	0
Tartar sauce (1T)	**0.6**	0.2	8.1
Thai peanut sauce (1T)	**4.0**	1.0	2.0
Vanilla, double strength (1t)	**3.0**	0	0
Vinegar:			
balsamic (1T)	**0.9**	0	0
cider (1T)	**0.9**	trace	(0)
tarragon (1T)	**0.9**	0	0
wine (1T)	**0.9**	0	0
White sauce, medium thick (1C)	**22.0**	9.8	31.3
Worcestershire sauce (1T)	**1.0**	0	0

DESSERTS AND SNACK FOODS

Food (Serving)	Carbo/gr	Protein/gr	Fat/gr
Brownies:			
dry mix, Duncan Hines:			
Chewy Fudge (1 sq.)	**25.0**	2.0	7.0
Double Fudge (1 sq.)	**29.0**	2.0	7.0
Cake:			
from mix w/moderate icing, 8" dia.			
angelfood (⅟₁₂)	**31.5**	3.0	0.1
chocolate (⅟₁₂)	**59.3**	3.0	7.7
devil's food (⅟₁₂)	**53.6**	4.0	11.3
gingerbread (2¾" sq.)	**32.2**	2.0	4.3
white (⅟₁₂)	**59.7**	3.7	10.2
yellow (⅟₁₂)	**53.0**	3.8	10.4
frozen			
Pepperidge Farm, 7" dia.			
Boston cream (⅛)	**42.0**	3.0	9.0
coconut (⅛)	**35.0**	2.0	11.0
devil's food (⅛)	**34.0**	2.0	12.0
vanilla (⅛)	**35.0**	2.0	11.0
Sara Lee, 8" dia.			
fudge golden (⅛)	**34.0**	3.0	13.0
German chocolate (⅛)	**34.0**	4.0	15.0
strawberry shortcake (⅛)	**27.0**	2.0	7.0
pound cake, 10.75 oz. loaf			
all butter (¼)	**38.0**	4.0	16.0
chocolate swirl (¼)	**42.0**	5.0	16.0
individually packaged snack cakes			
cupcakes, orange, Hostess			
(2 cakes)	**55.0**	2.0	10.0

Food (Serving)	Carbo/gr	Protein/gr	Fat/gr
Devil Dogs (1)	**28.0**	2.0	7.0
Ho Hos (3 cakes)	**50.0**	3.0	18.0
King Dons (2 cakes)	**45.0**	3.0	19.0
Ring Dings (2 cakes)	**43.0**	2.0	18.0
Snowballs (2 cakes)	**61.0**	3.0	11.0
Suzy Q's (2 cakes)	**70.0**	4.0	18.0
Twinkies (2 cakes)	**51.0**	3.0	9.0
Yodels (3 cakes)	**52.0**	3.0	24.0
Candy:			
Almond Joy (1.76 oz. bar)	**28.0**	2.0	13.0
Andes Creme de Menthe Thins (8)	**22.0**	2.0	13.0
Cadbury, 5 oz. bar			
Caramello (5 blocks)	**25.0**	2.0	9.0
Dairy Milk (9 blocks)	**24.0**	3.0	12.0
Fruit & Nut (9 blocks)	**24.0**	3.0	11.0
Krisp (9 blocks)	**25.0**	3.0	10.0
Roast Almond (9 blocks)	**21.0**	4.0	13.0
Chunky (1.4 oz. bar)	**22.0**	3.0	11.0
Crunch, Nestlé's (1.55 oz. bar)	**29.0**	2.0	12.0
Good & Plenty (35 pieces)	**35.0**	1.0	0
Gum Drops (1 oz.)	**24.8**	trace	0.2
hard candies:			
butterscotch (4)	**15.0**	0	0
peppermint (4)	**15.0**	0	0
sour balls (5)	**14.9**	0	0
Hershey Hugs (8 pieces)	**22.0**	3.0	12.0
w/almonds (9 pieces)	**23.0**	4.0	13.0
Hershey Kisses (8 pieces)	**23.0**	3.0	12.0
w/almonds (8 pieces)	**19.0**	4.0	13.0
jelly beans (10)	**26.4**	trace	0.1
Junior Mints (16)	**34.0**	<1.0	3.5
Kit Kat (1.5 oz. bar)	**26.0**	3.0	12.0
Mars Chocolate Almond (1.76 oz. bar)	**31.0**	3.0	13.0
M&M's			
almond (1.31 oz. pack)	**21.0**	3.0	11.0
peanut (1.74 oz. pack)	**30.0**	5.0	13.0
plain (1.69 oz. pack)	**34.0**	2.0	10.0

Food (Serving)	Carbo/gr	Protein/gr	Fat/gr
Candy (*continued*):			
milk chocolate			
Hershey (1.55 oz. bar)	**25.0**	3.0	13.0
w/almonds (1.45 oz. bar)	**20.0**	5.0	14.0
Nestlé's (1.45 oz. bar)	**23.0**	4.0	13.0
Milky Way (2.15 oz. bar)	**43.0**	2.0	11.0
Mounds (1.9 oz. bar)	**31.0**	2.0	13.0
Munch Peanut Bar (1.42 oz. bar)	**17.0**	6.0	15.0
Peanut Butter Cups, Reese's			
(1.6 oz. pack)	**25.0**	5.0	14.0
Peppermint Patty, York (1.5 oz.)	**34.0**	<1.0	3.0
Raisinets (1.58 oz. pack)	**31.0**	2.0	8.0
Skør (1.4 oz. bar)	**23.0**	2.0	13.0
Snickers (2.07 oz.)	**35.0**	5.0	14.0
3 Musketeers (2.13 oz. bar)	**46.0**	2.0	8.0
Toffee, English,			
Callard & Bowser (2)	**12.0**	0	4.0
Tootsie Roll Midgees (6)	**33.0**	<1.0	3.0
Twix (2 oz. bar)	**37.0**	3.0	14.0
Twizzlers, strawberry and			
licorice (2.5 oz. pack)	**54.0**	2.0	1.0
Cookies:			
animal crackers (15)	**23.0**	2.0	2.0
Arrowroot biscuits (4)	**26.0**	2.0	4.0
Butter, Danish (4)	**19.0**	2.0	8.0
Chip-A-Roos (2)	**18.0**	1.0	7.0
Chips Ahoy (3)	**23.0**	1.0	8.0
Chips Deluxe (1)	**9.0**	1.0	4.5
Dutch Apple, Archway (1)	**18.0**	1.0	3.5
Dutch Cocoa, Archway (1)	**18.0**	1.0	3.5
Fig Newtons (2)	**20.0**	1.0	2.5
Frookwich sandwich cookies,			
assorted flavors (2)	**14.0**	1.0	4.0
Fudge Grahams (3)	**19.0**	1.0	4.5
ginger snaps (4)	**22.0**	1.0	2.5
Hydrox (3)	**21.0**	2.0	7.0
Lorna Doones (4)	**19.0**	2.0	7.0
Milano (3)	**21.0**	2.0	10.0

Food (Serving)	Carbo/gr	Protein/gr	Fat/gr
Molasses, Archway (1)	18.0	1.0	3.5
Nilla Wafers (8)	24.0	2.0	5.0
Nutter Butter (2)	19.0	3.0	6.0
oatmeal			
plain, Archway (1)	16.0	1.0	3.5
plain, Nabisco (1)	12.0	1.0	3.0
apple-filled (1)	16.0	1.0	3.0
chocolate chip (3)	23.0	3.0	8.0
raisin (1)	17.0	1.0	3.5
Oreos			
traditional (3)	23.0	2.0	7.0
Double Stuf (2)	19.0	1.0	7.0
reduced fat (3)	25.0	2.0	3.5
Pecan Sandies (1)	11.0	<1.0	3.0
Rich Tea (4)	25.0	2.0	5.0
Shortbread, Walker's (1)	11.0	1.0	5.0
SnackWell's, chocolate or			
creme sandwich (2)	21.0	1.0	2.5
double fudge (1)	12.0	1.0	(3.0)
sugar wafers (10)	25.7	1.7	6.8
Sweetmeal (3)	24.0	2.0	7.0
Vienna Fingers (2)	21.0	2.0	6.0
Ice Cream and Frozen Treats:			
Ben & Jerry's ice cream			
butter pecan (½C)	20.0	5.0	25.0
Cherry Garcia (½C)	25.0	4.0	16.0
chocolate fudge brownie (½C)	33.0	4.0	14.0
Coffee Olé (½C)	22.0	4.0	16.0
vanilla (½C)	21.0	4.0	17.0
White Russian (½C)	21.0	3.0	16.0
Breyers ice cream			
butter almond (½C)	15.0	4.0	11.0
cherry vanilla (½C)	17.0	3.0	7.0
chocolate (½C)	19.0	3.0	8.0
coffee (½C)	15.0	3.0	8.0
mint chocolate chip (½C)	18.0	3.0	10.0
strawberry (½C)	15.0	3.0	6.0
vanilla (½C)	15.0	3.0	8.0

Food (Serving)	Carbo/gr	Protein/gr	Fat/gr
Ice Cream and Frozen Treats (*continued*):			
Breyers low fat ice cream			
brownie marble fudge (½C)	**23.0**	4.0	5.0
butter pecan (½C)	**19.0**	3.0	4.0
vanilla (½C)	**19.0**	3.0	4.0
Breyers fat free ice cream			
caramel praline crunch (½C)	**27.0**	3.0	0
chocolate (½C)	**20.0**	3.0	0
vanilla (½C)	**21.0**	3.0	0
vanilla fudge twirl (½C)	**24.0**	3.0	0
Häagen-Dazs ice cream			
butter pecan (½C)	**20.0**	5.0	23.0
chocolate (½C)	**22.0**	5.0	18.0
coffee (½C)	**21.0**	5.0	18.0
rum raisin (½C)	**22.0**	4.0	17.0
strawberry (½C)	**23.0**	4.0	16.0
vanilla (½C)	**21.0**	5.0	18.0
Frozen Yogurt:			
Ben & Jerry's low fat,			
Cherry Garcia (½C)	**31.0**	4.0	3.0
chocolate fudge brownie (½C)	**36.0**	6.0	3.0
English Toffee Crunch (½C)	**32.0**	4.0	6.0
Ben & Jerry's no fat,			
black raspberry swirl (½C)	**32.0**	3.0	0
coffee fudge (½C)	**31.0**	4.0	0
vanilla fudge (½C)	**32.0**	3.0	0
Crowley			
chocolate (½C)	**21.0**	3.0	2.5
peach (½C)	**24.0**	3.0	2.5
strawberry (½C)	**23.0**	3.0	2.0
vanilla (½C)	**21.0**	3.0	2.5
Sherbet:			
Breyer's sherbet, fruit flavors			
(½C)	**26.0**	1.0	1.0
Häagen-Dazs sorbet			
banana strawberry (½C)	**34.0**	<1.0	0
lemon (½C)	**31.0**	0	0
peach (½C)	**35.0**	<1.0	0

Food (Serving)	Carbo/gr	Protein/gr	Fat/gr
Individual bars and sandwiches			
Fudgsicle			
original (1)	**12.0**	2.0	1.0
fat free (1)	**13.0**	3.0	0
sugar free (1)	**8.0**	2.0	0.5
Good Humor			
Chocolate Eclair (1)	**21.0**	2.0	9.0
Strawberry Shortcake (1)	**23.0**	2.0	7.0
Toasted Almond (1)	**25.0**	2.0	8.0
Häagen-Dazs Sorbet Stick:			
chocolate (1)	**20.0**	1.0	0
Wild Berry (1)	**22.0**	0	0
Klondike Bar (1)	**24.0**	3.0	20.0
Popsicle			
original (1)	**18.0**	0	0
sugar free (1)	**3.0**	0	0
Weight Watchers			
Chocolate Dip Bar (1)	**11.0**	2.0	6.0
Chocolate Mousse Bar (1)	**18.0**	4.0	1.0
English Toffee Crunch Bar (1)	**12.0**	2.0	7.0
Orange Vanilla Treat (1)	**17.0**	4.0	1.0
Vanilla Sandwich Bar (1)	**30.0**	4.0	3.5
Welch's fruit juice bars:			
original (1)	**11.0**	0	0
no-sugar added (1)	**6.0**	0	0
Pies:			
Homemade, 9" dia.			
apple (⅛)	**45.0**	2.6	13.1
banana custard (⅛)	**35.0**	5.1	10.6
blueberry (⅛)	**41.2**	2.8	12.7
cherry (⅛)	**45.3**	3.1	13.3
chocolate meringue (⅛)	**38.2**	5.5	13.7
coconut custard (⅛)	**28.4**	6.8	14.3
lemon meringue (⅛)	**39.6**	3.9	10.7
mince (⅛)	**48.6**	3.0	13.6
pecan (⅛)	**52.8**	5.3	23.6
pumpkin (⅛)	**27.9**	4.6	12.8
rhubarb (⅛)	**45.1**	3.0	12.6

Food (Serving)	Carbo/gr	Protein/gr	Fat/gr
Pies (*continued*):			
Bake and Serve, Mrs. Smith's, 8" dia.			
apple (⅙)	**41.0**	2.0	11.0
apple cranberry (⅙)	**43.0**	2.0	11.0
blueberry (⅙)	**39.0**	2.0	11.0
cherry (⅙)	**41.0**	2.0	11.0
coconut custard (⅕)	**35.0**	7.0	12.0
Dutch apple crumb (⅙)	**48.0**	3.0	13.0
lemon meringue (⅕)	**56.0**	2.0	8.0
mince (⅙)	**48.0**	2.0	11.0
peach (⅙)	**38.0**	2.0	11.0
pumpkin custard, 9" dia (⅛)	**39.0**	5.0	8.0
Frozen, Sara Lee, 9" dia.			
chocolate cream pie (⅕)	**49.0**	4.0	32.0
Individually packaged,			
Table Talk, 5 oz.			
apple (1)	**59.0**	4.0	13.0
blueberry (1)	**53.0**	4.0	15.0
cherry (1)	**56.0**	4.0	14.0
lemon (1)	**58.0**	4.0	16.0
peach (1)	**54.0**	4.0	14.0
pineapple (1)	**53.0**	4.0	15.0
Puddings:			
chocolate, instant, made			
with milk (1C)	**63.4**	7.8	6.5
custard, baked (1C)	**29.0**	14.0	15.0
tapioca (1C)	**28.2**	8.3	8.4
pudding snacks, individual snack cups			
Jell-O, chocolate and vanilla,			
113 gr cup			
regular (1)	**28.0**	3.0	5.0
fat free (1)	**23.0**	2.0	0
Kozy Shack, 4 oz. cups			
flan or creme caramel (1)	**25.0**	4.0	3.5
rice (1)	**22.0**	4.0	3.0
Swiss Miss, 113 gr cup			
chocolate (1)	**26.0**	3.0	6.0
tapioca (1)	**24.0**	2.0	4.0

Food (Serving)	Carbo/gr	Protein/gr	Fat/gr
Puddings (*continued*):			
vanilla (1)	**24.0**	2.0	6.0
Snacks:			
cheese flavored:			
Cheese Doodles (1 oz.)	**16.5**	2.0	8.5
Cheese Nips (29 crackers)	**18.0**	3.0	6.0
Chee-tos (1 oz.)	**16.0**	2.0	9.5
Cheez-it (27 crackers)	**16.0**	4.0	8.0
corn chips:			
Doritos			
Cooler Ranch (12 chips)	**18.0**	2.0	7.0
Taco Supreme (12 chips)	**21.0**	2.0	7.0
Fritos			
original (32 chips)	**15.0**	2.0	10.0
Scoops (10 chips)	**16.0**	2.0	9.0
tortilla chips			
Guiltless Gourmet			
baked (20 chips)	**22.0**	2.0	1.0
baked white corn (20 chips)	**22.0**	3.0	1.0
Harry's Rio Grande			
blue corn (1 oz.)	**19.0**	2.0	6.0
guacamole (1 oz.)	**20.0**	2.0	7.0
Santitas (6 chips)	**19.0**	2.0	6.0
Tostitos (6 chips)	**19.0**	2.0	1.0
Cracker Jacks (⅔C)	**23.0**	1.0	2.0
onion rings, Wise (39 rings)	**20.0**	0	6.0
popcorn			
traditional popped, plain (1C)	**4.6**	0.8	0.8
microwave, Orville Redenbacher:			
butter (1C)	**15.0**	2.0	13.0
natural (1C)	**18.0**	2.0	11.0
pork rinds, fried (12)	**0**	9.0	4.0
potato chips			
Lay's (20 chips)	**15.0**	2.0	10.0
Pringles (14 chips)	**15.0**	1.0	11.0
Ruffles (17 chips)	**14.0**	2.0	10.0
Wise (16 chips)	**14.0**	2.0	10.0
potato sticks, French's (¾C)	**16.0**	2.0	12.0

Food (Serving)	Carbo/gr	Protein/gr	Fat/gr
pretzels, Bachman's			
hard sourdough (1)	**18.0**	2.0	0
rods (2)	**24.0**	3.0	0.5
stix (1 oz.)	**20.0**	2.0	1.0
twists (5)	**23.0**	3.0	1.0
vegetable chips:			
Harry's Garden (1 oz.)	**19.0**	2.0	7.0
Terra Chips (1 oz.)	**18.0**	1.0	7.0

FATS, OILS AND SALAD DRESSINGS

Food (Serving)	Carbo/gr	Protein/gr	Fat/gr
Lard (1T)	**0**	0	14.0
Oil, salad or cooking:			
corn (1T)	**0**	0	13.6
cottonseed (1T)	**0**	0	13.6
olive (1T)	**0**	0	13.5
peanut (1T)	**0**	0	13.5
safflower (1T)	**0**	0	13.6
sesame (1T)	**0**	0	13.6
soybean (1T)	**0**	0	13.6
soybean-cottonseed blend (1T)	**0**	0	13.6
Salad dressings:			
Kraft			
Catalina (2T)	**8.0**	0	11.0
fat free (2T)	**8.0**	0	0
Creamy Italian (2T)	**5.4**	0	11.0
fat free (2T)	**12.0**	0	0
French (2T)	**4.0**	0	12.0
fat free (2T)	**12.0**	0	0
Italian (2T)	**2.0**	0	11.0
fat free (2T)	**3.0**	0	0
Ranch (2T)	**2.0**	0	15.0
fat free (2T)	**11.0**	<1.0	0
Thousand Island (2T)	**5.0**	0	10.0
fat free (2T)	**9.0**	0	0
7 Seas			
Classic Caesar (2T)	**2.0**	<1.0	10.0
Creamy Italian (2T)	**2.0**	0	12.0

Food (Serving)	Carbo/gr	Protein/gr	Fat/gr
Salad dressings (*continued*):			
Herbs & Spices (2T)	**1.0**	0	9.0
Italian (2T)	**2.0**	0	9.0
fat free (2T)	**2.0**	0	0
Ranch, fat free (2T)	**11.0**	0	0
Red Wine Vinegar & Oil (2T)	**2.0**	0	9.0
fat free (2T)	**3.0**	0	0
Russian (2T)	**3.0**	0	16.0
Wishbone			
Blue Cheese (2T)	**2.0**	<1.0	17.0
lite (2T)	**2.0**	1.0	7.0
fat free (2T)	**7.0**	1.0	0
Caesar, fat free (2T)	**5.0**	1.0	0
Creamy Roasted Garlic (2T)	**3.0**	0	13.0
fat free (2T)	**9.0**	0	0
French (2T)	**5.0**	0	11.0
fat free (2T)	**7.0**	0	0
Honey Dijon (2T)	**9.0**	1.0	10.0
fat free (2T)	**10.0**	1.0	0
Italian (2T)	**3.0**	0	10.0
lite (2T)	**2.0**	0	0.5
Ranch (2T)	**1.0**	0	17.0
lite (2T)	**5.0**	0	9.0
Robusto Italian (2T)	**4.0**	1.0	10.0
Russian (2T)	**15.0**	0	6.0
Thousand Island (2T)	**7.0**	0	12.0
lite (2T)	**8.0**	0	5.0
Mayonnaise:			
Hellmann's			
original (1T)	**0**	0	11.0
light (1T)	**1.0**	0	5.0
low fat (1T)	**4.0**	0	1.0
Kraft			
original (1T)	**0**	0	11.0
light (1T)	**2.0**	0	5.0
fat free (1T)	**2.0**	0	0
Miracle Whip, Kraft			
original (1T)	**2.0**	0	7.0

Food (Serving)	Carbo/gr	Protein/gr	Fat/gr
light (1T)	**2.0**	0	3.0
Vegetable shortening, Crisco (1T)	**0**	0	12.0

FISH AND SHELLFISH

Food (Serving)	Carbo/gr	Protein/gr	Fat/gr
Bass:			
black sea (1 fillet)	0	23.6	19.4
stuffed (1 piece)	23.4	33.2	32.4
striped, oven fried (1 fillet)*	13.4	43.0	17.0
Blue fish:			
baked with butter (3 oz.)	0	22.0	4.0
fried (1 fillet)*	9.2	44.3	19.1
Clams:			
raw (4-5)	4.1	7.8	0.6
canned, minced (1C)	3.0	25.3	4.0
fried, Mrs. Paul's (28)*	28.0	8.0	15.0
smoked (½C)	3.0	9.0	9.0
stuffed, Matlaw's (2 lg.)	21.0	8.0	8.0
Cod:			
broiled (1 fillet)	0	18.5	3.4
dried, salted (1 piece)	0	23.2	0.6
Crab:			
canned (1C)	1.0	24.0	3.0
deviled (1C)	31.9	27.4	22.6
steamed, pieces (1C)	0.8	26.8	2.9
imitation, Sea Legs Supreme (½C)	8.0	9.0	1.0
Fish cakes:			
fried (1 regular/5 bite size)*	5.6	8.8	4.8
frozen, fried (1 regular/5 bite size)*	10.3	5.5	10.7
Fish sticks, breaded, frozen (1)	1.8	4.7	2.5
Flounder (1 fillet)	0	17.1	4.7
Gefilte fish, Manischewitz (1 ball)	5.0	5.0	4.0
Haddock (1 fillet)	0	20.1	6.6

Food (Serving)	Carbo/gr	Protein/gr	Fat/gr
Halibut (1 fillet)	0	31.5	8.8
Herring, Vita:			
in sour cream (¼C)	8.0	7.0	7.0
in wine sauce (¼C)	10.0	9.0	5.0
Lobster:			
cubed (1C)	0.4	27.1	2.2
Newburg (1C)	12.8	46.3	26.5
Ocean perch, fried (1 fillet)*	6.0	16.0	11.0
Oysters:			
raw (1C)	8.2	20.2	4.3
smoked (⅓C)	4.0	8.0	5.0
Salmon:			
canned (7.75 oz.)	0	47.7	26.8
steak, broiled (1)	0	34.5	9.4
smoked, Iceland Supreme			
Gravlox (2 oz.)	<1.0	21.0	12.0
Nova (2 oz.)	<1.0	12.0	4.0
Sardines, King Oscar:			
in spring water, 85 gr (1 tin)	<1.0	17.0	24.0
in oil, 85 gr (1 tin)	0	15.0	16.0
in mustard sauce, 106 gr (1 tin)	<1.0	16.0	17.0
in tomato sauce, 106 gr (1 tin)	2.0	15.0	18.0
Scallops:			
fried			
Mrs. Paul's (12)*	20.0	10.0	8.0
Morning Catch (8)*	22.0	6.0	7.0
ready to eat, Ocean Classic (3 oz.)	3.0	19.0	1.0
Shad (3 oz.)	0	20.0	10.0
Shrimp:			
breaded, Bee Gee (½C)	25.0	11.0	10.0
cocktail, SauSea, 113 gr (1 jar)	20.0	8.0	0
cooked			
Contessa Extra Jumbo (1C)	0	13.0	0
Ocean Classic (3 oz.)	0	8.0	0
Swordfish steak (1 med.)	0	38.2	8.2

*(An * after serving size indicates breaded.)*

Food (Serving)	Carbo/gr	Protein/gr	Fat/gr
Tuna, canned:			
in oil (3½ oz.)	**0**	24.0	7.0
in water (3½ oz.)	**0**	27.7	0.8
Tuna salad, w/mayo, celery,			
pickle, egg and onion (1C)	**7.0**	30.0	22.0

FRUIT

Food (Serving)	Carbo/gr	Protein/gr	Fat/gr
Acerola (10)	5.6	0.3	0.2
Apple:			
fresh, 2¾" dia. (1)	20.0	0.3	0.8
dried chips (12)	20.0	2.0	7.0
Apple sauce, unsweetened (1C)	26.4	0.5	0.5
Apricots:			
fresh (3)	13.7	1.1	0.2
canned in syrup (3 halves)	18.7	0.5	0.1
canned in water pack (3 halves)	8.1	0.6	0.1
dried (10 halves)	23.3	1.8	0.2
Avocado:			
California (½)	6.5	2.4	18.4
Florida (½)	13.5	2.0	16.8
Banana:			
whole (1 med.)	26.4	1.3	0.2
mashed (1C)	50.0	2.5	0.5
sliced (1C)	33.3	1.7	0.3
chips, dried			
sweetened (¼C)	20.0	1.0	8.0
unsweetened (¼C)	16.0	2.0	10.0
Blackberries:			
fresh (1C)	18.6	1.7	1.3
canned (1C)	22.0	2.0	1.5
Blueberries:			
fresh (1C)	22.2	1.0	0.7
frozen, unsweetened (1C)	22.4	1.2	0.8
Boysenberries:			
canned (1C)	22.2	1.7	0.2

Food (Serving)	Carbo/gr	Protein/gr	Fat/gr
Boysenberries (*continued*):			
frozen, unsweetened (1C)	**14.4**	1.5	0.4
Cantaloupe, 5" dia. (½)	**20.4**	1.9	0.3
Cherimoya (¼ med.)	**29.3**	1.6	0.5
Cherries:			
sour			
fresh (1C)	**14.7**	1.2	0.3
canned, water pack (1C)	**29.6**	2.2	0.5
sweet			
fresh (1C)	**20.4**	1.5	0.4
canned in syrup (1C)	**52.6**	2.3	0.5
canned, water pack (1C)	**26.1**	2.0	0.5
Cranberries, fresh (1C)	**10.3**	0.4	0.7
Dates, hydrated (10)	**58.3**	1.8	0.4
Figs:			
fresh (1 med.)	**10.2**	0.6	0.2
canned in syrup (3)	**18.5**	0.4	0.2
canned, water pack (3)	**9.9**	0.4	0.2
Fruit cocktail:			
canned in syrup (1C)	**50.2**	1.0	0.3
canned, water pack (1C)	**23.8**	1.0	0.2
Fruit salad:			
canned in syrup (1C)	**49.5**	0.8	0.3
canned, water pack (1C)	**22.3**	1.0	0.2
Gooseberries, fresh (1C)	**14.6**	1.2	0.3
Grapefruit:			
fresh, 3½" dia. (½)	**10.3**	0.5	0.1
canned in syrup (1C)	**45.2**	1.5	0.3
canned, water pack (1C)	**18.5**	1.5	0.2
Grapes, fresh:			
Thompson seedless (10)	**9.0**	trace	trace
Tokay and Emperor (10)	**10.0**	trace	trace
Honeydew, cubed (1C)	**13.1**	1.4	0.5
Kiwi (2 med.)	**18.0**	1.0	1.0
Kumquat, fresh (1 med.)	**3.2**	0.2	trace
Lemon:			
whole, med. (1)	**6.0**	0.8	0.2
juice (1C)	**19.5**	1.2	0.5

Food (Serving)	Carbo/gr	Protein/gr	Fat/gr
peel (1t)	**0.3**	trace	trace
Lime juice (1T)	**1.4**	trace	trace
Loganberries, fresh (1C)	**21.5**	1.4	0.9
Loquats, raw (10)	**15.3**	0.5	0.2
Lychees, raw (10)	**14.8**	0.8	0.3
Mango:			
fresh, diced (1C)	**27.7**	1.2	0.7
dried slices (3)	**36.0**	0	0
Nectarine, 2½" dia. (1)	**23.6**	0.8	trace
Orange:			
whole, 2⅝" dia. (1)	**16.0**	1.3	0.3
rind (1t)	**0.5**	trace	trace
Papaya:			
fresh (1 med.)	**30.4**	1.8	0.3
dried spears (40 gr)	**35.0**	0	0
Passion fruit or granadilla (1)	**3.9**	0.4	0.1
Peach:			
fresh (1 med.)	**9.7**	0.6	0.1
canned in syrup (½ med.)	**19.3**	0.4	0.1
canned, water pack (½ med.)	**7.4**	0.4	0.1
Pear:			
fresh			
Barlett, 2½" dia. (1)	**25.1**	1.1	0.7
Bosc, 2½" dia. (1)	**22.0**	1.0	1.0
D'Anjou, 3" dia. (1)	**31.0**	1.0	1.0
canned in syrup (½ med.)	**18.4**	0.2	0.2
canned, water pack (½ med.)	**7.6**	0.2	0.2
Pineapple:			
fresh, chunk (1C)	**21.2**	0.6	0.3
canned in syrup (1C)	**49.5**	0.8	0.8
canned, water pack (1C)	**25.1**	0.7	0.2
dried slices (40 gr)	**35.0**	0	0
Plum:			
Damson, 1" dia. (10)	**17.8**	0.5	trace
prune, 1½" dia. (1)	**5.6**	0.2	0.1
purple			
canned in syrup (3)	**28.7**	0.5	0.1
canned, water pack (3)	**11.3**	0.4	0.2

Food (Serving)	Carbo/gr	Protein/gr	Fat/gr
Pomegranate, 3½" dia. (1)	**25.3**	0.8	0.5
Prunes:			
cooked (1C)	**66.7**	2.1	0.6
dried (10)	**56.9**	1.8	0.5
Raisins (1T)	**7.0**	0.2	trace
Raspberries:			
fresh (1C)	**21.0**	2.0	1.9
canned, water pack (1C)	**21.4**	1.7	0.2
frozen (1C)	**61.5**	1.8	0.5
Rhubarb, cooked w/sugar (1C)	**97.2**	1.4	0.3
Strawberries:			
fresh, whole (1C)	**12.5**	1.0	0.7
frozen, sliced (1C)	**70.9**	1.3	0.5
Tangerine, 2½" dia. (1)	**11.7**	0.8	0.2
Watermelon, diced (1C)	**10.2**	0.8	0.3

GELATIN

Food (Serving)	Carbo/gr	Protein/gr	Fat/gr
Gelatin, unflavored (1 pack/7 gr)	**0**	6.0	0
Jell-O:			
from dry mix, most flavors			
regular (½C)	**19.0**	2.0	0
sugar free (½C)	**0**	1.0	0
individual snack cups, 99 gr			
regular (1)	**17.0**	1.0	0
sugar free (1)	**0**	1.0	0

MEAT, POULTRY AND EGGS

Food (Serving)	Carbo/gr	Protein/gr	Fat/gr
Bacon:			
regular, fried (2 strips)	**0.5**	3.8	7.8
Canadian, fried (1 slice)	**0.1**	5.7	3.7
Beef:			
ground, lean (3 oz. patty)	**0**	23.3	9.6
pot roast (3 oz.)	**0**	23.0	16.0
rib roast (3 oz.)	**0**	24.0	11.4
steak, broiled, lean only (2.4 oz.)	**0**	21.0	4.0
beef and vegetable stew, canned (1C)	**17.4**	14.2	7.6
creamed chipped (1C)	**17.4**	20.1	25.2
pot pie, Swanson's frozen, 7 oz. (1)	**39.0**	10.0	23.0
Chicken:			
breaded and baked, heat and serve:			
Perdue			
breaded breast cutlet (1)	**18.0**	10.0	13.0
breaded breast nuggets (4)	**15.0**	9.0	12.0
Weaver			
breaded breast patty (1)	**10.0**	10.0	10.0
honey batter breast tenders (5)	**12.0**	12.0	16.0
honey batter mini-drums (5)	**15.0**	14.0	13.0
broiled (½ bird)	**0**	42.0	7.0
fried			
breast (½)	**1.0**	26.0	5.0
drumstick (1)	**trace**	12.0	4.0
heat and serve, Swanson (3 oz.)	**12.0**	14.0	13.0
roasted			
light (3 oz.)	**0**	44.2	4.8
light, ground (1C)	**0**	34.8	3.7

Food (Serving)	Carbo/gr	Protein/gr	Fat/gr
dark, diced, no skin (1C)	0	39.2	8.8
heat and serve, Tyson			
breast (½)	1.0	34.0	13.0
thigh (1)	1.0	22.0	19.0
drumstick (1)	1.0	40.0	18.0
pot pie, Swanson's frozen, 7 oz. (1)	45.0	9.0	22.0
wings, hot, heat and serve, Weaver (4)	0	22.0	16.0
Corned beef, canned (3 oz.)	0	22.0	10.0
Corned beef hash, canned (1C)	23.5	19.4	24.9
Eggs, large:			
fried (1)	0.1	6.3	7.9
hard-boiled (1)	0.5	6.5	5.8
poached (1)	0.5	6.5	5.8
scrambled with milk (1)	1.5	7.2	8.3
Egg substitute, Egg Beaters (¼C)	1.0	6.0	0
Ham:			
baked (3 oz.)	0	17.8	18.8
steak (3 oz.)	0	11.0	7.0
deviled (¼C)	0	8.0	14.0
Goose, roasted, with skin (3 oz.)	0	25.2	21.9
Lamb:			
roasted, lean (3 oz.)	0	24.4	6.0
chop, broiled (2½ oz. chop)	0	15.6	20.9
Liver:			
beef (3 oz. slice)	4.5	22.4	9.0
chicken (1)	0.8	6.6	1.1
Paté:			
chicken liver, Chef Giovanni (2 oz.)	5.0	5.0	17.0
de campagne, Tour Eiffel (2 oz.)	2.0	7.0	15.0
Pork:			
roasted, lean, fat trimmed (3 oz.)	0	25.2	8.5
chop, broiled (2.7 oz.)	0	19.0	24.7
Sausage: *See* Sausage and Luncheon Meat			
Turkey, roasted:			
light, with skin (3 oz.)	0	28.6	8.3
dark, with skin (3 oz.)	0	27.5	11.1
ground (1C)	0	34.7	6.7
pot pie, Swanson's frozen, 7 oz. (1)	44.0	11.0	24.0

Food (Serving)	Carbo/gr	Protein/gr	Fat/gr
Veal:			
cutlet, broiled (3 oz.)	0	23.0	9.0
loin (3 oz.)	0	22.4	11.4

MILK AND MILK PRODUCTS

Food (Serving)	Carbo/gr	Protein/gr	Fat/gr
Butter:			
traditional			
pat (1)	trace	trace	4.1
tablespoon (1)	0.1	0.1	11.5
stick (4 oz.)	0.5	0.7	91.9
whipped			
pat (1)	trace	trace	3.1
tablespoon (1)	trace	0.1	7.6
stick (2⅔ oz.)	0.3	0.5	61.2
Buttermilk (1C)	12.5	8.8	0.2
Cheese:			
American (1 oz.)	trace	6.0	9.0
Boursin (2T)	1.0	2.0	13.0
Bleu or Roquefort (1 oz.)	0.6	6.1	8.6
Bonbel (1 oz.)	0	6.0	8.0
Brie (1 oz.)	0	5.0	9.0
Cabot (1 oz.)	1.0	7.0	9.0
Camembert (1 oz.)	0.5	5.0	7.0
cheddar (1 oz.)	0.6	7.1	9.1
Cheese Whiz (2T)	4.0	2.0	8.0
Cracker Barrel Cheddar (1 oz.)	<1.0	7.0	9.0
⅓ less fat (1 oz.)	<1.0	7.0	6.0
Edam (1 oz.)	0	8.0	7.0
feta (1 oz.)	<1.0	5.0	6.0
fontina (1 oz.)	0	8.0	8.0
goat (1 oz.)	0	5.0	6.0
Gorgonzola (1 oz.)	<1.0	6.0	8.0
Gouda (1 oz.)	0	7.0	8.0

Food (Serving)	Carbo/gr	Protein/gr	Fat/gr
Cheese (*continued*):			
Havarti (1 oz.)	**0**	6.0	10.0
Jarlsberg (1 oz.)	**0**	7.0	8.0
Laughing Cow, 1 oz. wedge (1)	**1.0**	4.0	6.0
marscarpone (1 oz.)	**1.0**		
mozzarella (1 oz.)	**1.0**	6.0	7.0
part skim (1 oz.)	**1.0**	8.0	5.0
Muenster (1 oz.)	**1.0**	7.0	8.0
Parmesan, grated (1T)	**0.2**	2.1	1.5
provolone (1 oz.)	**1.0**	7.0	8.0
ricotta (1C)	**7.0**	28.0	32.0
part skim (1C)	**13.0**	28.0	19.0
Romano (1 oz.)	**1.0**	9.0	8.0
Swiss (1 oz.)	**0.5**	7.8	7.9
Swiss Knight, 1 oz. wedge (1)	**0**	6.0	8.0
Velveeta (1 oz.)	**3.0**	4.0	6.0
Cottage Cheese:			
Friendship			
whole milk (½C)	**4.0**	14.0	5.0
California style (½C)	**4.0**	15.0	5.0
w/pineapple (½C)	**16.0**	16.0	4.0
2% milkfat (½C)	**4.0**	15.0	2.5
1% milkfat (½C)	**4.0**	16.0	1.0
w/pineapple (½C)	**17.0**	12.0	1.0
nonfat (½C)	**5.0**	15.0	0
w/peach (½C)	**15.0**	12.0	0
Light'n Lively			
1% milkfat w/peach and			
pineapple (½C)	**14.0**	12.0	1.0
Garden salad (½C)	**4.0**	13.0	1.5
low fat (½C)	**4.0**	14.0	1.0
fat free (½C)	**5.0**	15.0	0
Cream cheese:			
Philadelphia			
original (2T)	**1.0**	2.0	10.0
w/chive and onion (2T)	**2.0**	2.0	10.0
w/smoked salmon (3T)	**2.0**	2.0	9.0
w/strawberries (2T)	**5.0**	1.0	9.0

Food (Serving)	Carbo/gr	Protein/gr	Fat/gr
light (2T)	**2.0**	3.0	5.0
Cream:			
half-and-half (1T)	**0.7**	0.5	1.8
heavy, 37.6% fat (1T)	**0.5**	0.3	5.6
light, 20.6% fat (1T)	**0.6**	0.5	3.1
whipped (1 oz.)	**2.0**		
whipped toppings, prepared			
Cool Whip (2T)	**2.0**	0	1.5
RediWip, original (2T)	**<1.0**	0	2.0
Ice cream: *See* Desserts and Snacks			
Margarine:*			
traditional			
tablespoon (1)	**0.1**	0.1	11.5
stick (4 oz.)	**0.5**	0.7	91.9
whipped			
tablespoon (1)	**trace**	0.1	7.6
stick (2⅔ oz.)	**0.3**	0.5	61.2
Milk:			
whole (1C)	**11.0**	8.0	8.0
2% fat (1C)	**11.7**	8.1	4.7
1% fat (1C)	**11.7**	8.0	2.6
skim (1C)	**11.9**	8.4	0.4
chocolate, carton			
Hershey's (1C)	**28.0**	8.0	9.0
Nestlés Quik (1C)	**31.1**	7.0	9.0
See also Condiments,			
Seasonings and Sauces			
for chocolate syrups			
condensed (1 fl. oz.)	**20.7**	3.1	3.3
evaporated (1 fl. oz.)	**3.1**	2.2	2.5
Sour Cream, Breakstone:			
original (2T)	**1.0**	<1.0	5.0
⅓ less fat (2T)	**2.0**	1.0	3.5
Fat free (2T)	**6.0**	2.0	0

Margarine is an example of a low carbohydrate food not recommended by Dr. Atkins because its fats are in an unnatural and unhealthy form.

Food (Serving)	Carbo/gr	Protein/gr	Fat/gr
Yogurt:			
Breyers, 8 oz. cup			
black cherry (1)	**46.0**	9.0	2.5
blueberry (1)	**45.0**	9.0	2.5
lemon (1)	**38.0**	10.0	3.0
peach (1)	**45.0**	9.0	2.5
strawberry (1)	**44.0**	9.0	2.5
vanilla (1)	**38.0**	10.0	3.0
Breyers, fat free, 8 oz. cup			
most flavors (1)	**22.5**	9.0	0
Columbo, 8 oz. cup			
most single			
fruit flavors (1)	**36.0**	7.0	6.0
plain (1)	**13.0**	9.0	8.0
non-fat most single			
fruit flavors (1)	**43.0**	8.0	0
Dannon, 8 oz. cup			
light, most flavors (1)	**17.0**	8.0	0
low fat			
fruit on the bottom,			
most flavors (1)	**45.0**	9.0	3.0
plain (1)	**17.0**	13.0	4.0
vanilla (1)	**39.0**	11.0	3.5
fat free, plain (1)	**17.0**	13.0	0

Yogurt, frozen: *See* Desserts and Snacks

NUTS AND SEEDS

Food (Serving)	Carbo/gr	Protein/gr	Fat/gr
Almond paste (1 oz.)	14.5	3.1	9.1
Almonds:			
dried (1 oz.)	5.5	5.3	15.4
roasted (1 oz.)	5.5	5.3	16.4
Brazil (1 oz.)	3.1	4.1	19.0
Cashew nut butter (2T)	9.0	4.0	15.0
Cashews (1 oz.)	8.3	4.9	13.0
Chestnuts (1 oz.)	8.4	0.6	0.3
Coconut, fresh, shelled (1 oz.)	4.3	0.9	9.5
Hazelnuts or filberts (1 oz.)	4.7	3.6	17.7
Macadamia:			
raw (1 oz.)	4.5	2.2	20.3
dried, shelled (1 oz.)	3.9	2.4	20.9
Peanut butter: regular (1T)	3.0	4.0	8.1
Peanuts: roasted, shelled (1 oz.)	5.4	8.6	14.0
Pecans, shelled (1 oz.)	4.1	2.6	20.2
Pine nuts or pignolias (1 oz.)	3.3	8.8	13.4
Pistachios, shelled (1 oz.)	5.4	5.5	15.2
Pumpkin/squash seeds, hulled (1 oz.)	4.2	8.1	13.1
Sesame seeds (1T)	1.4	1.5	4.3
Soybeans, roasted (⅓C)	6.0	10.0	7.0
Sunflower seeds, hulled (1 oz.)	5.6	6.7	13.2
Walnuts (1 oz.)	4.2	5.8	16.8
Water chestnuts, fresh (1 oz.)	5.4	0.4	0.1

PASTA AND RICE

Food (Serving)	Carbo/gr	Protein/gr	Fat/gr
Macaroni, enriched, cooked (1C)	**39.1**	6.5	0.7
Macaroni and cheese:			
canned (1C)	**25.7**	9.4	9.6
dry mix, Kraft, prepared (1C)	**48.0**	11.0	18.5
frozen, Stouffer's (1C)	**29.0**	13.0	16.0
Noodles:			
chow mein, canned (1C)	**26.1**	5.9	10.6
egg, enriched, cooked (1C)	**37.3**	6.6	2.4
egg substitute (2 oz. dry)	**41.0**	9.0	0.5
lo mein (½C dry)	**45.0**	5.0	0
somen (2 oz. dry)	**41.0**	5.0	1.0
packaged mix, Golden Sauté, prepared			
Parmesan angel hair pasta (1C)	**42.0**	8.0	11.0
penne pasta (1C)	**44.0**	8.0	9.0
Ravioli in tomato sauce:			
canned, Chef Boyardee			
beef (1C)	**36.0**	9.0	5.0
cheese (1C)	**44.0**	7.0	(0)
frozen, Stouffer's: cheese (301 gr)	**51.0**	15.0	13.0
Rice:			
arborio (1C)	**40.0**	3.0	0
basmati, Fantastic Foods (¼C*)	**38.0**	3.0	0
brown (1C)	**49.7**	4.9	1.2
Jasmati, Rice Select (¼C*)	**34.0**	3.0	0
long grain and wild rice (1C)	**41.0**	6.0	1.0
risotto (¼C*)	**37.0**	3.0	0

An asterisk [*] by serving size indicates uncooked or dry measurement.

Food (Serving)	Carbo/gr	Protein/gr	Fat/gr
Texmati, Master Choice (¼C*)	**34.0**	3.0	0.5
wild rice (⅓C)	**14.0**	3.0	0
white (1C)	**49.6**	4.1	0.2
Rice, packaged mixes:			
Goya			
rice and red or black beans (¼C*)	**35.5**	5.0	(0)
yellow rice (¼C*)	**37.0**	4.0	0
Rice-a-Roni, prepared beef (1C)	**51.0**	7.0	8.0
chicken (1C)	**52.0**	7.0	9.0
rice pilaf (1C)	**53.0**	6.0	8.0
Spanish rice (1C)	**46.0**	6.0	7.0
Spaghetti, enriched, cooked (1C)	**39.1**	6.5	0.7
in tomato sauce w/cheese,			
canned (1C)	**38.5**	5.5	1.5
w/meatballs and tomato sauce,			
canned (1C)	**28.5**	12.8	10.8
Spaghetti and macaroni,			
specialty varieties, dry:			
brown rice, Pastario (2 oz.)	**43.0**	5.0	1.0
corn, DeBoles (2 oz.)	**45.0**	5.0	1.0
kamut spirals, Eden Organic (½C)	**33.0**	10.0	1.5
polenta pasta, Gabriele (2 oz.)	**35.0**	5.0	2.0
quinoa, Ancient Harvest (2 oz.)	**45.0**	5.0	1.0
semolina and spinach (2 oz.)	**41.0**	7.0	0.5
spelt rotini (2 oz.)	**40.0**	8.0	1.5
tomato and basil angel hair,			
DeBoles (2 oz.)	**41.0**	7.0	1.0
whole wheat (2 oz.)	**40.0**	7.0	1.0
Spaghetti sauces:			

See Condiments, Seasonings and Sauces

SAUSAGE AND PREPARED LUNCHEON MEATS

Food (Serving)	Carbo/gr	Protein/gr	Fat/gr
Bologna:			
regular, Oscar Mayer (1 slice)	**1.0**	3.0	8.0
beef, Oscar Mayer (1 slice)	**1.0**	3.0	8.0
turkey, Louis Rich (1 slice)	**1.0**	3.0	3.5
Braunschweiger, Oscar Mayer (2 oz.)	**1.0**	8.0	17.0
Chicken breast, Louis Rich (1 slice)	**1.0**	5.0	1.0
Frankfurters:			
regular, Hygrade (1)	**2.0**	6.0	16.0
beef, Ball Park (1)	**2.0**	6.0	16.0
Hygrade (1)	**4.0**	5.0	17.0
Oscar Mayer (1)	**1.0**	5.0	13.0
chicken, Wampler Longacre (1)	**0**	7.0	11.0
turkey, Wampler Longacre (1)	**0**	6.0	8.0
Ham:			
regular, Oscar Mayer (3 slices)	**0**	10.0	2.5
turkey, Louis Rich (1 slice)	**0**	5.0	1.0
Kielbasa, Hillshire Farms			
regular (2 oz.)	**2.0**	8.0	8.0
beef (2 oz.)	**1.0**	7.0	17.0
Olive loaf, Oscar Mayer (1 slice)	**2.0**	3.0	6.0
Pastrami, turkey, Louis Rich (1 slice)	**0**	5.0	1.0
Pepperoni, Hormel, 2½" dia. (15 slices)	**0**	5.0	13.0
Salami:			
Cotto, regular, Oscar Mayer (2 slices)	**0**	6.0	9.0
beef, Oscar Mayer (2)	**1.0**	6.0	7.0
hard, Oscar Mayer (3 slices)	**0**	6.0	9.0

Food (Serving)	Carbo/gr	Protein/gr	Fat/gr
turkey, Louis Rich (1)	**0**	4.0	2.5
Sausage:			
pork, traditional			
link (1)	**trace**	2.4	5.7
patty (2 oz.)	**trace**	4.9	11.9
brown and serve links			
regular, Swift (2)	**1.0**	6.0	12.0
beef			
Swift (3)	**1.0**	7.0	25.0
Jones (2)	**1.0**	6.0	17.0
Spiced loaf, Oscar Mayer (1 slice)	**2.0**	4.0	5.0
Turkey, honey roast, Louis Rich (1 slice)	**1.0**	5.0	0.5

SOUPS AND BROTHS

Food (Serving)	Carbo/gr	Protein/gr	Fat/gr
Bouillon (1 cube)	**0.2**	0.8	0.1
Soups, canned, condensed			
(diluted with water):			
asparagus, cream of (1C*)	**16.7**	6.9	5.9
bean w/pork (1C)	**21.8**	8.0	5.8
beef broth (1C)	**2.6**	5.0	0
beef noodle (1C)	**7.0**	3.8	2.6
celery, cream of (1C*)	**15.2**	6.4	9.3
clam liquor (1C)	**5.0**	5.5	0.2
chicken broth (1C)	**1.0**	1.0	1.5
chicken consommé (1C)	**1.9**	3.4	trace
chicken, cream of (1C*)	**14.5**	7.4	10.3
chicken gumbo (1C)	**7.4**	3.1	1.4
chicken noodle (1C)	**7.9**	3.4	1.9
chicken w/rice (1C)	**5.8**	3.1	1.2
chicken vegetable (1C)	**9.6**	4.2	2.5
clam chowder, Manhattan (1C)	**12.8**	2.2	2.5
minestrone (1C)	**14.2**	4.9	3.4
mushroom, cream of (1C*)	**16.2**	6.9	14.2
pea, split (1C)	**20.6**	8.6	3.2
tomato (1C*)	**15.7**	2.0	2.5
turkey w/rice (1C)	**10.0**		
vegetable beef (1C)	**9.6**	5.1	2.2
vegetarian vegetable (1C)	**13.2**	2.2	2.0

An asterisk [*] by the serving portion indicates diluted with milk.

Food (Serving)	Carbo/gr	Protein/gr	Fat/gr
Soups, canned, ready to serve:			
Campbell's Chunky			
beef w/vegetable (1C)	**18.0**	13.0	4.0
chicken, spicy and vegetable (1C)	**13.0**	7.0	1.0
chicken corn chowder (1C)	**18.0**	10.0	15.0
chicken noodle (1C)	**16.0**	9.0	3.0
chicken w/rice (1C)	**18.0**	9.0	3.0
clam chowder			
Manhattan (1C)	**21.0**	7.0	15.0
New England (1C)	**20.0**	6.0	4.0
minestrone (1C)	**22.0**	5.0	5.0
sirloin burger w/veg. (1C)	**20.0**	11.0	9.0
vegetable (1C)	**22.0**	3.0	3.0
Campbell's Healthy Request			
chicken noodle (1C)	**25.0**	9.0	3.0
chicken vegetable (1C)	**18.0**	7.0	2.0
clam chowder,			
New England (1C)	**15.0**	5.0	3.0
minestrone (1C)	**24.0**	4.0	2.0
pea, split, w/ham (1C)	**28.0**	9.0	2.0
penne, zesty, and vegetable (1C)	**17.0**	4.0	0.5
tomato vegetable w/pasta (1C)	**22.0**	4.0	2.0
turkey vegetable w/rice (1C)	**17.0**	7.0	2.5
vegetable, hearty (1C)	**20.0**	3.0	1.0
vegetable, Southwestern (1C)	**28.0**	5.0	1.0
Healthy Choice			
chicken Alfredo w/pasta (1C)	**17.0**	12.0	2.5
chicken corn chowder (1C)	**30.0**	8.0	3.0
chicken, hearty (1C)	**20.0**	8.0	2.5
chicken noodle (1C)	**20.0**	9.0	3.0
chicken pasta (1C)	**17.0**	8.0	2.5
chicken w/rice (1C)	**15.0**	7.0	3.0
clam chowder, New England (1C)	**23.0**	6.0	1.5
minestrone (1C)	**23.0**	6.0	1.0
pea, split, w/ham (1C)	**25.0**	11.0	2.0
Progresso			
beef barley (1C)	**13.0**	10.0	4.0
beef minestrone (1C)	**14.0**	12.0	4.0

Food (Serving)	Carbo/gr	Protein/gr	Fat/gr
Progresso (*continued*):			
beef noodle (1C)	**15.0**	13.0	3.5
chicken rice (1C)	**11.0**	6.0	3.0
chicken vegetable (1C)	**13.0**	7.0	2.0
clam chowder			
Manhattan (1C)	**11.0**	12.0	2.0
New England (1C)	**17.0**	6.0	10.0
escarole (1C)	**2.0**	2.0	1.0
lentil (1C)	**22.0**	9.0	2.0
minestrone (1C)	**22.0**	6.0	2.5
pea, green split (1C)	**25.0**	10.0	3.0
vegetable (1C)	**15.0**	4.0	2.0
vegetable, hearty w/rotini (1C)	**20.0**	4.0	1.0
Progresso, Healthy Classic			
beef vegetable (1C)	**25.0**	10.0	1.5
chicken noodle (1C)	**9.0**	6.0	1.5
chicken rice w/vegetables (1C)	**13.0**	6.0	1.5
clam chowder, New England (1C)	**21.0**	6.0	2.5
cream of broccoli (1C)	**13.0**	2.0	3.0
garlic and pasta (1C)	**18.0**	4.0	1.5
lentil (1C)	**20.0**	5.0	2.5
minestrone (1C)	**20.0**	8.0	1.5
tomato and garden vegetables (1C)	**19.0**	3.0	1.0
vegetable (1C)	**13.0**	4.0	1.5
dry mix			
beef noodle (1C)	**11.5**	2.4	1.2
chicken noodle (1C)	**7.7**	1.9	1.4
chicken rice (1C)	**8.4**	1.2	1.0
onion (1C)	**5.5**	1.4	1.2
pea, green (1C)	**20.6**	7.6	1.5
tomato (1C)	**12.2**	1.4	1.4
packaged			
Oriental noodle, Ramen			
all flavors (½ pack)	**27.0**	4.0	8.0

SWEETENERS

> NOTE: Although most published scientific studies proclaimed aspartame (Nutra-Sweet, Equal) to be safe, clinical experience often indicates otherwise. Headaches, irritability, failure to lose weight or to control blood glucose have all been reported and I have confirmed this in many patients. It is likely to cross-react with those who cannot tolerate MSG. The best advice is to use it sparingly, preferably by blending it with other sweeteners. Remember, too, that aspartame loses its sweetness when heated.

Food (Serving)	Carbo/gr	Protein/gr	Fat/gr
Honey (1T)	17.8	0.1	0
Molasses, light (1T)	13.0	—	—
Sugar:			
granulated (1T)	11.9	0	0
brown (1T)	13.4	0	0
confectioner's (1T)	10.9	0	0
maple (1 oz.)	25.5	—	—
Sugar substitutes:			
Equal (1 pkt.)	1.0	trace	0
Sweet'n Low (1 pkt.)	0.9	0	0
Syrups:			
chocolate, see Condiments, Seasonings and Gravies			
corn (1T)	15.4	0	0
maple, 100% pure (1T)	13.0	0	0
maple/cane blend (1T)	12.8	0	0

VEGETABLES

Food (Serving)	Carbo/gr	Protein/gr	Fat/gr
Artichoke, med. (1 bud)	**11.9**	3.4	0.2
Asparagus:			
fresh, med. (4 spears)	**2.2**	1.3	0.1
canned (4 spears)	**2.0**	1.4	0.2
canned, low sodium, cut (1C)	**6.5**	4.8	0.5
frozen, cut (1C)	**6.3**	5.8	0.4
Bamboo shoots (1C)	**7.9**	3.9	0.5
Bean sprouts (1C)	**5.6**	6.5	1.5
Beans:			
baby lima (1C)	**32.5**	10.2	0.2
green snap (1C)	**6.8**	2.0	0.3
yellow snap (1C)	**5.8**	1.8	0.3
See also Beans and Legumes			
Beets (1C)	**12.2**	1.9	0.2
Broccoli:			
raw (1C)	**7.0**	4.8	0.5
cooked (1C)	**8.5**	5.4	0.6
in cheese sauce, Green Giant (⅔C)	**9.0**	3.0	2.5
Brussels sprouts (1C)	**9.9**	6.5	0.6
Cabbage, shredded:			
raw (1C)	**4.9**	1.2	0.2
cooked (1C)	**6.2**	1.6	0.3
Carrots:			
raw (1 lg.)	**7.0**	0.8	0.1
cooked (1C)	**11.0**	1.4	0.3
Cauliflower:			
raw (1C)	**4.4**	2.3	0.2
cooked (1C)	**5.1**	2.9	0.3

Food (Serving)	Carbo/gr	Protein/gr	Fat/gr
in cheese sauce, Green Giant (½C)	**8.0**	2.0	2.5
Celery:			
raw silk (1)	**1.6**	0.4	trace
cooked, diced (1C)	**4.7**	1.2	0.2
Chard, Swiss (1C)	**4.8**	2.6	0.3
Chinese cabbage (1C)	**2.3**	0.9	0.1
Cole slaw w/dressing (1C)	**8.5**	1.4	9.5
Collards, cooked (1C)	**9.8**	5.4	1.2
Corn:			
fresh on the cob (1)	**16.2**	2.5	0.8
fresh kernels (1C)	**31.0**	5.3	1.7
canned (1C)	**43.1**	5.3	1.1
canned, creamed (1C)	**51.2**	5.4	1.5
Cucumber, sliced (1C)	**3.6**	0.9	0.1
Dandelion greens (1C)	**6.7**	2.1	0.6
Eggplant (1C)	**8.2**	2.0	0.4
Endive or escarole (1C)	**2.1**	0.9	0.1
Garlic, raw (1 clove)	**0.9**	0.2	trace
Kale (1C)	**6.7**	(5.0)	(0.8)
Kohlrabi (1C)	**8.7**	2.8	0.2
Lettuce, chopped or shredded:			
Boston or Bibb (1C)	**1.4**	0.7	0.1
romaine (1C)	**1.9**	0.7	0.2
iceberg (1C)	**1.6**	0.5	0.1
Mushrooms:			
regular (1C)	**3.1**	1.9	0.2
porcini (1C)	**4.0**		
shiitake (1C)	**4.0**		
Mustard greens (1C)	**5.6**	3.1	0.6
Okra (1C)	**9.6**	3.2	0.5
Onions (1C)	**14.8**	2.6	0.2
Parsley (1T)	**0.3**	0.1	trace
Parsnip:			
diced (1C)	**23.1**	2.3	0.8
mashed (1C)	**31.3**	3.2	1.1
Peas (1C)	**19.4**	8.6	0.6
Pepper, raw:			
green, diced (1C)	**7.2**	1.8	0.3

Food (Serving)	Carbo/gr	Protein/gr	Fat/gr
Pepper, raw (*continued*):			
red, diced (1C)	**10.7**	2.1	0.5
Plantain (1 lg.)	**82.0**	2.9	1.1
Potato salad w/mayo and eggs (1C)	**33.5**	7.5	23.0
Potatoes:			
au gratin (1C)	**33.3**	13.0	19.4
baked (1)	**32.8**	4.0	0.2
boiled (1)	**38.9**	4.8	0.2
french fried (10)	**18.0**	2.2	6.6
hashed brown, frozen (1C)	**45.0**	3.0	18.0
instant			
flake, prepared (1C)	**30.5**	4.0	6.7
granules, prepared (1C)	**30.2**	4.2	7.6
mashed (1C)	**25.8**	4.4	9.0
scalloped (1C)	**36.0**	7.4	9.6
Pumpkin:			
fresh (3½ oz.)	**7.0**		
canned (1C)	**19.4**	2.5	0.7
Radishes, large (10)	**2.9**	0.8	0.1
Rutabagas, mashed (1C)	**19.7**	2.2	0.2
Sauerkraut (1C)	**9.4**	2.4	0.5
Scallions (1T)	**0.5**	0.1	trace
Spinach:			
raw (1C)	**2.4**	1.8	0.2
cooked (1C)	**6.5**	5.4	0.5
creamed, Seabrook (½C)	**10.0**	4.0	6.0
Squash			
summer:			
raw (1C)	**5.5**	1.4	0.1
cooked (1C)	**6.5**	1.9	0.2
winter			
acorn, baked (½C)	**21.8**	3.0	0.2
butternut, mashed (1C)	**25.5**	2.7	0.2
hubbard, mashed (1C)	**16.9**	2.7	0.7
Sweet potatoes:			
baked (1)	**37.0**	2.4	0.6
boiled (1)	**39.8**	2.6	0.6
candied (1 piece)	**29.1**	2.8	1.1

Food (Serving)	Carbo/gr	Protein/gr	Fat/gr
mashed (1C)	**67.1**	4.3	1.0
Tomatoes:			
fresh, 2.6" dia. (1)	**5.8**	1.4	0.2
cooked (1C)	**13.3**	3.1	0.5
paste (¼C)	**12.2**	2.2	0.5
sauce (¼C)	**4.0**	<1.0	0
spaghetti sauce, *see* Condiments, Seasonings and Sauces			
sun-dried (average)	**5.0**		
Turnip greens (1C)	**5.2**	3.2	0.3
Turnip:			
raw (1C)	**8.6**	1.3	0.3
mashed (1C)	**11.3**	1.8	0.5

SAMPLES OF CARBOHYDRATE-RICH "FATTENING" ITEMS

Food (Serving)	Carbo/gr
Banana split	91.0
Burrito, bean	48.0
Cheeseburger (¼ pounder)	33.0
Chicken salad sandwich	26.6
Corn bread stuffing (¼C)	69.0
Egg roll, Empire miniature (6)	43.0
Hot dog with bun (1)	24.0
Ice cream soda (1C)	49.0
Onion rings (fast food order)	33.0
Pizza, frozen:	
Celeste Pizza for One, 7 oz.	
4 cheese (1)	47.0
sausage (1)	52.0
Stouffer's French Bread	
deluxe (1)	42.0
double cheese (1)	46.0
Shake (medium)	90.0
Vanilla shake (1 average)	50.0
Whaler	64.0

SOURCES

Sources of data for this guide:

Nutritive Value of American Foods in Common Units, *Agriculture Handbook* No. 456, U.S. Dept. of Agriculture

Nutritive Value of Foods, *Home and Garden Bulletin* No. 72, U.S. Dept. of Agriculture

Nutritional values listed on manufacturer's labels

Food Values of Portions Commonly Used, Jean A.T. Pennington and Helen Nichols Church, Harper and Row, NY, NY 14th Ed.